UCLA Symposia on Molecular and Cellular Biology, New Series

Series Editor, C. Fred Fox

RECENT TITLES

Volume 56
Cellular and Molecular Biology of Tumors and Potential Clinical Applications, John Minna and W. Michael Kuehl, *Editors*

Volume 57
Proteases in Biological Control and Biotechnology, Dennis D. Cunningham and George L. Long, *Editors*

Volume 58
Growth Factors, Tumor Promoters, and Cancer Genes, Nancy H. Colburn, Harold L. Moses, and Eric J. Stanbridge, *Editors*

Volume 59
Chronic Lymphocytic Leukemia: Recent Progress and Future Direction, Robert Peter Gale and Kanti R. Rai, *Editors*

Volume 60
Molecular Paradigms for Eradicating Helminthic Parasites, Austin J. MacInnis, *Editor*

Volume 61
Recent Advances in Leukemia and Lymphoma, Robert Peter Gale and David W. Golde, *Editors*

Volume 62
Plant Gene Systems and Their Biology, Joe L. Key and Lee McIntosh, *Editors*

Volume 63
Plant Membranes: Structure, Function, Biogenesis, Christopher Leaver and Heven Sze, *Editors*

Volume 64
Bacteria–Host Cell Interaction, Marcus A. Horwitz, *Editor*

Volume 65
The Pharmacology and Toxicology of Proteins, John S. Holcenberg and Jeffrey L. Winkelhake, *Editors*

Volume 66
Molecular Biology of Invertebrate Development, John D. O'Connor, *Editor*

Volume 67
Mechanisms of Control of Gene Expression, Bryan Cullen, L. Patrick Gage, M.A.Q. Siddiqui, Anna Marie Skalka, and Herbert Weissbach, *Editors*

Volume 68
Protein Purification: Micro to Macro, Richard Burgess, *Editor*

Volume 69
Protein Structure, Folding, and Design 2, Dale L. Oxender, *Editor*

Volume 70
Hepadna Viruses, William Robinson, Katsuro Koike, and Hans Will, *Editors*

Volume 71
Human Retroviruses, Cancer, and AIDS: Approaches to Prevention and Therapy, Dani Bolognesi, *Editor*

Volume 72
Molecular Biology of the Human Brain, Edward G. Jones, *Editor*

Volume 73
The T-Cell Receptor, Mark M. Davis and John Kappler, *Editors*

Volume 74
Growth Regulation of Cancer, Marc E. Lippman, *Editor*

Volume 75
Steroid Hormone Action, Gordon Ringold, *Editor*

Volume 76
Molecular Biology of Intracellular Protein Sorting and Organelle Assembly, Ralph A. Bradshaw, Lee McAlister-Henn, and Michael G. Douglas, *Editors*

Volume 77
Signal Transduction in Cytoplasmic Organization and Cell Motility, Peter Satir, John Condeelis, and Elias Lazarides, *Editors*

Volume 78
Tumor Progression and Metastasis, Garth J Nicolson and Isaiah J. Fidler, *Editors*

Volume 79
Altered Glycosylation in Tumor Cells, Ser Itiroh Hakomori, Donald M. Marcus, and Christopher L. Reading, *Editors*

Please contact the publisher for information about previous titles in this series.

UCLA Symposia Board

C. Fred Fox, Ph.D., Director
Professor of Microbiology, University of California, Los Angeles

Charles J. Arntzen, Ph.D.
Director, Plant Science and Microbiology
E.I. du Pont de Nemours and Company

Floyd E. Bloom, M.D.
Director, Preclinical Neurosciences/
Endocrinology
Scripps Clinic and Research Institute

Ralph A. Bradshaw, Ph.D.
Chairman, Department of Biological
Chemistry
University of California, Irvine

Francis J. Bullock, M.D.
Vice President, Research
Schering Corporation

Ronald E. Cape, Ph.D., M.B.A.
Chairman
Cetus Corporation

Ralph E. Christoffersen, Ph.D.
Executive Director of Biotechnology
Upjohn Company

John Cole, Ph.D.
Vice President of Research
and Development
Triton Biosciences

Pedro Cuatrecasas, M.D.
Vice President of Research
Glaxo, Inc.

Mark M. Davis, Ph.D.
Department of Medical Microbiology
Stanford University

J. Eugene Fox, Ph.D.
Vice President, Research
and Development
Miles Laboratories

J. Lawrence Fox, Ph.D.
Vice President, Biotechnology Research
Abbott Laboratories

L. Patrick Gage, Ph.D.
Director of Exploratory Research
Hoffmann-La Roche, Inc.

Gideon Goldstein, M.D., Ph.D.
Vice President, Immunology
Ortho Pharmaceutical Corp.

Ernest G. Jaworski, Ph.D.
Director of Biological Sciences
Monsanto Corp.

Irving S. Johnson, Ph.D.
Vice President of Research
Lilly Research Laboratories

Paul A. Marks, M.D.
President
Sloan-Kettering Memorial Institute

David W. Martin, Jr., M.D.
Vice President of Research
Genentech, Inc.

Hugh O. McDevitt, M.D.
Professor of Medical Microbiology
Stanford University School of Medicine

Dale L. Oxender, Ph.D.
Director, Center for Molecular Genetics
University of Michigan

Mark L. Pearson, Ph.D.
Director of Molecular Biology
E.I. du Pont de Nemours and Company

George Poste, Ph.D.
Vice President and Director of Research
and Development
Smith, Kline and French Laboratories

William Rutter, Ph.D.
Director, Hormone Research Institute
University of California, San Francisco

George A. Somkuti, Ph.D.
Eastern Regional Research Center
USDA-ARS

Donald F. Steiner, M.D.
Professor of Biochemistry
University of Chicago

Tumor Progression and Metastasis

Tumor Progression and Metastasis

Proceedings of a Triton Biosciences—
Smith, Kline & French—UCLA
Symposium Held in Keystone, Colorado
April 6–12, 1987

Editors

Garth L. Nicolson
Department of Tumor Biology
The University of Texas MD Anderson Cancer Center
Houston, TX

Isaiah J. Fidler
Department of Cell Biology
The University of Texas MD Anderson Cancer Center
Houston, TX

Alan R. Liss, Inc. • New York

Address all Inquiries to the Publisher
Alan R. Liss, Inc., 41 East 11th Street, New York, NY 10003

Copyright © 1988 Alan R. Liss, Inc.

Printed in the United States of America

Under the conditions stated below the owner of copyright for this book hereby grants permission to users to make photocopy reproductions of any part or all of its contents for personal or internal organizational use, or for personal or internal use of specific clients. This consent is given on the condition that the copier pay the stated per-copy fee through the Copyright Clearance Center, Incorporated, 27 Congress Street, Salem, MA 01970, as listed in the most current issue of "Permissions to Photocopy" (Publisher's Fee List, distributed by CCC, Inc.), for copying beyond that permitted by sections 107 or 108 of the US Copyright Law. This consent does not extend to other kinds of copying, such as copying for general distribution, for advertising or promotional purposes, for creating new collective works, or for resale.

Library of Congress Cataloging-in-Publication Data

Tumor progression and metastasis.

(UCLA symposia on molecular and cellular biology ; new ser., v. 78)
  Includes bibliographies and index.
  1. Metastasis—Congresses. 2. Tumors—Growth—Congresses. 3. Cancer—Genetic aspects—Congresses.
I. Nicolson, Garth L.   II. Fidler, Isaiah J., 1936–   .   III. Triton Biosciences, Inc.   IV. Smith, Kline & French Laboratories. V. University of California, Los Angeles. VI. Series.   [DNLM: 1. Neoplasm Invasiveness—congresses. 2. Neoplasm Metastasis—congresses. W3 U17N new ser. v.78 / QZ 202 T9238 1987]
RC269.5.T85 1988   616.99′4071   88-9120
ISBN 0-8451-2677-6

Pages 1–126 of this volume are reprinted from the Journal of Cellular Biochemistry, Volumes 35 and 36. The Journal is the only appropriate literature citation for the articles printed on these pages. The page numbers in the table of contents, contributors list, and index of this volume correspond to the page numbers at the foot of these pages.

The table of contents does not necessarily follow the pattern of the plenary sessions. Instead, it reflects the thrust of the meeting as it evolved from the combination of plenary sessions, poster sessions, and workshops, culminating in the final collection of invited papers, submitted papers, and workshop summaries. The order in which articles appear in this volume does not follow the order of citation in the table of contents. Many of the articles in this volume were published in the Journal of Cellular Biochemistry, and they are reprinted here. These articles appear in the order in which they were accepted for publication and then published in the Journal. They are followed by papers which were submitted solely for publication in the proceedings.

Contents

Contributors xiii
Preface
Garth L. Nicolson and Isaiah J. Fidler xix

I. TUMOR PROGRESSION AND DIVERSIFICATION: GENETIC ASPECTS

In Vivo Metastatic Progression of an H-*ras* Transformed Mouse 10T1/2 Cell Line
M.-C. Gingras, L. Jarolim, J.A. Wright, and A.H. Greenberg 127

Application of Gene Transfer to the Study of Tumor Progression and Metastasis
Carol Waghorne, Martin L. Breitman, and Robert S. Kerbel 135

Cytogenetic Diversity in Primary Human Tumors
Sandra R. Wolman, Patricia M. Camuto, and Mary Ann Perle 39

Simultaneous Transfer of Tumorigenic and Metastatic Phenotypes by Transfection With Genomic DNA From a Human Cutaneous Squamous Cell Carcinoma
Honnavara N. Ananthaswamy, Janet E. Price, Leonard H. Goldberg, and
Elise S. Bales 29

Malignant Progression of Human Breast Cancer
Helene S. Smith, Charles M. Dollbaum, Britt-Marie Ljung, Brian Mayall, and
Adeline J. Hackett 143

II. TUMOR PROGRESSION AND DIVERSIFICATION: HOST ASPECTS

Role of Inflammatory Cells in Tumor Progression and Diversification
Gloria H. Heppner 151

Heterogeneity of Fibroblast Response in Host-Tumor Cell-Cell Interactions in Metastatic Tumors
Mustafa Kh. Dabbous, Lena Haney, Lee M. Carter, A.K. Paul, and James Reger . . . 1

Interactions Between Genetic Constitution of Metastatic Tumour Cells and Host Factors
D. Tarin 157

Differences Among Endothelial Cells: Their Relation to Tumor Growth and Metastasis
Marek Kaminski and Robert Auerbach 161

Immunologic Factors Influencing the Metastasis of Skin Cancers
Margaret L. Kripke and Cynthia A. Romerdahl 167

III. GENE EXPRESSION AND METASTASIS

Mechanism of Induction of Class I Major Histocompatibility Antigen Expression by Murine Leukemia Virus
Douglas V. Faller, Lise D. Wilson, and David C. Flyer 61

Gene Expression and Tumor Cell Escape From Host Effector Mechanisms in Murine Large Cell Lymphoma
Ronald A. LaBiche, Mitsuzi Yoshida, Gary E. Gallick, Tatsuro Irimura, Donald L. Robberson, Jim Klostergaard, and Garth L. Nicolson 103

ERV3 Human Endogenous Provirus mRNAs Are Expressed in Normal and Malignant Tissues and Cells, But Not in Choriocarcinoma Tumor Cells
Maurice Cohen, Nobuyuki Kato, and Erik Larsson 13

DNA Methylation Patterns and Tumor Heterogeneity
Peter A. Jones, Lois A. Chandler, Hamid Ghazi, Thomas Ahlering, and Louis Dubeau 173

IV. REGULATION OF THE METASTATIC PHENOTYPE

Spontaneous Fusion Between Metastatic Mammary Tumor Subpopulations
Fred R. Miller, Donna McInerney, Clare Rogers, and Bonnie E. Miller 21

Isolation and Visualization of Met-72-Positive, Metastatic Variants Present in B16 Melanoma Tumor Masses
Nanette P. Parratto and Arthur K. Kimura 75

Spontaneous and Oncogene-Mediated Acquisition of the Invasive Phenotype by Cells in Culture
Marc Mareel, Peter Coopman, Chris Dragonetti, Walter Fiers, Jin Gao, Ludwine Messiaen, and Frans Van Roy 179

Prostate Cancer and the Invasive Phenotype: Application of New In Vivo and In Vitro Approaches
James M. Kozlowski, Robert McEwan, Harold Keer, Julia Sensibar, Edward R. Sherwood III, Chung Lee, John T. Grayhack, Adriana Albini, and George R. Martin 189

V. TUMOR INVASION AND DISSEMINATION

Lymphatic Metastasis
Ian Carr and Norman Pettigrew 233

Tumor Cell Surface Lectins and Metastasis
Avraham Raz and Reuben Lotan 237

Expression of Cell Adhesion Molecules During Embryogenesis and Malignancy
Robert Brackenbury and Gerald M. Edelman 245

Interactions of Human Carcinoma Cells With Extracellular Matrix
R.J. Bernacki, K. Pavelic, C.L. Sullivan, G. Leto, M.A. Bulbul, Y.M. Rustum, M.J. Niedbala, and K. Crickard 251

VI. TUMOR IMPLANTATION AND GROWTH

Heparanases and Tumor Metastasis
Motowo Nakajima, Tatsuro Irimura, and Garth L. Nicolson 49

Basement Membranes, Reconstituted to Assess the Invasiveness of Tumor Cells
Adriana Albini, Sharon L. Aukerman, Antonella Melchiori, Eric W. Thompson, Reuven Reich, Thomas B. Shima, George R. Martin, and Yukihide Iwamoto 261

Interactions Between Tumor Cells and Liver Cells During Liver Metastasis Formation
    Ed Roos, John G. Collard, Folkert F. Roossien, and Geertje La Rivière 271

Increased Content of Chondroitin Sulfate Proteoglycan in Human Colorectal Carcinoma Metastases Compared With the Primary Tumor as Determined by an Anti-Chondroitin-Sulfate Monoclonal Antibody
    Takao Yamori, David M. Ota, Karen R. Cleary, and Tatsuro Irimura 115

Use of the Nude Mouse Model to Investigate Human Colorectal Cancer Metastases
    Raffaella Giavazzi 279

VII. FUTURE PERSPECTIVES FOR THERAPY OF METASTASIS

New Approaches to Achieve Systemic Activation of Macrophages for Destruction of Disseminated Cancer Cells
    Isaiah J. Fidler 285

Correlation of Immunomodulatory and Therapeutic Activities of Interferon and Interferon Inducers in Metastatic Disease
    Paul L. Black, Hamblin Phillips, Henry R. Tribble, Robin Pennington, Mark Schneider, and James E. Talmadge 87

Use of a Virus-Modified Tumor Cell Vaccine for Postoperative Immunotherapy of Metastases in an Animal Model System
    Volker Schirrmacher, Paul von Hoegen, and Rüdiger Heicappell 293

Index 297

Contributors

Thomas Ahlering, Urological Cancer Research Laboratory, USC Cancer Center, Los Angeles, CA 90033 [173]

Adriana Albini, Laboratory of Developmental Biology and Anomalies, National Institute of Dental Research and National Eye Institute, National Institutes of Health, Bethesda, MD 20892 [189, 261]

Honnavara N. Ananthaswamy, Department of Immunology, The University of Texas M.D. Anderson Cancer Center, Houston, TX 77030 [29]

Robert Auerbach, Laboratory of Developmental Biology, Department of Zoology, University of Wisconsin, Madison, WI 53706 [161]

Sharon L. Aukerman, Department of Cell Biology, The University of Texas M.D. Anderson Cancer Center, Houston, TX 77030 [261]

Elise S. Bales, Department of Immunology, The University of Texas M.D. Anderson Cancer Center, Houston, TX 77030 [29]

R.J. Bernacki, Department of Experimental Therapeutics, Grace Cancer Drug Center, Roswell Park Memorial Institute, Buffalo, NY 14263 [251]

Paul L. Black, Preclinical Evaluation Laboratory, PRI, National Cancer Institute-Frederick Cancer Research Facility, Frederick, MD 21701 [87]

Robert Brackenbury, The Rockefeller University, Laboratory of Developmental and Molecular Biology, New York, NY 10021 and Department of Anatomy and Cell Biology, University of Cincinnati College of Medicine, Cincinnati, OH 45267 [245]

Martin L. Breitman, Division of Cancer and Cell Biology, Mount Sinai Hospital Research Institute and Department of Medical Genetics, University of Toronto, Toronto, Ontario M5G 1X5, Canada [135]

M.A. Bulbul, Department of Experimental Therapeutics, Grace Cancer Drug Center, Roswell Park Memorial Institute, Buffalo, NY 14263 [251]

Patricia M. Camuto, Department of Pathology, New York University School of Medicine, New York, NY 10016 [39]

Ian Carr, Department of Pathology, University of Manitoba and St. Boniface General Hospital, Winnipeg, Manitoba R2A 2A6, Canada [233]

Lee M. Carter, Department of Biochemistry, The University of Tennessee, Memphis, The Health Science Center, Memphis, TN 38163 [1]

Lois A. Chandler, Urological Cancer Research Laboratory, USC Cancer Center, Los Angeles, CA 90033 [173]

Karen R. Cleary, Department of Pathology, The University of Texas M.D. Anderson Cancer Center, Houston, TX 77030 [115]

Maurice Cohen, BRI Basic Research Program, National Cancer Institute-Frederick Cancer Research Facility, Frederick, MD 21701 [13]

John G. Collard, Division of Cell Biology, Antoni van Leeuwenhoek Huis, The Netherlands Cancer Institute, 1066 CX Amsterdam, The Netherlands [271]

The number in brackets is the opening page number of the contributor's article.

Contributors

Peter Coopman, Laboratory of Experimental Cancerology, Department of Radiotherapy and Nuclear Medicine, University Hospital, State University Ghent, B-9000 Ghent, Belgium [179]

K. Crickard, Department of Gynecology and Obstetrics, Buffalo General Hospital, Buffalo, NY 14263 [251]

Mustafa Kh. Dabbous, Departments of Biochemistry, Periodontics, and U.T. Memphis Cancer Center, The University of Tennessee, Memphis, The Health Science Center, Memphis, TN 38163 [1]

Charles M. Dollbaum, Peralta Cancer Research Institute, Oakland, CA 94609 [143]

Chris Dragonetti, Laboratory of Experimental Cancerology, Department of Radiotherapy and Nuclear Medicine, University Hospital, State University Ghent, B-9000 Ghent, Belgium [179]

Louis Dubeau, Urological Cancer Research Laboratory, USC Cancer Center, Los Angeles, CA 90033 [173]

Gerald M. Edelman, The Rockefeller University, Laboratory of Developmental and Molecular Biology, New York, NY 10021 [245]

Douglas V. Faller, Division of Pediatric Oncology, Dana Farber Cancer Institute and Department of Pediatrics, Harvard Medical School and Childrens Hospital Medical Center, Boston, MA 02115 [61]

Isaiah J. Fidler, Department of Cell Biology, The University of Texas M.D. Anderson Cancer Center, Houston, TX 77030 [xix, 285]

Walter Fiers, Laboratory of Molecular Biology, State University Ghent, B-9000 Ghent, Belgium [179]

David C. Flyer, Department of Microbiology, Milton S. Hershey Medical Center, Hershey, PA 17033 [61]

Gary E. Gallick, Department of Tumor Biology, The University of Texas M.D. Anderson Cancer Center, Houston, TX 77030 [103]

Jin Gao, Chinese Academy of Basic Medical Sciences, Beijing, China [179]

Hamid Ghazi, Urological Cancer Research Laboratory, USC Cancer Center, Los Angeles, CA 90033 [173]

Raffaella Giavazzi, Mario Negri Institute for Pharmacological Research, 24100 Bergamo, Italy [279]

M.-C. Gingras, Manitoba Institute of Cell Biology, University of Manitoba, Winnipeg, Manitoba R3E 0V9, Canada [127]

Leonard H. Goldberg, Department of Dermatology, Baylor College of Medicine, Houston, TX 77030 [29]

John T. Grayhack, Department of Urology, Northwestern University Medical School, Chicago, IL 60611 [189]

A.H. Greenberg, Manitoba Institute of Cell Biology, University of Manitoba, Winnipeg, Manitoba R3E 0V9, Canada [127]

Adeline J. Hackett, Peralta Cancer Research Institute, Oakland, CA 94609 [143]

Lena Haney, Department of Periodontics, The University of Tennessee, Memphis, The Health Science Center, Memphis, TN 38163 [1]

Rüdiger Heicappell, Institut für Immunologie und Genetik, Deutsches Krebsforschungszentrum, D-6900 Heidelberg and Urologische Universitätsklinik, D-4000 Düsseldorf, Federal Republic of Germany [293]

Gloria H. Heppner, Michigan Cancer Foundation, Detroit, MI 48201 [151]

Tatsuro Irimura, Department of Tumor Biology, The University of Texas M.D. Anderson Cancer Center, Houston, TX 77030 [49,103,115]

Yukihide Iwamoto, Laboratory of Developmental Biology and Anomalies, National Institute for Dental Research, National Institutes of Health, Bethesda, MD 20892 [261]

L. Jarolim, Manitoba Institute of Cell Biology, University of Manitoba, Winnipeg, Manitoba R3E 0V9, Canada [127]

Peter A. Jones, Urological Cancer Research Laboratory, USC Cancer Center, Los Angeles, CA 90033 [173]

Marek Kaminski, Laboratory of Developmental Biology, Department of Zoology, University of Wisconsin, Madison, WI 53706 [161]

Nobuyuki Kato, BRI Basic Research Program, National Cancer Institute-Frederick Cancer Research Facility, Frederick, MD 21701 [13]

Harold Keer, Department of Urology, Northwestern University Medical School, Chicago, IL 60611 [189]

Robert S. Kerbel, Division of Cancer and Cell Biology, Mount Sinai Hospital Research Institute and Department of Medical Genetics, University of Toronto, Toronto, Ontario M5G 1X5, Canada [135]

Arthur K. Kimura, Department of Pathology, University of Florida College of Medicine, Gainesville, FL 32610 [75]

Jim Klostergaard, Department of Tumor Biology, The University of Texas M.D. Anderson Cancer Center, Houston, TX 77030 [103]

James M. Kozlowski, Department of Urology, Northwestern University Medical School, Chicago, IL 60611 [189]

Margaret L. Kripke, Department of Immunology, The University of Texas M.D. Anderson Cancer Center, Houston, TX 77030 [167]

Ronald A. LaBiche, Department of Tumor Biology, The University of Texas M.D. Anderson Cancer Center, Houston, TX 77030 [103]

Geertje La Rivière, Division of Cell Biology, Antoni van Leeuwenhoek Huis, The Netherlands Cancer Institute, 1066 CX Amsterdam, The Netherlands [271]

Erik Larsson, Department of Pathology, Uppsala University, Uppsala, Sweden [13]

Chung Lee, Department of Urology, Northwestern University Medical School, Chicago, IL 60611 [189]

G. Leto, Department of Experimental Therapeutics, Grace Cancer Drug Center, Roswell Park Memorial Institute, Buffalo, NY 14263 [251]

Britt-Marie Ljung, Department of Pathology, University of California, San Francisco, San Francisco, CA 94143 [143]

Reuben Lotan, Department of Tumor Biology, The University of Texas M.D. Anderson Cancer Center, Houston, TX 77030 [237]

Marc Mareel, Laboratory of Experimental Cancerology, Department of Radiotherapy and Nuclear Medicine, University Hospital, State University Ghent, B-9000 Ghent, Belgium [179]

George R. Martin, Laboratory of Developmental Biology and Anomalies, National Institute of Dental Research, National Institutes of Health, Bethesda, MD 20892 [189, 261]

Brian Mayall, Department of Laboratory Medicine, University of California, San Francisco, San Francisco, CA 94143 [143]

Robert McEwan, The Upjohn Company, Molecular Biology Research, Kalamazoo, MI 49001 [189]

Donna McInerney, E. Walter Albachten Department of Immunology, Michigan Cancer Foundation, Detroit, MI 48201 [21]

Antonella Melchiori, Istituto Scientifico Tumori, 16132 Genova, Italy [261]

Ludwine Messiaen, Laboratory of Experimental Cancerology, Department of Radiotherapy and Nuclear Medicine, University Hospital, State University Ghent, B-9000 Ghent, Belgium [179]

Bonnie E. Miller, E. Walter Albachten Department of Immunology, Michigan Cancer Foundation, Detroit, MI 48201 [21]

Fred R. Miller, E. Walter Albachten Department of Immunology, Michigan Cancer Foundation, Detroit, MI 48201 [21]

Motowo Nakajima, Department of Tumor Biology, The University of Texas M.D. Anderson Cancer Center, Houston, TX 77030 [49]

Garth L. Nicolson, Department of Tumor Biology, The University of Texas M.D. Anderson Cancer Center, Houston, TX 77030 [xix, 49, 103]

Contributors

M.J. Niedbala, Department of Experimental Therapeutics, Grace Cancer Drug Center, Roswell Park Memorial Institute, Buffalo, NY 14263 [251]

David M. Ota, Department of Surgery, The University of Texas M.D. Anderson Cancer Center, Houston, TX 77030 [115]

Nanette P. Parratto, Department of Pathology, University of Florida College of Medicine, Gainesville, FL 32610 [75]

A.K. Paul, Department of Biochemistry, The University of Tennessee, Memphis, The Health Science Center, Memphis, TN 38163 [1]

K. Pavelic, Department of Experimental Therapeutics, Grace Cancer Drug Center, Roswell Park Memorial Institute, Buffalo, NY 14263 [251]

Robin Pennington, Preclinical Evaluation Laboratory, PRI, National Cancer Institute-Frederick Cancer Research Facility, Frederick, MD 21701 [87]

Mary Ann Perle, Department of Pathology, New York University School of Medicine, New York, NY 10016 [39]

Norman Pettigrew, Department of Pathology, University of Manitoba, Winnipeg, Manitoba R3E 0W2, Canada [233]

Hamblin Phillips, Preclinical Evaluation Laboratory, PRI, National Cancer Institute-Frederick Cancer Research Facility, Frederick, MD 21701 [87]

Janet E. Price, Department of Cell Biology, The University of Texas M.D. Anderson Cancer Center, Houston, TX 77030 [29]

Avraham Raz, Department of Cell Biology, The Weizmann Institute of Science, Rehovot 76100, Israel and Metastasis Research Program, Michigan Cancer Foundation, Detroit, MI 48201 [237]

James Reger, Department of Anatomy, The University of Tennessee, Memphis, The Health Science Center, Memphis, TN 38163 [1]

Reuven Reich, Laboratory of Developmental Biology and Anomalies, National Institute for Dental Research, National Institutes of Health, Bethesda, MD 20892 [261]

Donald L. Robberson, Department of Genetics, The University of Texas M.D. Anderson Cancer Center, Houston, TX 77030 [103]

Clare Rogers, E. Walter Albachten Department of Immunology, Michigan Cancer Foundation, Detroit, MI 48201 [21]

Cynthia A. Romerdahl, Department of Immunology, The University of Texas M.D. Anderson Cancer Center, Houston, TX 77030 [167]

Ed Roos, Division of Cell Biology, Antoni van Leeuwenhoek Huis, The Netherlands Cancer Institute, 1066 CX Amsterdam, The Netherlands [271]

Folkert F. Roossien, Division of Cell Biology, Antoni van Leeuwenhoek Huis, The Netherlands Cancer Institute, 1066 CX Amsterdam, The Netherlands [271]

Y.M. Rustum, Department of Experimental Therapeutics, Grace Cancer Drug Center, Roswell Park Memorial Institute, Buffalo, NY 14263 [251]

Volker Schirrmacher, Institut für Immunologie und Genetik, Deutsches Krebsforschungszentrum, D-6900 Heidelberg, Federal Republic of Germany [293]

Mark Schneider, Preclinical Evaluation Laboratory, PRI, National Cancer Institute-Frederick Cancer Facility, Frederick, MD 21701 [87]

Julia Sensibar, Department of Urology, Northwestern University Medical School, Chicago, IL 60611 [189]

Edward R. Sherwood III, Department of Urology, Northwestern University Medical School, Chicago, IL 60611 [189]

Thomas B. Shima, Laboratory of Developmental Biology and Anomalies, National Institute for Dental Research, National Institutes of Health, Bethesda, MD 20892 [261]

Helene S. Smith, Peralta Cancer Research Institute, Oakland, CA 94609 [143]

C.L. Sullivan, Department of Experimental Therapeutics, Grace Cancer Drug Center, Roswell Park Memorial Institute, Buffalo, NY 14263 [251]

James E. Talmadge, Preclinical Evaluation Laboratory, PRI, National Cancer Institute-Frederick Cancer Research Facility, Frederick, MD 21701 **[87]**

D. Tarin, Nuffield Department of Pathology, John Radcliffe Hospital, Oxford University, Oxford OX3 9DU, England **[157]**

Erik W. Thompson, Laboratory of Developmental Biology and Anomalies, National Institute for Dental Research, National Institutes of Health, Bethesda, MD 20892 **[261]**

Henry R. Tribble, Preclinical Evaluation Laboratory, PRI, National Cancer Institute-Frederick Cancer Research Facility, Frederick, MD 21701 **[87]**

Frans Van Roy, Laboratory of Molecular Biology, State University Ghent, B-9000 Ghent, Belgium **[179]**

Paul von Hoegen, Institut für Immunologie und Genetik, Deutsches Krebsforschungszentrum, D-6900 Heidelberg, Federal Republic of Germany and Department of Medicine, Division of Immunology, Medical Center, Stanford University, Stanford, CA 94305 **[293]**

Carol Waghorne, Division of Cancer and Cell Biology, Mount Sinai Hospital Research Institute, Toronto, Ontario M5G 1X5, Canada and Department of Pathology, Dalhousie University, Halifax, Nova Scotia B3H 4H7, Canada **[135]**

Lise D. Wilson, Division of Pediatric Oncology, Dana Farber Cancer Institute and Department of Pediatrics, Harvard Medical School and Childrens Hospital Medical Center, Boston, MA 02115 **[61]**

Sandra R. Wolman, Department of Pathology, New York University School of Medicine, New York, NY 10016 **[39]**

J.A. Wright, Manitoba Institute of Cell Biology, University of Manitoba, Winnipeg, Manitoba R3E 0V9, Canada **[127]**

Takao Yamori, Department of Tumor Biology, The University of Texas M.D. Anderson Cancer Center, Houston, TX 77030 **[115]**

Mitsuzi Yoshida, Department of Tumor Biology, The University of Texas M.D. Anderson Cancer Center, Houston, TX 77030 **[103]**

Preface

Dramatic advances in patient care and cancer therapy have led to more favorable clinical results for many patients, but many others die from cancer metastases that are refractory to therapy. The realization that some of the most common forms of cancer cannot be adequately treated once the primary tumor metastasizes led to the organization of a conference held in Keystone, Colorado, April 6–12, 1987. The meeting was devoted to the exchange of new information on various cancers and their metastatic processes. This proceedings volume is derived from the conference presentations.

Successful diagnosis and treatment of metastatic cancers can only advance with growing knowledge of the pathogenesis of metastasis and the unique properties of highly malignant cells and their host microenvironments, as well as the development of new approaches for the treatment of metastases. A basic goal of the meeting was to bring together scientists and clinicians from a variety of disciplines to explore these areas. This resulted in interactions between basic scientists involved in studying the biochemistry, molecular biology, immunology, cell biology, and genetics of experimental and clinical metastasis with physicians involved in the pathology, radiotherapy, chemotherapy, and biological therapy of metastases in cancer patients. Such interactions gave rise to lively discussions and increased planning of interdisciplinary studies.

This volume is organized roughly along the lines of the meeting. It begins with presentations on the genetics of metastasis and ends with contributions on future perspectives for the clinical therapy of metastases. The sections that intervene deal with host aspects of tumor heterogeneity, progression and metastasis, gene expression and regulation of the metastatic phenotype, and tumor invasion, dissemination, implantation, and growth of metastatic cells in specific organ environments. New technologies, such as gene and chromosome transfer, gene expression analysis, cell surface biochemical characterization, and the use and delivery of biological response modifiers, were prominent throughout the meeting and form the basis for many of the contributions to this volume. We feel that readers of this volume, like the conference attendees, will come away with the realization that new and better approaches for the diagnosis, treatment, and ultimately the understanding of cancer metastasis will be forthcoming only when we gain greater insight into the biology of cancer metastasis and begin to elucidate the molecular mechanisms by which malignant cells proliferate, diversify, invade, disseminate, implant, survive, and grow in distant organs.

We are extremely grateful to Robin Yeaton, who performed a tremendous service and rendered much assistance during the organization of the meeting and during its sessions in Keystone. We are also indebted to Dharm Darshan Khalsa for her help with the manuscripts and the editing and review process.

Preface

We wish to thank Triton Biosciences, Inc., and Smith, Kline & French Laboratories for their generous cosponsorship of this meeting. We gratefully acknowledge additional support from Pfizer Central Research, Pfizer, Inc. Further financial support was received from USHHS grant R13 CA44477-01.

Garth L. Nicolson
Isaiah J. Fidler

Heterogeneity of Fibroblast Response in Host-Tumor Cell-Cell Interactions in Metastatic Tumors

Mustafa Kh. Dabbous, Lena Haney, Lee M. Carter, A.K. Paul, and James Reger

Departments of Biochemistry (M.K.D., L.M.C, A.K.P.), Periodontics (L.H., M.K.D.), Anatomy (J.R.), and U.T. (M.K.D.), Memphis Cancer Center, The University of Tennessee, Memphis, The Health Science Center, Memphis, Tennessee 38163

The spread and invasion of tumor cells into host tissues are associated with the release of elevated levels of collagenolytic activity of both host and tumor cell origins. However, the mechanisms of regulation of the enzyme activity is still unresolved. Histological examination of human and animal tumors revealed morphological changes in stromal fibroblasts and mast cells at the tumor periphery. Numerous mast cells appeared at microfoci along the tumor: host tissue junction and mast cell degranulation were associated with collagenolysis. In vitro studies, using rat mammary adenocarcinoma and human lung adenocarcinoma cells, showed that both tumor cells and host fibroblasts participate in matrix degradation. Tumor-associated stromal fibroblasts released higher levels of enzyme activity than normal fibroblasts and were more responsive to stimulation by tumor-conditioned media and soluble mast cell products. Host fibroblasts appear to be heterogeneous populations of responsive and nonresponsive subpopulations based on their response to tumor- or mast-cell-mediated stimulation of collagenase release. Fibroblast subpopulations were obtained by density fractionation of serum-deprived, synchronized confluent fibroblasts on discontinuous Percoll gradient. Density-fractionated fibroblast subpopulations differed in their response to stimulation by mast cell products and tumor-cell-conditioned media. The stimulatory activity of tumor-cell-conditioned media also varied as a function of the metastatic potential of the tumor cells. The data suggest that cellular interactions between tumor cells and select subpopulations of host fibroblasts at the tumor periphery play a key role in host tissue degradation. However, heterogeneity of stromal fibroblasts may determine the site and extent of the tissue damage at foci of tumor invasion.

Key words: tumor invasion, cell-cell interaction, fibroblast response, collagenolytic activity, mast cell products

Received April 12, 1987; accepted June 30, 1987.

© 1987 Alan R. Liss, Inc.

Invasive neoplasms and metastatic tumor cells may be confronted by a variety of natural tissue barriers in vivo, especially connective tissue stroma and basement membrane structures. As collagen represents the major structural protein of all tissues and provides the chief obstacle to passive migration of tumor cells [1], it has been postulated that collagenolytic enzymes are required to facilitate the spread and invasion of tumor cells into host tissues [for reviews see 2-7]. There is now substantial evidence to support this hypothesis; collagen degradation has been observed at the outer margin of some invasive tumors [7-9], and immunolocalization studies have demonstrated the enzyme collagenase at similar sites [11-14]. The expression of collagen-degrading enzymes is invariably microenvironmental in nature, often occurring at microfoci around the tumor periphery [11], and it seems likely that local host tumor cell interactions are important in modulating collagenolytic activity [15-19]. Work in this laboratory and others showed the enhanced release of collagenolytic activity in cultures of stromal fibroblasts stimulated by tumor cells or their conditioned media [15-17]. Furthermore, mast cell accumulation in increased numbers and degranulation at the tumor periphery in association with stromal lysis have been recently reported [20]. Stromal response at the tumor:host junction, however, appears to be variable [9,20]. Tumor-associated fibroblasts, presumably at the invasion zone, appear to be more responsive to stimulation by tumor cell conditioned media [16] and by mast cell products (MCP), than normal host fibroblasts [20]. It is not known whether the difference in fibroblast response is due to tumor-derived modulation of fibroblast behavior, or to the presence of responsive and nonresponsive fibroblast subpopulations. Because of our interest in the mechanism of tumor invasion and metastasis, especially the cellular interactions involved in matrix degradation, we have focused our attention on stromal fibroblast interactions at the host:tumor interface "invasion zone." In this report, we present data which suggest the heterogeneity of stromal fibroblasts and the presence of subpopulations within apparently homogeneous cell lines which vary in their response to both host- and tumor-derived modulators of collagenolytic activity at the invasion zone. This phenotypic variability may be one of several factors which play a significant role in determining the preferred direction of the invasive tumor growth in vivo.

MATERIALS AND METHODS
Fibroblast Cultures

Normal rat skin fibroblasts (NRS) and rat mammary adenocarcinoma-associated fibroblasts (Ln2-F, Ln3-F) were grown and maintained as described previously [20]. Human fibroblasts from normal lung (LT7, LT9, LT10), embryonal testis (HET1), gingiva (GH8), and basal cell carcinoma-associated fibroblasts (BCE5) were established from explants prepared from surgical specimen provided by the Department of Pathology, University of Tennessee (Memphis, TN). BCE5, HET1, GN32, and GH8 subpopulations were obtained by the Percoll density gradient method and by selective detachment by brief trypsinization. All fibroblasts except rat were grown in Alpha-minimum essential medium (AMEM) supplemented with 10% fetal calf serum (FCS) (Grand Island Biological Co., Grand Island, NY). Rat fibroblasts were cultured in the presence of 10% heat-inactivated fetal calf serum and without antibiotics.

Tumor Cells

Human breast scirrhous (MCF7) and infiltrating ductal (BT20) carcinoma cells were obtained from the EG & G Mason Research Institute (Rockville, MD). Human lung adenocarcinoma (CaLu6) was kindly provided by Dr. Nathan Sloane, Department of Biochemistry, University of Tennessee (Memphis, TN). MTLn2, MTF7, and MTLn3 clones, derived from the rat mammary adenocarcinoma 13762NF, were provided by Dr. Garth Nicolson, Department of Tumor Biology, University of Texas, M.D. Anderson Hospital and Tumor Institute (Houston, TX). All cells were grown and maintained in the same growth media as described above.

Tumor-Cell-Conditioned Medium

Serum-free conditioned media were collected after 24 hr from tumor cells incubated at 5×10^5 cells per ml of medium. The media were sterilized through a Millex-GS filter unit and stored at $-20°C$. Each conditioned medium was diluted (1:3) with serum-free AMEM before incubating with the fibroblasts.

Mast Cell Products (MCP)

Mast cell products were derived from purified rat peritoneal mast cells collected from rats bearing mammary adenocarcinoma tumors. Enriched mast cell fractions were obtained by Percoll discontinuous density gradient as described previously [21]. The isolated mast cells were adjusted to 4×10^6 cells per ml in 1 M NaCl, extracted overnight at $4°C$, and sonicated for 10 sec. The preparation was centrifuged at 16,000 rpm for 1 hr and the resulting supernatant (MCP) was stored at $-20°C$.

Histology

Rat and human tumor specimen with surrounding host tissues were fixed in 1% formaldehyde and 0.25% glutaraldehyde in 0.1 M sodium cacodylate buffer (pH 7.4) at $4°C$ and embedded in JB-4 plastic. Sections (2 μm) were stained according to the method of Bromley et al [22].

Collagenase Activity

For assays, fibroblast cultures were each seeded at 10^5 cells per well in multiwell trays containing growth medium. After 24 hr, the media were removed and replaced with serum-free AMEM with and without a supplement of MCP (10%) or tumor-cell-conditioned medium. Media were collected from triplicate wells at day 3 and stored at $-20°C$. For protein determination, total cell densities were dissolved in 500 μl 0.1 N NaOH per well. Protein concentrations were determined by the method of Lowry et al [23]. Collagenase activity in the serum-free media was assayed by measuring the release of soluble radioactive peptides from 30 μl [^{14}C]-glycine-labeled reconstituted collagen fibril gels after 18 hr at $35°C$ as described earlier [16]. One unit of collagenase degrades 1 μg of collagen per min at $35°C$. Latent collagenase was activated by incubating 20 min with 25 μg trypsin followed by fivefold concentration of soybean trypsin inhibitor.

Fibroblast Subpopulation

BCE5, GH8, and HET1 explants were prepared from the fresh tissue and maintained in AMEM supplemented with 10% FCS. After initial growth, the fibroblasts were harvested and purified using a 2%, 6%, 10%, 14%, 18%, 24%, 30%, 35%, and 40% Percoll discontinuous density gradient. The isolated cells were collected at each interface, washed twice in D-PBS, and plated for growth at $37°C$ in a

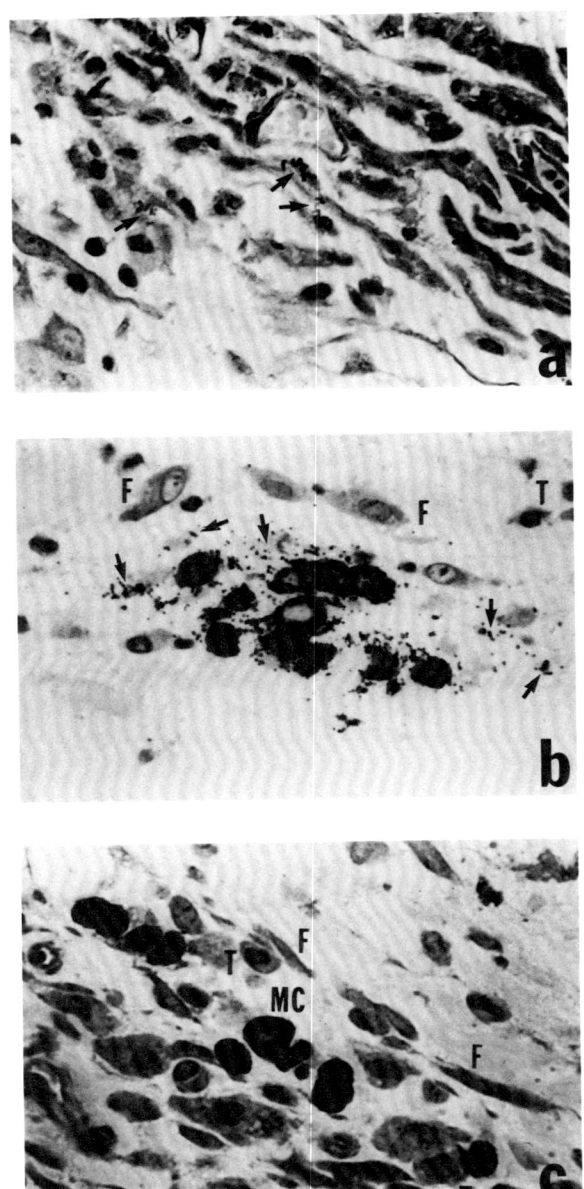

Fig. 1. Photomicrographs of (a) stromal connective tissue with mast cells and mast cell granules (arrows); (b) a group of mast cells showing degranulation adjacent to enlarged fibroblasts; (c) coexistence of intact mast cells (MC), fibroblasts (F), and tumor cells (T). ×360.

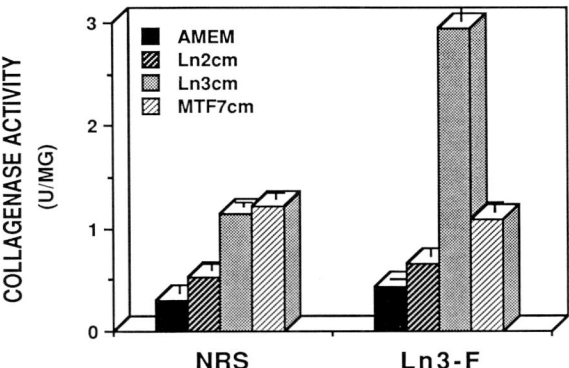

Fig. 2. Effect of tumor-cell-conditioned media on the collagenolytic activity of normal rat fibroblast (NRS), and Ln3 tumor-derived fibroblast (Ln3-F). 24-Hr serum-free conditioned media were derived as described in the text and incubated with fibroblasts for 3 days. Collagenase assay was carried out using 200 μl of medium by the collagen fibril assay using [^{14}C]-labeled collagen.

5% CO_2 humidified atmosphere. Subpopulations were also derived by trypsinization using the method of Hassell and Stanek [24].

RESULTS

Histologic examination of MTLn3 tumor specimens revealed increased number of fibroblasts and mast cells in localized areas of the stroma adjacent to the invading tumor cells. Fibroblasts appeared remarkably large, and mast cell degranulation was often seen associated with foci of matrix degradation along the host:tumor interface (Fig. 1). Similar observations were made in the human tumor specimens (data not shown).

Tumor Cell-Fibroblast Interactions

Normal fibroblasts release very low levels of latent collagenase activity in vitro [16,20]. Tumor cells also release negligible amounts of enzyme activity in the culture media [20]. However, cocultures of the highly metastatic cell variant MTLn3 (Ln3) of rat mammary adenocarcinoma, and normal rat fibroblast (NRS) stimulated the release of relatively higher levels of enzyme activity. The stimulatory effect was not dependent on direct cell-cell contact since media conditioned by the tumor cells (Ln3cm) enhanced the release of fibroblast collagenolytic activity (Fig. 2). The enhancement of in vitro enzyme release was dependent on the nature of the target fibroblast and the metastatic potential of the effector (tumor cell). Thus, stromal fibroblasts derived from the tumor periphery (Ln3-F) were more responsive than normal fibroblasts (NRS), and media conditioned by the highly metastatic clone MTLn3 cells (Ln3cm) were more effective than those of the low metastatic clone variant MTLn2 (Ln2cm). Conditioned media derived from the tumor clone MTF7 (with metastatic potential intermediate between Ln2 and Ln3) appeared to have no differential effect on either normal (NRS) or tumor-derived (Ln3-F) fibroblasts. In this respect, MTF7 and MTLn2 tumor-cell-conditoned media had similar effects. The response of stromal fibroblasts associated with the low metastatic variant MTLn2 (Ln2-F) was not significantly different from that of normal fibroblasts NRS when stimulated by Ln2 conditioned media (Ln2cm) (Fig. 3). The enhancement of enzyme activity of tumor-associated fibroblasts appeared to be tumor specific and varied with the metastatic potential of the tumor cells.

Fibroblast Heterogeneity

Fibroblast heterogeneity has been examined by density-fractionation of apparently homogeneous population of fibroblasts. Several human fibroblast cell lines were grown to confluence and then serum-deprived to obtain a nongrowing population synchronized in the G1/G0 phase of the cycle [25]. Based on differences in cell density, cells were fractionated into distinct zones at 2–10%, 18%, 24%, and 35% Percoll. These distinct bands were recovered from the gradient centrifugation of several cell lines examined. Differences were observed, however, in the extent and distribution of cell populations among the different zones. The cells removed by aspiration and grown as described in Materials and Methods showed distinct differences in growth rates.

Density-fractionated fibroblast subpopulations differed in size and in morphology (Fig. 4). The fraction separating at 2–10% (B) contained small spindle-shaped cells (major); large, flat, and thin cells (minor); and dendritic cells with long processes (minor). The fraction C, separating at 24%, represents the major population and contains a uniform cell type—mainly short, broad cells with uniform size. The density fraction D, separated at 35% Percoll zone, contained mainly long, spindle-shaped densely packed cells with ruffled edges and long processes. Staining fixed cells with fluorescein-labeled anti-actin stained the cytoskeletal elements in most of the cells in the subpopulations. However, fraction C (24%) was poorly stained with anti-actin antibodies. Staining fixed cells with fluorescein-labeled antimyosin antibody showed no significant labeling of the 24% (C) fraction, while a large number of cells in the 35% (D) fraction were densely labeled, suggesting increased content of myosin-containing structural components in these cells (Fig. 4E,F). The heterogeneity observed in antimyosin staining of cells in this subpopulation may be due to variation in the myofibrillar content or due to microheterogeneity among cells in this subpopulation.

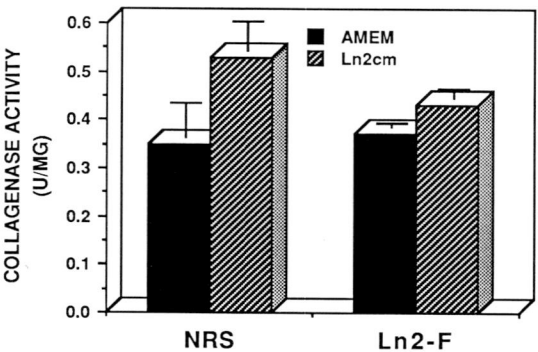

Fig. 3. Effect of MTLn2 tumor-cell-conditioned media on the collagenolytic activity of normal rat fibroblasts (NRS) and Ln2 tumor-derived fibroblasts (Ln2-F). Experimental conditions as in Figure 2.

Heterogeneity of Tumor Cell-Host Fibroblast Interactions

We have previously shown that tumor-associated fibroblasts (TAF) differ in their phenotype from normal fibroblasts [16]. It was suggested that TAF may represent a select subpopulation of responsive fibroblasts or that they may be simply tumor-activated stromal fibroblasts. The response of various fibroblast cell lines and their density-fractionated subpopulations to tumor-cell-conditioned media has been examined. Human fibroblast cell lines HET1, GH8, and BCE and their subpopulations were stimulated by incubation with media conditioned by human lung adenocarcinoma cells (CaLu6) or by basal cell carcinoma cells (BCE). The parental cell line (P) of HET1 did not show any significant effect in the collagenolytic activity after 3 days of incubation with CaLu6-conditioned medium (CaLu6-cm) (showed 5% decrease). However, subpopulations A and C showed significantly high responses, D showed a decrease, while the collagenolytic activity of B, E, and F was nearly unaffected by CaLu6-cm (Fig. 5). The decrease in enzyme activity of subpopulation D in presence of conditioned medium compared to AMEM may be due to a certain degree of inhibition.

The gingival fibroblast cell line GH8 (P), on the other hand, was responsive to stimulation by the lung tumor-cell-conditioned medium (CaLu6) as shown in Figure 5 (bottom l). The relative response of the parental population (P) and its subpopulations when stimulated by CaLu6-cm is also depicted in Figure 5. The pattern of response, in general, differed significantly from that of HET1. While the collageno-

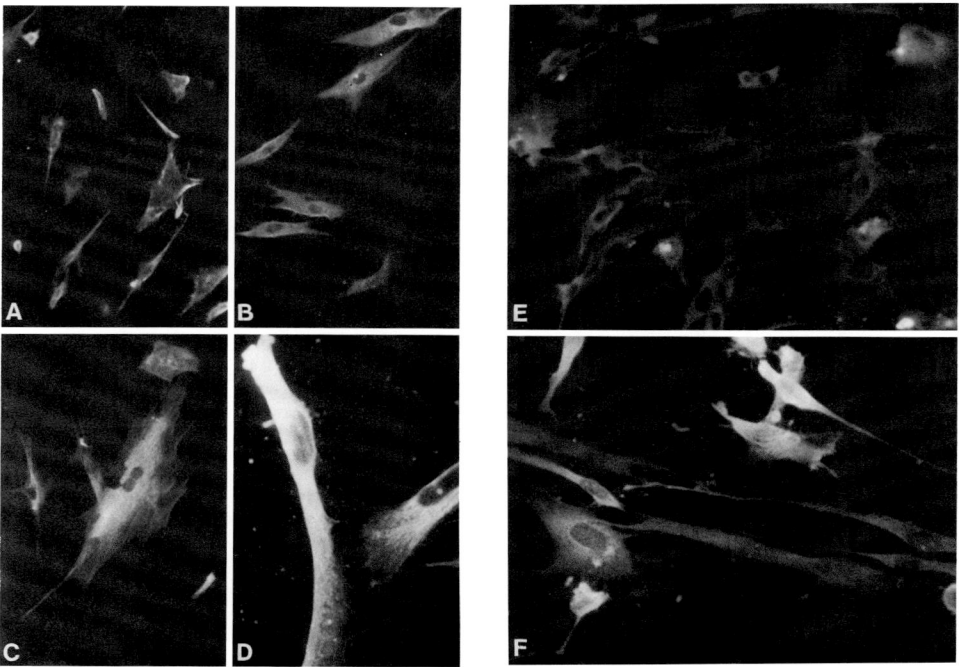

Fig. 4. Fluorescence photomicrographs of human basal cell epithelioma-associated fibroblasts showing in vitro identification of actin and myosin proteins. Indirect immunofluorescence staining with anti-actin: **A**: tumor-associated fibroblast (TAF). Fibroblasts obtained from Percoll gradient zones. **B**: 2–10%. **C**: 24%. **D**: 35%. **E**: 24%. **F**: 35%. (All stained with antimyosin.) A,B,E, ×160. C,D,F, ×400.

lytic activity of subpopulations A, B, and E was enhanced, that of subpopulations C and D slightly decreased while that of F was unchanged (Fig. 5). The data indicated that fibroblast heterogeneity does not appear to be tissue-specific. The presence of certain subpopulations of fibroblasts that are responsive and others that are nonresponsive to tumor-derived soluble factor(s), was also demonstrated among the apparently homogeneous gingival fibroblast cell line GH8 (Fig. 5, bottom).

Tumor-associated fibroblasts (TAF) in the stromal tissue represent the fraction most intimately associated with the tumor cells and appear to play a significant role during invasion and tumor progression. The question of heterogeneity of stromal fibroblasts adjacent to the invading tumor mass was also examined. These fibroblasts appeared to be heterogeneous in their response to tumor-derived soluble factor(s). The enzyme activity of tumor-associated fibroblasts (TAF) derived from basal cell carcinoma was significantly enhanced by BCE-derived conditioned media (Fig. 6). However, only select subpopulations of the density-fractionated tumor-associated fibroblasts were responsive to the BCE tumor-conditioned medium. These responsive subpopulations represented a major portion of the TAF cell population (approximately 60%).

Cellular interactions between tumor cells and host fibroblasts, leading to en-

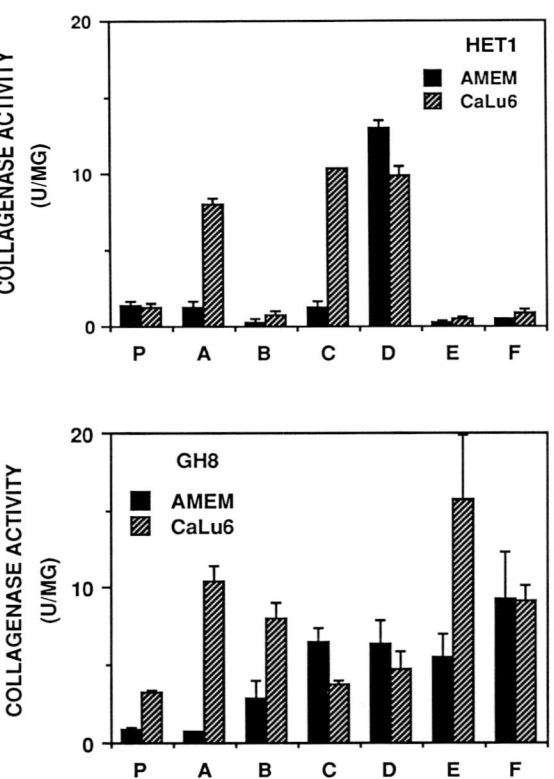

Fig. 5. Effect of human lung adenocarcinoma (CaLu6)-conditioned medium on the collagenase activity of human embryonal testis (HET1) and gingival (GH8) fibroblasts and their subpopulations. Control cultures contained serum-free AMEM. **P** represents the parental cell line and **A–F** represent density-fractionated cell subpopulations separated at 6%, 10%, 14%, 18%, 24%, and 35% Percoll gradient interfaces, respectively. Bars represent the mean values of triplicate assays ± SD.

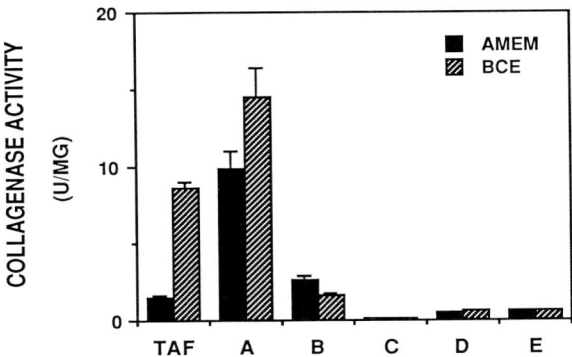

Fig. 6. The effect of basal cell carcinoma (BCE) on tumor-associated stromal fibroblasts (TAF), and density-fractionated subpopulations derived from TAF cells separated at (A) 2–10%; (B) 18%; (C) 24%; (D) 30%; and (E) 35% on Percoll gradient as described in the text. 24-Hr serum-free medium was collected from BCE tumor cell cultures, incubated with BCE-derived fibroblast subpopulations, then media were collected after 3 days and assayed as described in the text.

hanced collagenolysis, may depend to a certain extent on the type of tumor cells from which the conditioned medium was derived and appear to be tumor-specific. Using GH8 fibroblasts and their density-fractionated subpopulations as target cells, it was found that tumor modulation of collagenolytic activity varies with the type of tumor cells (Fig. 7). Less dense fibroblast subpopulations appeared to be more responsive to lung adenocarcinoma CaLu6-cm than to breast carcinoma. High-density subpopulations, except for subpopulation E, appeared to be more responsive to both tumor cell types. Fibroblast subpopulations appear to be selective in their response to tumor-derived soluble factor(s).

DISCUSSION

The spread and invasion of tumor cells into host tissues appear to be facilitated by the release of elevated levels of collagenolytic enzymes [2–6]. The enhanced release of these enzymes appears to be responsible for most of the stromal tissue damage frequently observed at the tumor periphery [1–9,26]. The enzyme production is microenvironmental in nature [11], often occurring at microfoci along the tumor periphery, and it is likely that host-tumor cell interactions play a major role in modulating the collagenolytic activity [15–17,28–32]. It has been previously demonstrated that tumor cells or their conditioned media stimulated the collagenolytic activity in cultures of host fibroblasts [15–17]. Epithelial-mesenchymal interactions have been described earlier [29]. Although Gross et al suggested that tumor products may mediate the interaction between tumor cells and host cells [30], a mechanism for in vivo modulation of collagenase synthesis is as yet not known. It may be postulated to occur through elaboration of a factor, possibly by the tumor acting directly to increase synthesis of collagenolytic enzymes or through a decrease in suppressor mechanisms for active enzyme synthesis. Stimulation of collagenase release by basal cell carcinoma-derived fibroblasts [15], rabbit synovial fibroblasts in response to both animal and human tumor cells [17], and by VX-2-derived fibroblast-like cells (F-cells) stimulated by homologous tumor-conditioned medium [16], demonstrated the importance of tumor cell-host fibroblast interactions in the collagenolysis of host tissues.

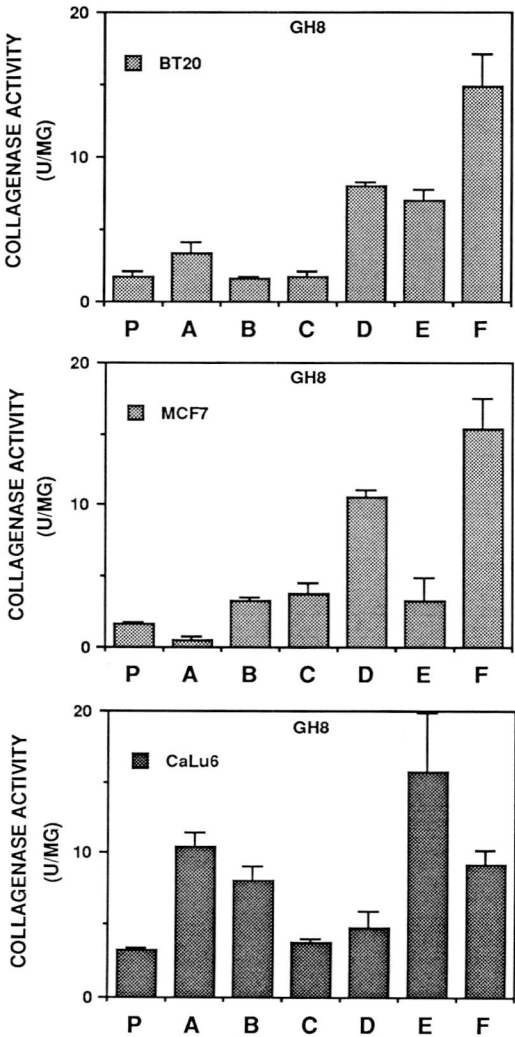

Fig. 7. Response of human fibroblast (GH8) and subpopulations to human breast (BT20, MCF7) and lung (CaLu6) carcinomas. Fibroblast subpopulations **A–F** were produced and maintained as described in the text. 24-Hr serum-free media were collected and incubated with the target cells in multiwell trays for 3 days, as described in the text.

Using rabbit VX-2 carcinoma and associated rabbit fibroblasts, we have reported that both tumor cells and host fibroblasts were capable of releasing collagenase activity in vitro [16]. Data presented in this report showed that, although the level of collagenolytic activity produced by in vitro cultures of rat mammary adenocarcinomas was relatively low, media conditioned by these cells had the potential to stimulate the enzyme activity of syngeneic host fibroblasts. The stimulation was dependent on the metastatic potential of the tumor cells, thus Ln3cm was more effective than Ln2cm. Although MTF7 had metastatic potential intermediate between that of MTLn3 and MTLn2, its ability to stimulate fibroblast collagenase activity was higher than predicted in comparison with Ln3cm and Ln2cm. However, MTF7 is a clone derived from the parental cell population at the primary site and differs from the lung metastasis variants Ln3 and Ln2 [31]. Media conditioned by the low metastatic variant MTLn2 or by MTF7 cells appeared to have no differential effect on either NRS or Ln3F. Furthermore, MTLn2-associated fibroblasts Ln2-F did not differ significantly from NRS in their response to tumor-derived conditioned media. These observations suggest that tumor cell-host fibroblast interactions appear to be tumor specific. The stimulatory activity depends also on the nature of the target fibroblasts, as histologic observations suggested the unique morphology of fibroblasts at the tumor periphery. Biochemical data showed that MTLn3 tumor-associated fibroblasts (Ln3-F) were more responsive to stimulation by Ln3cm than normal syngeneic fibroblasts (NRS).

Host tissue degradation appears to be localized at certain foci along the tumor periphery. Selectivity in interactions at the site of tumor invasion or preferred collagenolysis site may indicate specificity in tumor cell-host cell interactions. Such interactions may depend on the distribution of cell populations at the invasion zone [18]. Tumor-associated stromal fibroblasts may represent activated fibroblasts or a select subpopulation of responder cells at the invasion zone. The data indicated that certain stromal fibroblasts appear to be activated by adjacent tumor cells or their products, and hence are more responsive to tumor-mediated stimulation than normal fibroblasts. Alternatively, host fibroblasts are heterogeneous and tumor cells or their products may change the microenvironment in their vicinity to become more selective for a given subpopulation of fibroblasts which is more responsive to tumor-derived stimulation. The concept of responder and nonresponder fibroblast subpopulations in an apparently homogeneous mass culture is well supported in the literature [32–35]. Phenotypic variability in fibroblast cultures has been recently described, and density fractionated fibroblasts were shown to consist of distinct cell fractions [36] which were morphologically and biochemically different. Our biochemical and morphological data showed phenotypic variability among density-fractionated subpopulations of stromal fibroblasts. The fibroblast subpopulations showed selectivity and varied in their response to tumor-derived soluble factors (conditioned media). Preliminary binding studies with a partially characterized, tumor-derived cytokine, suggested that tumor-derived subpopulations of fibroblasts showed different specific binding properties towards the cytokine (unpublished data).

The role of fibroblasts in tumor invasion and progression does not appear to be a passive one. It has been recently reported that stromal fibroblasts facilitate tumor take and engraftment [27] and shorten the lag period for tumor growth and increase the growth rate. These authors showed that the addition of fibroblasts to tumor cells was necessary for tumor growth when the number of tumor cells alone was insufficient to produce tumors. Interactions between tumor cells and fibroblasts may be necessary in order for tumor-derived cells to initiate a tumor graft in the host. Certain subpopulations of stromal fibroblasts may play a significant role in tumor invasion, in response to tumor-mediated changes in the microenvironment. Fibroblast heterogeneity and selectivity in the response of morphologically and functionally different subpopulations appear to play a key role in local host-tumor interactions modulating collagenolysis at sites of matrix degradation in the invasion zone.

ACKNOWLEDGMENTS

The authors are grateful to Dr. Garth Nicolson, Department of Tumor Biology, The University of Texas System Cancer Center, M.D. Anderson Hospital and Tumor

Institute, Houston, Texas, for making the rat mammary adenocarcinoma 13762NF model available for these studies and for the valuable discussions and suggestions. The authors are also grateful to Dr. David Woolley, The University of Manchester, University Research Laboratories, University Hospital of South Manchester, Manchester, England, for his valuable input.

This work was supported by PHS Grant from NCI CA-25617.

REFERENCES

1. Hay ED: "Cell Biology of Extracellular Matrix." New York: Plenum, 1982.
2. Sugarbaker EV, Weingard DN, Roseman JM: In Liotta LA, Hart IR (eds): "Cancer Metastasis." Boston: Martinus Nijhoff, 1982, pp 427–465.
3. Liotta LA, Thorgeirsson UP, Garbisa S: Cancer Metastasis Rev 1:277, 1982.
4. Woolley DE: In Marcel MM, Calman KC (eds): "Invasion." Oxford: University Press, 1985, pp 228–251.
5. Strauli P: In Strauli P, Barrett AJ, Boici A (eds): "Proteinases and Tumor Invasion." EORTC Monograph series, vol 6, New York: Raven Press, 1980, pp. 1–15.
6. Wirl G, Frick J: Urol Res 7:103, 1979.
7. Hashimoto K, Yamanishi Y, Dabbous MKh: Cancer Res 32:2561, 1972.
8. Yamanishi Y, Dabbous MKh, Hashimoto K: Cancer Res 32:2551, 1972.
9. Van den Hooff A, Tigchelaar-Guttar W: Proc of the Konink, Nederlandse Akad van Westen, series C: Biol Med Sci 86:179, 1983.
10. Bauer EA, Gordon JM, Reddick ME, Eisen AZ: J Invest Dermatol 69:363, 1977.
11. Woolley DE: In Liotta LA, Hart IR (eds): "Cancer Invasion and Metastasis." Boston: Martinus, Nijhoff, 1980, pp 391–404.
12. Woolley DE, Tetlow LC, Mooney CJ, Evanson JM: In Strauli P (ed): "Proteinases in Tumor Invasion." New York: Raven Press, 1980, pp 97–115.
13. Woolley DE, Grafton CA: Br J Cancer 42:260, 1980.
14. Barsky SH, Togo S, Garbisa S, Liotta LA: Lancet 1:296, 1983.
15. Bauer EA, Uitto J, Walters, RC, Eisen AZ: Cancer Res 39:4594, 1979.
16. Dabbous MKh, El-Torky M, Haney L, Brinkley SrB, Sobhy N: Int J Cancer 31:357, 1983.
17. Biswas C: Biochem Biophys Res Commun 109:1026, 1982.
18. Woolley DE: Cancer Metastasis Rev 3:361, 1984.
19. Gebbert H: Cancer Metastasis Rev 4:293, 1985.
20. Dabbous MKh, Woolley DE, Haney L, Carter LM, Nicolson GL: Clin Exp Metastasis 4:141, 1986.
21. Darzynkiewiez Z, Sharpless T, Staino-Coico L, Melarned MR: Proc Natl Acad Sci USA 77:6696, 1980.
22. Bromley M, Woolley DE: Arthritis Rheum 27:857, 1984.
23. Lowry OH, Rosenbrough NJ, Farr AL, Randall RJ: J Biol Chem 193:265, 1951.
24. Hassell TM, Stanek EJ: Arch Oral Biol 28:617, 1983.
25. Declerck YA, Lang WE: Cancer Res 46:3580, 1986.
26. Picard O, Rolland Y, Popoun MF: Cancer Res 46:3290, 1986.
27. Knudson W, Biswas C, Toole BP: Proc Natl Acad Sci USA 81:6769, 1984.
28. Lynett-Wilson E, Gartner M, Campbell: 4th International Workshop on Immunodeficient Animals in Experimental Research, Chexbres, Switzerland: Karger, 1982.
29. Grillo HC, Gross J: Dev Biol 15:300, 1967.
30. Gross J, Azizkhan RG, Biswas C, Bruns RR, Hsieh DST, Folkman J: Proc Natl Acad Sci USA 78:1176, 1981.
31. Neri A, Welch D, Kwaguchi T, Nicolson GL: J Natl Cancer Inst 68:507, 1982.
32. Mitsui Y, Schneide EL: Exp Cell Res 103:23, 1976.
33. Bordin S, Page RC, Narayanan AS: Science 223:171, 1984.
34. Korn J, Torres D, Downie E: Arthritis Rheum 27:174, 1984.
35. Ko SD, Page RC, Narayanan AS: Proc Natl Acad Sci USA 74:3429, 1977.
36. Elias JA, Rossman MD, Zurier RB, Daniele RP: Am Rev Respir Dis 131:94, 1985.

ERV3 Human Endogenous Provirus mRNAs Are Expressed in Normal and Malignant Tissues and Cells, But Not in Choriocarcinoma Tumor Cells

Maurice Cohen, Nobuyuki Kato, and Erik Larsson

BRI Basic Research Program, National Cancer Institute Frederick Cancer Research Facility, Frederick, Maryland 21701 (M.C., N.K.); Department of Pathology, Uppsala University, Uppsala, Sweden (E.L.)

Messenger RNA expression of a human endogenous provirus, ERV3, has been characterized in 170 specimens of normal and malignant human tissues and cells. In contrast to the high expression in first-trimester and full-term placental chorionic villi, most other human tissues expressed ERV3 mRNAs at a level of 2–30% of placenta. However, ERV3 mRNAs were not detected in choriocarcinoma tumor cell lines. These studies suggest that the ERV3 provirus may have been preempted for a biological function and disruption of its mRNA expression results in choriocarcinoma.

Key words: human endogenous provirus, choriocarcinoma, proviral mRNA expression

Human DNA contains many integrated copies of retrovirus genomes that are related to the more widely characterized murine- and primate-type C retroviruses. Although a few of these human endogenous proviruses have been molecularly cloned and analyzed at the nucleotide sequence level [1], very little is known about their evolutionary origin or biological function(s). Recently, investigators described the RNA expression of a human type C-related provirus family that is present in human DNA in 70–100 copies per haploid genome [2].

We previously characterized another human endogenous provirus, ERV3, which was isolated from a human recombinant library by hybridization with the *pol* gene of an endogenous retroviral clone from chimpanzee and the baboon endogenous retrovirus long terminal repeat (LTR) [3]. ERV3 is a full-length provirus that contains a nondefective *env* glycoprotein gene [4] and functional promoters in the LTRs [5]

Nobuyuki Kato's present address is National Cancer Center Research Institute, Tsukiji 5-chome, Cho-ku, Tokyo, Japan.

Received May 6, 1987; revised and accepted July 28, 1987.

© 1988 Alan R. Liss, Inc.

(unpublished studies). In addition, the LTRs contain two glucocorticoid regulatory element sequences upstream from the promoter [5]. Because only a single copy of ERV3 is present in human DNA, ERV3 is useful for studying the expression and potential function of a specific human provirus. ERV3 was localized to human chromosome 7 [3].

To determine whether the ERV3 provirus is expressed in humans, we isolated RNA from various tissues of first-trimester abortuses and analyzed the RNAs by Northern blot hybridization [6]. We found that three major ERV3 mRNAs of 9, 7.3, and 3.5 kilobases (kb) were expressed in first-trimester placental chorionic villi but that only the 9-kb and low amounts of the 3.5-kb mRNAs were expressed in the embryo. RNA of full-term placental chorionic villi revealed a pattern identical with that of first-trimester placenta. We showed by Northern blot and S1 nuclease mapping analyses that the three ERV3 mRNAs were all spliced, *env*-containing RNAs [6]. The 9- and 7.3-kb mRNAs extended through the ERV3 3' LTR to a second splice donor site approximately 370 nucleotides (nt) downstream from the 3' LTR and contained, respectively, 5.5 or 3.8 kb of human genomic sequences [6]. The nature of these human sequences is presently under investigation. The 3.5-kb ERV3 mRNA was characterized by Northern blot analysis, S1 mapping, and sequence analysis of a cDNA clone isolated from a human 20-week-old fetal liver library [4,6]. The 3.5-kb mRNA was a typical subgenomic, spliced proviral message containing *env* but not *gag* or *pol* sequences and terminating in the 3' LTR.

We have undertaken an intensive investigation of ERV3 mRNA expression in human specimens to determine whether and to what extent normal expression is altered in malignant tissues and cells. In this study, we noted a dramatic absence of ERV3 mRNA expression in choriocarcinoma tumor cells.

MATERIALS AND METHODS
Tissue and Cells

Full-term human placentas were obtained from Frederick Memorial Hospital (Frederick, MD). Other human tissues were obtained from the Department of Pathology, University of Uppsala (Uppsala, Sweden). Human cell lines were obtained from Sloan-Kettering Institute for Cancer Research (Rye, NY). Choriocarcinoma cell lines ElFa and DoSmi were the kind gift of Dr. Roland Pattillo, Medical College of Wisconsin, (Milwaukee, WI). The MCF-7 cell line was kindly furnished by Dr. Sam C. Brooks, Michigan Cancer Foundation (Detroit, MI). The U-937 cell line was the kind gift of Dr. Kenneth Nilsson, University of Uppsala (Uppsala, Sweden). The choriocarcinoma cell line, GCC-SV, was kindly provided by Dr. Wolfgang Rettig, Memorial Sloan-Kettering Cancer Center (New York, NY).

Preparation of Nucleic Acids

Total RNA from tissues was prepared by the lithium chloride-urea method as previously described [6] with the modification that the first RNA pellet was washed with 3 M lithium chloride to remove contaminating DNA. Total RNA from tissue culture cells was also prepared by the lithium chloride-urea method, as above, except that cells were homogenized by vortexing. DNA was isolated from the supernatant fluid of the same preparation after the first RNA centrifugation. DNA was precipitated with ethanol, dissolved in TE (10 mM Tris, pH 7.5, 1 mM EDTA), treated with phenol-CHCl$_3$, and reprecipitated with ethanol. High-molecular-weight DNA from tissues was prepared in the standard manner [7].

Northern and Southern Blot Hybridization

Northern blot hybridization was as previously described [6,8]. For Southern analysis, 5 μg of DNA was digested with a restriction enzyme, and fragments were separated by electrophoresis in an agarose gel and transferred to nitrocellulose [9]. Hybridization conditions were the same as that for Northern blot hybridization [6]. After hybridization, the filters were washed twice with 2 × SSC, 0.1% SDS at room temperature for 10 min, in 1 × SSC, 0.1% SDS at 68°C for 1 hr, and finally in 0.1 × SSC, 0.1% SDS at 68°C for 1 hr. The filters were dried and autoradiographed with Kodak XAR-5 film with intensifying screens for 2 days.

RESULTS

To determine whether transcription of the human endogenous provirus, ERV3, is tissue specific and to compare the transcriptional levels of ERV3 in normal and malignant tissues, we surveyed ERV3 expression in 158 specimens of 31 different tissues, including 52 specimens from malignant tissues. Total RNA was isolated from each tissue and initially tested for ERV3 mRNAs by dot blot hybridization with a plasmid probe containing the entire ERV3 *env* glycoprotein and a portion of the transmembrane protein-coding sequence (Fig. 1). The highest level of expression was observed in the placental chorionic villi [6]. ERV3 transcripts represented 0.03–0.05% of the total mRNA in first-trimester and full-term placenta [6]. The composition of these mRNAs is summarized in Figure 1.

The level of ERV3 mRNA expression in most other human tissues was 10% or less than that of chorionic villi. However, several specimens revealed higher levels of expression including normal thymus, breast, testis, and gallbladder tissues and malignant breast, glioma, pancreas, stomach polyp, lung, rhabdomyosarcoma, and Wilms' tumor tissues. ERV3 expression in these specimens was 10–30% of that in placental chorionic villi (Table I). RNA from some of these tissues was analyzed by Northern blot hybridization using the ERV3 *env* probe as described above (Fig. 2). Each lane of the formaldehyde-agarose gel was loaded with 10 μg of total cellular

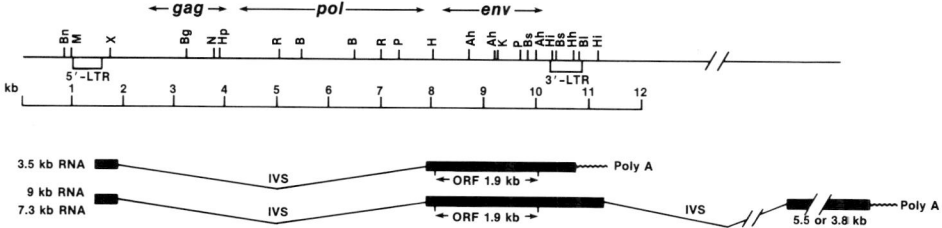

Fig. 1. Structure of the three ERV3 mRNAs. **Top:** Genetic and partial restriction map of the ERV3 provirus. **Bottom:** Exons are represented by thick bars; intervening sequences (IVS) by lines. Abbreviations: ORF, open reading frame; Ah, *Aha*III; Av, *Ava*I; B, *Bam*HI; Bg, *Bgl*II; Bl, *Bal*I; Bn, *Ban*I, Bs, *Bst*NI; H, *Hin*dIII; Hh, *Hha*I; Hi, *Hin*fI; Hp, *Hpa*I; K, *Kpn*I; M, *Mnl*I; N, *Nru*I; P, *Pst*I; R, *Eco*RI; X, *Xma*I.

TABLE I. ERV3 mRNA Expression in Human Tissues and Cells

Normal tissue
  Placental chorion — 40 first trimester, 6 term
  High-expression group (10–20% of placental chorion) — 4 gallbladder, 1 thymus, 1 testis, 1 breast
  Low-expression group (2–10% of placental chorion) — 11 endometrium, 10 stomach, 3 liver, 3 small intestine, 2 ovary, 2 myometrium, 2 epididymis, 2 prostate, 2 thyroid gland, 2 colon, 1 spleen, 1 lymph node, 1 skin, 1 pancreas, 1 bladder, 1 duodenum, 1 parotid, 1 testis

Malignant tissue
  High-expression group (10–30% of placental chorion) — 8 breast, 2 glioma, 2 pancreas, 1 stomach polyp, 1 lung (small cell), 1 rhabdomyosarcoma, 1 Wilms' tumor
  Low-expression group (2–10% of placental chorion) — 11 lung, 6 lymphoma, 4 stomach, 2 rectum, 2 kidney, 2 colon, 1 liver, 1 prostate, 1 gallbladder, 1 parotid, 1 bile duct, 1 duodenum, 1 bladder, 1 invasive hydatidiform mole

Cultured cells
  High-expression group (10–30% of placental chorion) — Monocytic leukemia, U937; 2 endometrial carcinoma, 2 cervical carcinoma, 1 breast carcinoma, MCF-7
  Low-expression group (<2% of placental chorion) — 6 choriocarcinoma

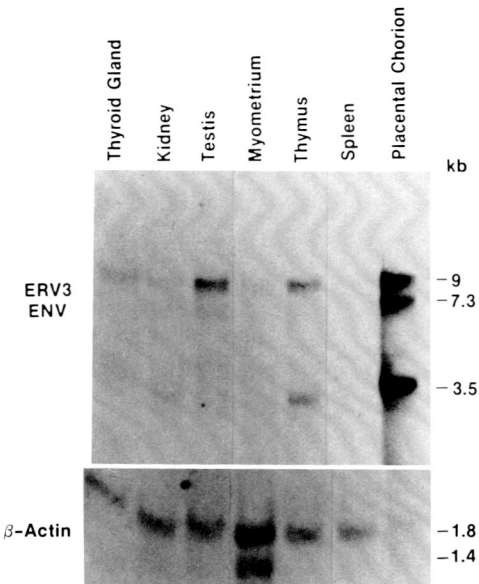

Fig. 2. Northern analysis of ERV3 mRNAs in human tissues. **Top:** Hybridization with ERV3 isolated 1.75-kb *env*-containing fragment, *Hin*dIII-*Pst*I; map position 8-9.7 (see Fig. 1). **Bottom insert:** Rehybridization of filter with chicken β-actin plasmid probe.

RNA. As a control, gels were stained with ethidium bromide before transfer to nitrocellulose to visualize the ribosomal RNAs. This provided a reliable means of estimating the relative quantity and quality of each RNA. In addition, filters were rehybridized with a chicken β-actin probe without removal of the ERV3 probe. The presence of the 1.8-kb β-actin mRNA and in some tissues the 1.4-kb β-actin mRNA, provided an independent assessment of RNA quality, although some differences in expression were noted among various tissues (Fig. 2). RNA from normal testis, thymus, and breast tissues and malignant breast, glioma, rhabdomyosarcoma, and Wilm's tumor tissues contained high levels of ERV3 mRNAs (Figs. 2, 3). In contrast, RNA from normal thyroid gland, kidney, myometrium, and spleen tissues and several malignant tissues, including leiomyosarcoma and sarcoma, contained low levels of ERV3 mRNAs. A striking feature of ERV3 expression in all these tissues was the absence of the 7.3-kb mRNA that was observed in the placental chorionic villi (Figs. 2, 3). Expression of the 7.3-kb mRNA is apparently specific for the placental chorion.

A high level of ERV3 mRNAs was also noted in some of the 12 human cell lines tested including the monocytic leukemia line, U937; breast cancer, MCF-7; two endometrium carcinomas, HEC-1B and An3CA; and two carcinomas of the cervix, C-33A and SiHa (Table 1). When analyzed by Northern blot hybridization, HEC-1B, AN3CA, and C-33A cells expressed the 9- and 3.5-kb ERV3 mRNAs, whereas SiHa cells expressed only the 3.5-kb mRNA (Fig. 4). Like nonplacental tissues, these human cell lines did not express the 7.3-kb mRNA. In contrast to endometrial and cervical carcinoma cells, two choriocarcinoma cell lines, BeWo and JAR, expressed almost no ERV3 mRNAs (Fig. 4). It is clear from the ethidium bromide-stained

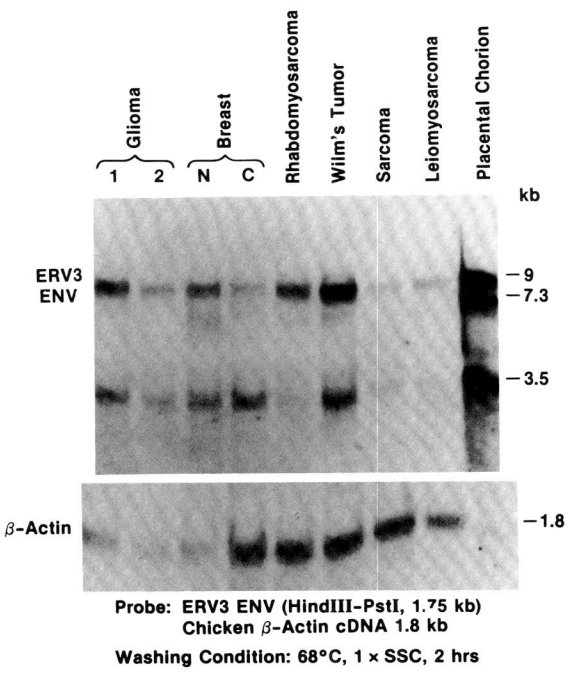

Fig. 3. Northern analysis of ERV3 mRNAs in human tissues. **Top:** hybridization with ERV3 1.75-kb *env* fragment. **Bottom insert:** Rehybridization of filter with chicken β-actin plasmid probe.

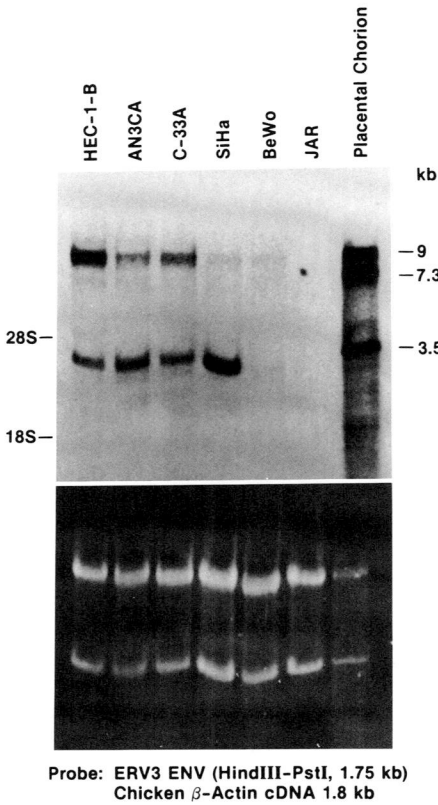

Fig. 4. Northern analysis of ERV3 mRNAs in human cells. **Top:** Hybridization with ERV3 1.75-kb *env* fragment. **Bottom:** Ethidium bromide staining of ribosomal RNAs in gel before transfer of RNA to nitrocellulose filter.

fluorescence pattern of the ribosomal RNAs (Fig. 4, bottom) that the absence of ERV3 mRNAs was not the result of differences in the amounts of RNA present in those lanes, nor to RNA degradation. To determine whether the absence of ERV3 mRNAs is a general feature of choriocarcinomas, we examined the RNA of four other choriocarcinoma cell lines, ElFa, DoSmi, GCC-SV, and JEG-3. Like JAR and BeWo, these choriocarcinoma lines also expressed almost no ERV3 mRNAs as determined by Northern and dot blot analysis, although long autoradiographic exposure revealed very low levels of ERV3 mRNAs in the ElFa line [6]. We were unable to obtain choriocarcinoma tumors; however, we obtained an invasive hydatidiform mole tissue. Invasive moles, moles that penetrate deep into the myometrium beyond their usual decidual implantation site, frequently occur following a molar pregnancy. Analysis of RNA from the invasive hydatidiform mole revealed a similar absence of ERV3 mRNA expression [6].

DISCUSSION

Three mRNAs of the human endogenous provirus, ERV3, are highly expressed in the human chorionic villi throughout development [6]. The abrogation of this expression in choriocarcinoma cells in culture and in an invasive hydatidiform mole tissue may represent the primary etiologic defect in these tumors. In other studies, we found that the absence of ERV3 mRNA expression is not the result of homozygous deletion of the proviral locus as shown by the finding that the ERV3 genome is present and unrearranged in the DNA of 5 choriocarcinoma cell DNAs [6].

Human gestational choriocarcinoma is a malignancy containing trophoblastic cells but no placental villi. The risk of choriocarcinoma is significantly elevated in women with a previous molar pregnancy: In several studies, 29–83% of choriocarcinomas were preceded by complete hydatidiform moles [10]. Complete hydatidiform moles usually result from elimination of the maternal nuclear component and duplication of the paternal chromosomes such that complete moles are homozygous with a 46,XX androgenous karyotype. Occasional dispermic fertilization of an empty egg results in 46,XY or 46,XX genetically heterozygous moles. However, all the choriocarcinomas that have been analyzed are heterozygous, suggesting that choriocarcinoma either does not directly descend from a complete mole, or it results only from the rare heterozygous moles.

Two classes of cellular genes have been associated with various cancers. One class, termed proto-oncogenes, is dominantly associated with malignancies. These elements can cause cellular transformation by disrupting normal growth processes and often result from chromosomal rearrangements or mutations that allow their aberrant expression. A second class of cellular genes may represent recessive suppressors of specific malignancies. These genes were discovered because their chromosomal loci are sometimes deleted in the resulting tumor. The prototype of this gene is a locus in chromosome region 11p13. Homozygous deletion or mutation of this locus can result in any of three embryonal tumors: Wilm's tumor, hepatoblastoma, or rhabdomyosarcoma [11–13]. The presence of immature cells in these childhood tumors suggested that the locus is required for normal differentiation [12]. Another member of this class of genes is the human retinoblastoma-susceptibility gene locus (RB) located in chromosome region 13q14. The gene is abnormally transcribed in retinoblastoma tumors [14, 15]. Because retinoblastoma is primarily a childhood cancer and has characteristics of an embryonal cancer, the RB locus may play a role in normal development [15]. Other recessive loci that may control specific malignancies include bladder cell carcinoma [16], uveal melanoma [17], and bilateral acoustic neurofibromatosis [18].

Although little is known about the molecular basis of choriocarcinoma, this malignancy may not derive from proto-oncogene activation resulting from a specific chromosomal rearrangement. Although several proto-oncogenes were found to be expressed in choriocarcinoma and hydatidiform mole cells, including c-*myc* and c-*ras* [19], and c-*fos* in the BeWo choriocarcinoma cell line [20], normal first-trimester trophoblast cells also express c-*myc* [21] and c-*sis* [22] mRNAs. Furthermore, no consistent chromosomal abnormalities were detected in four choriocarcinoma cell lines [23] or in three choriocarcinoma tumors [24].

The high level of ERV3 mRNA expression in normal placental chorionic villi throughout gestation, and the absence of ERV3 expression in choriocarcinoma cells suggests a possible biological function for an ERV3 gene product. Similar to the functions postulated for the Wilm's tumor and retinoblastoma loci, a possible function of the ERV3 provirus may be to act as a suppressor of tumorigenicity in the placenta. Loss of ERV3 mRNA expression would thus result in choriocarcinoma. Another possibility is that abrogation of ERV3 mRNA expression and choriocarcinoma susceptibility are pleiotropic effects of another defect, perhaps in a transcription factor. A third possibility is that loss of ERV3 expression may be an effect rather than a cause of choriocarcinoma. These possibilities are currently under investigation.

ACKNOWLEDGMENTS

These studies were supported by the National Cancer Institute under contract NO1-CO-2399 with Bionetics Research, Inc.; by the Japanese Overseas Cancer Fellowship of the Foundation for Promotion of Cancer Research, and by grants from the Swedish Cancer Society, project No. 2037-B87-03XA.

REFERENCES

1. Stoye J, Coffin J: In Weiss R, Teich N, Varmus H, Coffin J (eds): "RNA Tumor Viruses," Vol 2. Cold Spring Harbor, NY: Cold Spring Harbor Monograph Series, 1985, pp 357–404.
2. Martin MA, Bryan T, Rasheed S, Khan AS: Proc Natl Acad Sci USA 78:4892, 1981.
3. O'Connell CD, O'Brien SJ, Nash WG, Cohen M: Virology 138:225, 1984.
4. Cohen M, Powers M, O'Connell C, Kato N: Virology 147:449, 1985.
5. O'Connell C, Cohen M: Science 226:1204, 1984.
6. Kato N, Pfeifer-Ohlsson S, Kato M, Larsson E, Rydnert J, Ohlsson R, Cohen M: J Virol 61:2182, 1987.
7. Maniatis T, Fritsch EF, Sambrook J: "Molecular cloning: A Laboratory Manual." Cold Spring Harbor, NY: Cold Spring Harbor Laboratory, 1982.
8. Thomas PS: Proc Natl Acad Sci USA 77:5201, 1980.
9. Southern EM: J Mol Biol 98:503, 1975.
10. Rustin GJ, Bagshawe KD: CRC Crit Rev Oncol Hematol 3:103, 1985.
11. Solomon E: Nature 309:11, 1984.
12. Koufos A, Hansen MF, Copeland NG, Jenkins NA, Lampkin BC, Cavenee WK: Nature 316:330, 1985.
13. Weissman BE, Saxon PJ, Pasquale SR, Jones GR, Geiser AG, Stanbridge EJ; Science 236:175, 1987.
14. Friend SH, Bernards R, Rogel S, Weinberg RA, Rapaport JM, Albert DM, Dryja TP: Nature 323:643, 1986.
15. Lee W-H, Bookstein R, Hong F, Young L-J, Shew J-Y, Lee EY-HP: Science 235:1394, 1987.
16. Fearon ER, Feinberg AP, Hamilton SH, Vogenstein B: Nature 318:377, 1985.
17. Mukai S, Dryja TP: Cancer Genet Cytogenet 22:45, 1986.
18. Seizinger BR, Rouleau G, Ozelius LJ, Lane AH, St George-Hyslop P, Huson S, Gusella JF, Martuza RL: Science 236:317, 1987.
19. Sakar S, Kacinski BM, Kohorn EI, Merino MJ, Carter D, Blakemore KJ: Am J Obstet Gynecol 154:390, 1986.
20. Muller R, Tremblay JM, Adamson ED, Verman IM: Nature 304:484, 1983.
21. Pfeifer-Ohlsson S, Goustin AS, Rydnert J, Bjersing L, Wahlstrom T, Stehelin D, Ohlsson R: Cell 38:585, 1984.
22. Goustin AS, Betsholtz C, Pfeifer-Ohlsson S, Persson H, Rydnert J, Bywater M, Holmgren G, Heldin C-H, Westermark B, Ohlsson R: Cell 41:301, 1985.
23. Sheppard DM, Fisher RA, Lawler SD: Cancer Genet Cytogenet 16:251, 1985.
24. Wake N, Tanaka K, Chapman V, Matsui S, Sandberg AA: Cancer Res 41:3137, 1981.

Spontaneous Fusion Between Metastatic Mammary Tumor Subpopulations

Fred R. Miller, Donna McInerney, Clare Rogers, and Bonnie E. Miller

E. Walter Albachten Department of Immunology, Michigan Cancer Foundation, Detroit, Michigan 48201

This study describes a differential frequency of spontaneous fusion between metastatic and nonmetastatic subpopulations derived from a single mouse mammary tumor. Subpopulations 66, 66cl4 (a variant of 66 which is resistant to both thioguanine and ouabain), 410.4, and 44FTO (a thioguanine-resistant, ouabain-resistant derivative of 410.4) spontaneously metastasize from subcutaneous and mammary fatpad sites. Subpopulations 168, 168FARO (a diaminopurine-resistant, ouabain-resistant derivative of 168), 67, 68H, and 410 do not. The ability of these subpopulation lines to fuse spontaneously in vitro was determined after coculturing a drug-resistant line with a wild-type line in nonselective media. After 16–20 h of coculture, cells were plated in the appropriate media to select for fusion products—either HAT (hypoxanthine, aminopterin, thymidine) plus ouabain or AA (alanosine, adenine) plus ouabain—to determine the number of colony-forming cells (fusion products) present per 10^4 cells plated. When both subpopulations of the pair in the fusion mixture were metastatic, a significantly greater number of fusion products was recovered than if one or both of the subpopulations in the fusion mixture was nonmetastatic, with one exception: line 410 readily fused with both 66cl4 and 44FTO. Subline 410 was highly metastatic when originally isolated but lost its metastatic competence after a brief time in tissue culture.

Key words: hybrid cells, metastasis, heterogeneity, generation of aneuploidy

Cells from metastatic lesions are frequently more aneuploid than cells from primary tumors [1–4]. The mechanisms by which cells become aneuploid are unclear, but such cells could result from endoreduplication or by cell fusion, which might then be followed by asymmetric segregation. Cell fusion could play a significant role in progression by allowing the rapid assimilation of multiple properties from various subpopulations rather than requiring a single cell lineage to undergo sequential mutagenic alterations. Furthermore, asymmetric segregation subsequent to cell fusion offers a mechanism by which heterogeneity might be rapidly generated.

In many instances hybrids of nonmetastatic lymphatic tumor cells and normal host cells, usually macrophages or lymphocytes, have been found to be metastatic [5–

Received May 5, 1987; revised and accepted July 9, 1987.

© 1988 Alan R. Liss, Inc.

9]. It is not perfectly clear from those studies whether the fusion of tumor cell with one of these normal cells results in a more metastatic cell or if a rare metastatic subset of tumor cells is more likely to fuse. In experiments designed to study growth interactions between normal mammary gland cultures and metastatic mammary tumor cells in vitro, we were surprised to find that a significant number of hybrid cells formed. The purpose of the present investigation was to determine, utilizing subpopulations of a mouse mammary carcinoma, the extent to which these carcinoma cells spontaneously fuse and whether metastatic subpopulations are more likely to fuse than are nonmetastatic subpopulations.

MATERIALS AND METHODS
Cells

Tumor cell lines 66, 67, 168, 410, and 410.4 were isolated from a single, spontaneously arising mammary tumor from a BALB/cfC$_3$H mouse [10,11]. The thioguanine-resistant, ouabain-resistant cell lines 66c14 and 44FTO were isolated from lines 66 and 410.4, respectively, as previously described [12]. The 2,6-diaminopurine (DAP), ouabain-resistant cell line 168FARO was derived from line 168 by sequential selection in increasing concentrations of DAP until resistance had increased from 2 μg/ml to 100 μg/ml, followed by selection for resistance to 3 mM ouabain. When transplanted to subcutaneous sites in syngeneic mice, all of these cell lines form tumors but only lines 66, 66c14, 410.4, and 44FTO regularly form metastases [13–15]. Lines 67, 168, and 168FARO very rarely metastasize from the subcutis. Line 410 was originally isolated from a lung metastasis but lost metastatic potency after a brief time in tissue culture [13]. Occasionally, metastases do form in the lungs of a mouse bearing tumor 410. All lines were found to be free of mycoplasma contamination by the Hoechst staining method [16] and were free of mouse pathogenic viruses (PVM, Reo3, Sendai, GDVII, K, Polyoma, MVM, MAD, MHV, LCM, and Ectromelia) as determined by MAP tests performed by Microbiological Associates (Bethesda, MD).

Media and Drugs

The tumor cell lines 168, 410, and 410.4 were maintained in monolayer culture at 37°C in 5%– CO_2 in air atmosphere in Waymouth's Medium MB752/1 supplemented with 2 mM glutamine, penicillin (100 units/ml), streptomycin (100 μg/ml), and 10% fetal bovine serum. Lines 66, 66c14, 168FARO, and 44FTO were maintained in monolayer culture at 37°C in 10% CO_2 in air atmosphere in Dulbecco's Modified Eagle medium supplemented with 2 mM glutamine, penicillin (100 units/ml), streptomycin (100 μg/ml), mixed nonessential amino acids (1 mM), and 10% fetal bovine serum (DME-10).

Adenine, ouabain, 6-thioguanine, 2,6-diaminopurine, and a concentrated HAT mixture were purchased from Sigma Chemical Co. (St. Louis, MO). Alanosine was provided by the Drug Synthesis and Chemistry Branch, Division of Cancer Treatment, National Cancer Institute (Bethesda, MD). The final concentrations of selective drugs in DME-10 used were as follows: for HAT medium, hypoxanthine, 100 μM, aminopterin, 0.4 μM, thymidine, 16 μM; for thioguanine medium, 60 μM; for ouabain, 3 mM; for DAP, 250 μM; and for AA medium, alanosine, 50 μM, adenine, 50 μM.

Fusion In Vitro

To determine the ability of cell lines to spontaneously form cell hybrids, 5×10^5 cells of a cell line with drug-resistant phenotypes (66c14, 44FTO, or 168FARO) were mixed with 5×10^5 cells of a nonresistant wild-type line in DME-10 in a T-25 flask. After 16–20 h at 37°C in 10% CO_2 in air atmosphere, the cells were suspended with a solution of trypsin and EDTA. A single-cell suspension was formed by vigorously pipetting the cells and then passing the cell suspension two or three times through a 25-gauge needle. The cells were counted by hemacytometer and plated at 10^4 cells per 600-mm dish in DME-10 media containing selective drugs permissive only to the growth of fusion products. Medium containing HAT plus ouabain was used to select for fusion products between HGPRT$^-$(deficient in the enzyme hypoxanthine, guanine-phosphoribosyltransferase), ouabain-resistant cells and HGPRT$^+$, ouabain-sensitive cells. Medium containing AA plus ouabain was used to select for fusion products between APRT$^-$(deficient in the enzyme adenine phosphoribosyltransferase), ouabain-resistant cells and APRT$^+$, ouabain-sensitive cells [17, 18]. After 10 days incubation at 37°C in 10% CO_2 in air atmosphere, resulting colonies (>32 cells) were counted after fixing with Carnoy's solution and staining with crystal violet [19].

Fusion In Vivo

Cells from monolayer culture were injected into syngeneic BALB/c mice in a volume of 0.1 ml. Tumors were removed when they reached a mean diameter of 10 mm. Cell suspensions were made from the tumors using collagenase type III, hyaluronidase, and protease type IX as previously described [15] and plated in selective media to determine the cellular composition of the tumors.

Analysis of DNA Content

Cells were fixed and stained with propidium iodide as previously described [19] and analyzed for DNA content with a Becton-Dickenson FACS 440 flow cytometer.

RESULTS

The ability of the subpopulations to form colonies in various selective media is given in Table I. Only 66c14 and 44FTO grew in media containing thioguanine and ouabain and failed to grow in HAT. Only 168FARO grew in media containing both DAP and ouabain; 168FAR and 168FARO were uniquely unable to grow in AA. None of the subpopulations was able to grow in HAT plus ouabain or in AA plus ouabain.

To test the tendency of two nonmetastatic cell lines to fuse spontaneously in vitro we cocultured 168FARO with line 67, 168, or 410. Few fusion products were subsequently recovered by incubating the cell mixtures in AA plus ouabain (Table II). Typically, less than one colony-forming hybrid cell could be detected per 10^4 cells in the fusion mixtures.

If one cell line in the fusion mixture was metastatic, either 66c14 or 44FTO, and the other cell line was nonmetastatic, fusion was still a rare event. Typical experimental data are given in Table III. Lines 67, 168, and 168FAR did not readily fuse with either 66c14 or 44FTO as determined by the recovery of colonies growing in HAT plus ouabain. However, line 410, which is only sporadically metastatic,

TABLE I. Growth of Mouse Mammary Tumor Cell Lines in Selective Media

Cell line	Frequency of survival[a] in					
	HAT	T+O	HAT+O	AA	DAP+O	AA+O
66	.48	$<2 \times 10^{-5}$[b]	$<2 \times 10^{-5}$	.41	$<2 \times 10^{-5}$	$<2 \times 10^{-5}$
66c14	$<2 \times 10^{-5}$	.40	$<2 \times 10^{-5}$	.36	$<2 \times 10^{-5}$	$<2 \times 10^{-5}$
410.4	.23	$<2 \times 10^{-5}$	$<2 \times 10^{-5}$	.25	$<2 \times 10^{-5}$	$<2 \times 10^{-5}$
44FTO	$<2 \times 10^{-5}$	.32	$<2 \times 10^{-5}$	.29	$<2 \times 10^{-5}$	$<2 \times 10^{-5}$
410	.29	$<2 \times 10^{-5}$	$<2 \times 10^{-5}$	.34	$<2 \times 10^{-5}$	$<2 \times 10^{-5}$
67	.12	$<2 \times 10^{-5}$	$<2 \times 10^{-5}$	.16	$<2 \times 10^{-5}$	$<2 \times 10^{-5}$
168	.41	$<2 \times 10^{-5}$	$<2 \times 10^{-5}$	.38	$<2 \times 10^{-5}$	$<2 \times 10^{-5}$
168FAR	.40	$<2 \times 10^{-5}$	$<2 \times 10^{-5}$	$<2 \times 10^{-5}$	$<2 \times 10^{-5}$	$<2 \times 10^{-5}$
168FARO	.37	$<2 \times 10^{-5}$	$<2 \times 10^{-5}$	$<2 \times 10^{-5}$	.60	$<2 \times 10^{-5}$

[a]Frequency of survival = $\frac{\text{total number of colonies}}{\text{total number of cells plated}}$.

[b]Five dishes were plated with 1×10^4 cells each and no colonies grew; thus the frequency of survival is unknown but less than 2×10^{-5}.

TABLE II. Colony Formation in Selective Media by Fusion Mixtures of Paired Nonmetastatic Cell Lines

Cell lines in fusion mixture	Frequency of survival in		
	AA	DAP+O	AA+O
168FARO + 67	.27	.21	4×10^{-5}
168FARO + 168	.20	.11	5×10^{-5}
168FARO + 410	.24	.21	9×10^{-5}

TABLE III. Colony Formation in Selective Media by Fusion Mixtures of Paired Metastatic and Nonmetastatic Cell Lines

Cell lines in fusion mixture	Frequency of survival in		
	HAT	T+O	HAT+O
66c14 + 67	.18	.17	1.2×10^{-4}
66c14 + 168	.21	.14	$<2 \times 10^{-5}$
66c14 + 168FAR	.17	.27	1.3×10^{-5}
44FTO + 67	.23	.21	7×10^{-5}
44FTO + 168	.23	.22	1.8×10^{-4}
44FTO + 168FAR	.23	.26	5×10^{-5}
66c14 + 410	.19	.25	3.3×10^{-3}
44FTO + 410	.22	.25	5.5×10^{-3}

readily fused as evidenced by the recovery of 55 and 33 colony-forming cells per 10^4 cells of the fusion mixtures with 44FTO and 66c14, respectively. The ability of 410 to fuse was equal to that of the metastatic lines.

If both cell lines in the fusion mixture were metastatic, fusion products were readily obtained (Table IV). Both wild-type and drug-resistant forms of the metastatic subpopulations 66 and 410.4 were matched in each possible pairing with equivalent results. Data from all 39 experiments are shown in Figure 1. When both lines of the pair in the fusion mixture were metastatic, a significantly greater ($P < .002$) number of hybrids was recovered (median of 18 per 10^4 cells for 18 experiments) than if one of the lines in the fusion mixture was nonmetastatic (median of 0.6 per 10^4 cells for 15 experiments).

TABLE IV. Colony Formation in Selective Media by Fusion Mixtures of Paired Metastatic Cell Lines

Cell lines in fusion mixture	Frequency of survival in		
	HAT	T+O	HAT+O
66 + 66c14	.19	.14	8.2×10^{-3}
66c14 + 410.4	.30	.24	7.1×10^{-3}
66 + 44FTO	.17	.23	1.3×10^{-3}
410.4 + 44FTO	.33	.23	5.6×10^{-3}

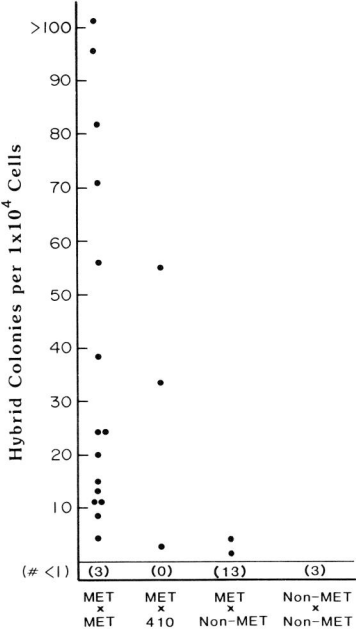

Fig. 1. Fusion frequency between paired tumor subpopulations. Each symbol represents the mean of five replicate wells for an individual experiment. The numbers of experiments in which the mean of five replicates indicated that fewer than one hybrid cell existed per 1×10^4 cells plated from a fusion mixture is also given.

Of 16 clones selected with HAT plus ouabain medium, 15 have displayed the DNA content expected by summing the DNA content of the parental cell lines in the fusion mixture. Figure 2 shows the DNA histograms for the parental lines and a hybrid clone from one such experiment. The one exception arose from a mixture of 66c14 and 66; this 2n clone was presumably either a revertant HGPRT$^-$, ouabain-resistant cell to HGPRT$^+$, a spontaneous mutation of HGPRT$^+$, ouabain-sensitive cell to ouabain resistant, or a spontaneous mutation of a HGPRT$^-$, ouabain-resistant cell to an increased resistance to aminopterin.

Colonies were not formed in HAT plus ouabain by cells from dissociated tumors arising in mice after SC injection of either 66c14 or 66 alone. However, tumors consisting of a mixture of 66 and 66c14 contained a significant number of hybrid cells. The data of Table V indicate that 98% of the clonogenic cells recovered from a tumor resulting from the injection of 66c14 cells grew in media selective for 66c14.

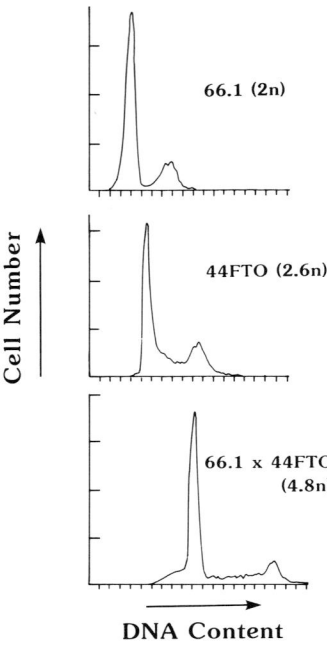

Fig. 2. Verification of the hybrid nature of a selected clone. The DNA histograms for the parental cells in the fusion mixture (66.1 and 44FTO) and the cell selected by growth in HAT plus ouabain (66.1 × 44FTO) are illustrated. Vertical and horizontal scales are identical for the three histograms.

TABLE V. In Situ Fusion: Colony Formation in Selective Media by Cells From Dissociated Tumors

Cells injected to form tumors	Percent of recovered cells which grew in[a]		
	HAT	T+O	HAT+O
1×10^5 line 66c14	2 (0-4)	98 (96-100)	0
1×10^5 line 66	100	0	0
2×10^4 66 + 1.8×10^5 66c14	71 (68-79)	21 (16-25)	8 (4-10)

[a]Six replicates were plated in each media for each tumor. Numbers given are the medians of the mean of the six replicates for five individual tumors. Figures in parenthesis represent the range of the means.

An additional 2% which grew in HAT were most likely host cells (fibroblasts?) rather than fusion products, because no colonies formed in HAT plus ouabain. Cells from dissociated tumors resulting from SC injection of line 66 cells grew only in HAT as expected. This indicates only that the rate of spontaneous mutation to ouabain resistance was too low to be detected. However, tumors formed by a mixture of 66 and 66c14, with 66c14 in excess to compensate for the tendency of 66 to overgrow 66c14 in mixtures, consisted of 8% (median of five tumors) hybrid cells.

DISCUSSION

The frequency with which the mammary tumor subpopulations fuse with one another is much higher than that described for various other cell types. Even the nonmetastatic subpopulations spontaneously form hybrid cells at a frequency of about 5×10^{-5}, which is greater than the range reported in the literature for other cell types: for example, 1×10^{-5} for spontaneous hybrid formation between mouse CI-Id cells and human WI-18Va2 cells [20], 4×10^{-6} between 3T3 cells and Chinese hamster cells [21], and less than 2×10^{-7} between mouse leukemia cells or mouse leukemia and Chinese hamster fibroblasts [22]. The frequency with which the metastatic subpopulations fuse (a median frequency of 2×10^{-3} with 1×10^{-2} being observed in one experiment) exceeds those reported for induced fusion by Sendai virus (5×10^{-5}, ref. [20]) or polyethylene glycol (2×10^{-4}, ref. [21] 3×10^{-4} to 4×10^{-5}, ref. [22]). The subpopulations were all derived from a BALB/cfC$_3$H mammary tumor and express the mouse mammary tumor virus (MMTV) to varying degrees [23]. MMTV has been reported to increase the frequency of hybridization [24] much like other enveloped viruses. However, the effect was seen with a cell line derived from mink lung but not with a mouse mammary tumor line or a line derived from normal mouse mammary gland [24]. Furthermore, the increase in spontaneous fusion of the mink lung cells was on the same order of magnitude as Sendai and Semliki Forest virus and was only seen at pH below 6. Therefore, it is unlikely that the frequency of hybridization seen with our cell lines can be attributed to MMTV infection. Roos and Choppin [25] found that mouse L fibroblast cells selected for resistance to PEG-induced fusion were more malignant, more metastatic, than the original L cells which readily formed hybrids following PEG treatment. The ability to fuse correlated with the lipid content of the L cell variants. We have not, as yet, determined the lipid content of our cell lines. The apparent discrepancy between our results, in which metastatic cells spontaneously fuse more readily, and the results of Roos and Choppin, in which metastatic cells fuse less frequently in response to PEG, might be due to a difference in cell systems or be because different mechanisms are responsible for spontaneous and PEG-induced fusion. Indeed, metastatic L cells concurrently demonstrated resistance to PEG-induced fusion and increased fusion rates induced by enveloped viruses [25].

A membrane property which might be important in fusion, and itself might be dependent upon lipid composition, is membrane fluidity. It has been reported that metastatic cell membranes are more fluid, or easily deformed, than membranes of nonmetastatic cells [26, 27].

Cells of our metastatic mammary tumor subpopulations may share a unique adhesion molecule [28] which allows them to adhere and fuse. Although expression of normal cell adhesion molecules may be reduced in cancer cells [29], Raz et al [30] have reported that the expression of a cell-surface lectin important in cell aggregation correlates with transformation and the acquisition of the metastatic phenotype.

Regardless of the mechanistic explanation, because the metastatic cells clearly fused spontaneously in situ, an important consequence of spontaneous fusion of tumor subpopulations is the potential for metastatic cells to rapidly acquire population characteristics such as resistance to chemotherapy. The occurrence of 8% hybrid cells in a metastatic tumor is not unprecedented; Hart described a similar frequency in B16-F10 tumors [31]. It remains to be seen whether the hybrid tumor-tumor cells are stable or rapidly generate heterogenous subpopulations. Chromosome loss is very rapid after the fusion of Eb tumor cells with normal host cells [9], but that probably reflects, in part, the necessity for loss of the tumor suppressor genes from the normal cells [32–35]. Our initial experiences with the tumor-tumor hybrids indicate that they are relatively stable, as assessed by total DNA content. However, unlike a tumor-normal cell hybrid, there is no strong selective pressure elicited against the tumor-tumor hybrid cells. Future experiments may elucidate the impact of spontaneous fusion on progression and the generation of heterogeneity.

ACKNOWLEDGMENTS

We thank Margaret Peterson for typing the manuscript. We wish to thank the Ben Kasle Laboratory for Flow Cytometry and the Comprehensive Cancer Center of Metropolitan Detroit, USPHS grant CA22453, for the FACS analysis.

This research was supported by USPHS grants CA28366 and CA27419 awarded by the National Cancer Institute.

REFERENCES

1. Mark J: Hereditas 65:59, 1970.
2. Mittelman F: Acta Pathol Microbiol Scand [A] 80:313, 1972.
3. Isaacs JT, Wake N, Coffey DS, Sandberg AA: Cancer Res 42:2353, 1982.
4. Wolman SR: Cancer Metastasis Rev 2:257, 1983.
5. DeBaetselier P, Gorelik E, Eshar Z, Ron Y, Katzav S, Feldman M, Segal S: J Natl Cancer Inst 67:1079, 1981.
6. Dennis JW, Donaghue TP, Florian M, Kerbel RS: Nature 292:242, 1981.
7. Lagarde AE, Donaghue TP, Dennis JW, Kerbel RS: J Natl Cancer Inst 71:183, 1983.
8. DeBaetselier P, Roos E, Brys L, Remels L, Feldman M: Int J Cancer 34:731, 1984.
9. Larizza L, Schirrmacher V: Cancer Metastasis Rev 3:193, 1984.
10. Dexter DL, Kowalski HM, Blazar BA, Fligiel Z, Vogel R, Heppner GH: Cancer Res 38:3174, 1978.
11. Blazar BA, Laing CA, Miller FR, Heppner GH: J Natl Cancer Inst 65:405, 1980.
12. Miller BE, McInerney D, Jackson D, Miller FR: Cancer Res 46:89, 1986.
13. Miller FR, Miller BE, Heppner GH: Invasion Metastasis 3:22, 1983.
14. Miller BE, Roi LD, Howard LM, Miller FR: Cancer Res 43:4102, 1983.
15. Miller FR, McInerney DJ, Rogers C, Aitken DR, Wei WZ: Invasion Metastasis 6:197, 1986.
16. Chen TR: Exp Cell Res 104:255, 1977.
17. Littlefield JW: Science 145:709, 1964.
18. Chan T, Creagan RP, Reardon, MP: Somat Cell Genet 4:1, 1978.
19. Miller BE, Miller FR, Heppner GH: Cancer Res 45:4200, 1985.
20. Poste G, Papahadjopoulos D: Methods Cell Biol 14:23, 1976.
21. Pontecorvo G: Somat Cell Genet 1:397, 1975.
22. Vaughan VL, Hansen D, Stadler J: Somat Cell Genet 2:537, 1976.
23. Hager JC, Heppner GH: Cancer Res 42:4325, 1982.
24. Redmond S, Peters G, Dickson C: Virology 133:393, 1984.
25. Roos DS, Choppin PW: Proc Natl Acad Sci (USA) 81:7622, 1984.
26. Sato H, Suzuki M: In Weiss L (ed): "Fundamental Aspects of Metastasis." Amsterdam: North-Holland Publ., 1976, pp 311-317.
27. Weiss L, Dimitrov DS: Cell Biophys 6:9, 1984.
28. Edelman GM: Science 219:450, 1983.
29. Hixson DC, McEntire KD, Obrink B: Cancer Res 45:3742, 1985.
30. Raz A, Meromsky L, Lotan R: Cancer Res 46:3667, 1986.
31. Hart IR: In Nicolson GL, Milas L (eds): "Cancer Invasion and Metastasis: Biological and Therapeutic Aspects." New York: Raven Press, 1984, pp 133-143.
32. Lagarde AE, Kerbel RS: Biochim Biophys Acta 823:81, 1985.
33. Stanbridge EJ: Nature 260:17, 1976.
34. Harris H, Miller OJ, Klein G, Worst P, Tachibana T: Nature 223:363, 1969.
35. Craig RW, Sager R: Proc Natl Acad Sci (USA) 82:2062, 1985.

Simultaneous Transfer of Tumorigenic and Metastatic Phenotypes by Transfection With Genomic DNA From a Human Cutaneous Squamous Cell Carcinoma

Honnavara N. Ananthaswamy, Janet E. Price, Leonard H. Goldberg, and Elise S. Bales

Departments of Immunology (H.N.A., E.S.B.) and Cell Biology (J.E.P.), The University of Texas M.D. Anderson Hospital and Tumor Institute at Houston, and Department of Dermatology (L.H.G.), Baylor College of Medicine, Houston, Texas 77030

High-molecular-weight genomic DNA isolated from a human cutaneous squamous cell carcinoma (AS) was assayed for its ability to induce tumorigenic transformation of NIH 3T3 cells. Subcutaneous injection of NIH 3T3 cells cotransfected with DNAs from AS tumor and pSV2-*neo* plasmid not only induced tumors at the site of injection, but also metastasized spontaneously to the lungs in 100% of nude mice injected. DNA isolated from a representative primary tumor and a metastasis was again used in a second round of transfection. Injection of secondary transfectants into nude mice again resulted in induction of both subcutaneous tumors and spontaneous long metastases. Southern blot hybridization with *ras*-specific probes revealed that DNA from both primary tumors and metastases induced by AS tumor DNA contained highly amplified Ha-*ras* oncogene. Furthermore, DNAs from secondary tumors and metastases induced by DNA from a primary tumor and a metastasis also contained similar highly amplified Ha-*ras* oncogene. These results suggest that the amplified Ha-*ras* oncogene may be responsible for induction of both tumorigenic and metastatic phenotypes in NIH 3T3 cells transfected with DNA from AS tumor.

Key words: tumorigenicity, metastasis, ha-*ras*, oncogene, gene transfer, skin cancer

Numerous studies have shown that cellular DNA from a variety of human and rodent tumors contain oncogenes capable of inducing morphologic and tumorigenic transformation when introduced into NIH 3T3 cells by DNA-mediated gene transfer [1–12]. Many normal cells also express oncogenes, which in this case are termed protooncogenes; these genes may play a role in the growth and differentiation of normal embryonic and adult tissues [13,14]. However, exposure of cells to carcinogenic agents may activate the normal genes into pathologic ones by causing them to

Received May 22, 1987; revised and accepted July 1, 1987.

© 1988 Alan R. Liss, Inc.

produce higher levels of their normal protooncogene product or by inducing structurally aberrant oncogene products [15–19]. A majority of the oncogenes so far identified in solid tumors belong to members of the *ras* gene family (designated Ha-*ras*, Ki-*ras*, and N-*ras*) [20–25]. Although the cellular *ras* protooncogenes are normally not active in the NIH 3T3 transforming assay, mutations that cause a single amino acid change in the 12th, 13th, or 61st codon or that increase the level of expression of unmutated *ras* can result in transformation of NIH 3T3 cells [17,18,26–30].

Although many different types of human tumors and tumor cell lines have been examined for the presence of activated oncogenes, most of the tumors originated in lung, colon, bladder, or other internal organs. We have found no published reports on oncogenes activated in nonmelanoma human skin cancers that originated on sun-exposed body sites. Epidemiological and clinical studies indicate that ultraviolet (UV) radiation present in sunlight is responsible for the induction of most skin cancers in humans [31,32]. Since cancers of the skin are the most prevalent form of human cancer, it is important to determine whether they contain specific transforming genes. Therefore, we began a series of experiments to determine whether DNA from fresh human skin cancers occurring on sun-exposed body sites contain oncogenes capable of inducing tumorigenic transformation when introduced into NIH 3T3 cells by DNA-mediated gene transfer. We report here that DNA isolated from a human primary squamous cell carcinoma induced tumorigenic transformation of NIH 3T3 cells. Interestingly, we also found that NIH 3T3 cells transfected with this human skin cancer DNA not only induced subcutaneous tumors at the site of injection, but also metastasized spontaneously to the lungs in 100% of mice injected. Both subcutaneous tumors and lung metastases induced in nude mice contained highly amplified Ha-*ras* oncogene.

MATERIALS AND METHODS
Tumor

The primary tumor used in this study originated on the left temple of a 67-year-old male Caucasian patient. The tumor (designated "AS") was diagnosed as a poorly differentiated squamous cell carcinoma. Untreated by prior chemotherapy or radiation, it was obtained at the time of surgical resection and immediately frozen at $-70°C$ until processed for DNA extraction.

Preparation of Cellular DNA

High-molecular-weight genomic DNA was isolated by the phenol extraction method described by Wigler et al [33], with slight modifications. The frozen tumor tissue was minced thoroughly with dissection scissors on ice and washed twice with ice-cold phosphate-buffered saline. The minced tissue was resuspended in buffer A (150 mM NaCl:10 mM Tris-HCl (pH 8.0):5 mM EDTA (pH 8.0)) (1 ml/100 mg tissue); proteinase K was added to a final concentration of 200 μg/ml; and the cells were lysed by adding sodium dodecyl sulfate (SDS) to 1%. The lysed preparation was heated at 65°C for 15 min to inactivate endogenous nucleases and then incubated at 37°C overnight with gentle shaking. An equal volume of 650 mM NaCl:10 mM Tris-HCl (pH 8.0):10 mM EDTA solution was added to the lysate and then extracted twice with an equal volume of buffer-saturated phenol. The aqueous phase was again extracted once with a mixture of phenol, chloroform, and isoamyl alcohol (25:24:1) and once with a mixture of chloroform and isoamyl alcohol (24:1). The DNA was precipitated from the aqueous phase by adding two volumes of cold absolute ethanol. The DNA precipitate was removed with a Pasteur pipette and washed successively with two changes of 70% ethanol and two changes of 100% ethanol. The precipitate was air-dried and dissolved in sterile 10 mM Tris-HCl (pH 8.0):1 mM EDTA. The cellular DNA was sized by gel electrophoresis in 0.8% agarose gels. Uncut and *Hind*III restriction enzyme-cut lambda DNAs were used as size markers.

DNA from pSV2-*neo* plasmids was isolated according to the procedure described by Maniatis et al [34]. Supercoiled plasmid DNA was purified on a CsCl gradient.

DNA Transfection

NIH 3T3 cells were used as recipients for DNA transfection. For best results, the cells were kept subconfluent by twice weekly subculturing in Dulbecco's medium (Grand Island Biological Co., Grand Island, NY) containing 10% calf serum (Hyclone). A cotransfection protocol [10] using pSV2-*neo* DNA [35], which confers resistance to the antibiotic G418, was employed to select cells that had taken up the foreign DNA. The calcium phosphate precipitate, which contained 120 μg of tumor DNA plus 2 μg of pSV2-*neo* DNA, was transfected onto four 60-mm plates containing 4×10^5 NIH 3T3 cells/plate. As controls, NIH 3T3 cells were transfected with pSV2-*neo* DNA alone or cotransfected with human placental DNA and pSV2-*neo* DNA. Twenty-four hours after transfection, cells from each dish were trypsinized and transferred to two 100-mm dishes. After another 16–20 hr, G418 was added to the medium at a concentration of 400 μg/ml. The cells were fed with fresh medium containing G418 every 3 or 4 days. The colonies, of which there were about 250 on each plate, reached confluency in 14–16 days.

Tumorigenicity Assay

G418-resistant colonies from sets of two 100-mm plates corresponding to one original 60-mm transfected plate were trypsinized, pooled, and centrifuged at 1,000 rpm for 5 min. The cell pellet was resuspended in Hanks' balanced salt solution and 5×10^6 cells were injected s.c. into 5–6-week-old, athymic nude Nu/Nu mice. Tumor growth was monitored weekly. When the tumor reached 15–20 mm in diameter, the mice were sacrificed and the tumor tissue was resected, established as cell lines, and subjected to G418 selection to eliminate contaminating host cells (which should be G418 sensitive). All tumor-bearing mice were examined for lung, liver, and lymph node metastasis following surgical resection of s.c. tumors. Visible colonies were excised and established as cell lines as described above.

Southern Blot Hybridization

DNA isolated from various tumors and metastases induced in nude mice were digested with restriction endonucleases and electrophoresed through a 0.8% agarose gel. DNA fragments that had been separated according to size by electrophoresis were denatured, blotted onto nitrocellulose filters, and immobilized by the method of Southern [36]. The DNA attached to the filter was prehybridized and then hybridized for about 24 hr with ^{32}P-labeled, nick-translated probes under stringent conditions according to manufacturer's instructions. The labeled Ha-*ras*, Ki-*ras*, and *alu* probes were obtained from Oncor, Inc. (Gaithersberg, MD). After hybridization, the filters were washed four times for 5 min each at room temperature with 2× standard saline citrate (SSC) (300 mM sodium chloride, 30 mM sodium citrate)-0.5% SDS and then three times for 20 min each at 56°C with 0.1% SSC-0.1% SDS. After being blot-dried, the filters were exposed at −70°C for 24–72 hr to Kodak XAR-5 film with intensifying screens.

RESULTS

High-molecular-weight DNA isolated from a primary human squamous cell carcinoma (AS) was assayed for transforming activity by cotransfection of NIH 3T3 cells. About 2 weeks after transfection, G418-resistant colonies were pooled and injected s.c. into nude mice. The time of first appearance of tumors and their subsequent growth were noted. The results shown in Table I indicate that all four mice injected with NIH 3T3 cells transfected with AS tumor DNA developed tumors within 4 weeks after injection. In contrast, untransfected NIH 3T3 cells or NIH 3T3 cells transfected with pSV2-*neo* DNA alone did not induce tumors. However, two of four mice injected with NIH 3T3 cells transfected with human placental DNA developed tumors 6–8 weeks after injection. Thus, the NIH 3T3 "tumor assay" employed by us and by Fasano et al [10] for detecting transforming genes has an intrinsic background of tumor induction when tested with normal DNA.

When the mice were autopsied following surgical resection of s.c. tumors, we were surprised to find lung metastasis in all four mice injected with AS DNA transfectants. Although these lung colonies were few (1–14), they were very large (Fig. 1). Contrarily, the two mice in the control group that had tumors induced by human placental DNA transfectants did not have any macroscopic or microscopic lung colonies. The primary tumors and lung metastases induced by AS DNA transfectants were designated as AS-1T, AS-2T, AS-3T, AS-4T and AS-1M, AS-2M, AS-3M and AS-4M, respectively.

DNAs prepared from primary tumor and metastasis cell lines were analyzed by Southern blotting for the presence of human repetitive sequences. All the primary

TABLE I. Tumorigenicity of DNA-Transfected NIH 3T3 Cells*

Donor DNA	Group	Tumor diameter (mm) on week				Metastasis	Tumor designation[a]
		1	2	3	4		
AS	1	0	0	4.5	17.0	Yes	AS-1T, AS-1M
	2	0	0	7.5	15.0	Yes	AS-2T, AS-2M
	3	0	7.0	18.0	25.5	Yes	AS-3T, AS-3M
	4	0	7.0	16.0	20.5	Yes	AS-4T, AS-4M
Human placenta	1	0	0	0	0	—	—
	2	0	0	0	0	—	—
	3	0	0	0	0	—	—
	4	0	0	0	0	—	—
None	1	0	0	0	0	—	—
	2	0	0	0	0	—	—
	3	0	0	0	0	—	—
	4	0	0	0	0	—	—

*About 2 weeks after transfection, G418-resistant colonies were pooled and injected s.c. into nude mice. Each group represents a pool of G418-resistant colonies and each line a nude mouse injected with 5 × 10^6 cells from two plates.
[a]Subcutaneous tumors are designated with a suffix "T" and lung metastases with an "M."

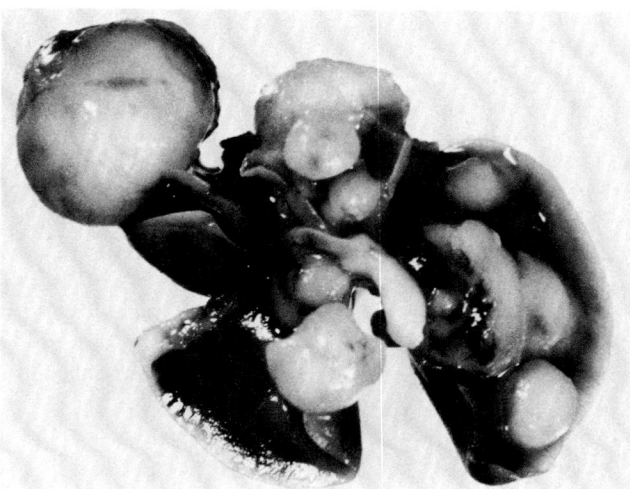

Fig. 1. Spontaneous lung metastases induced in nude mice by injection of NIH 3T3 cells transfected with AS DNA.

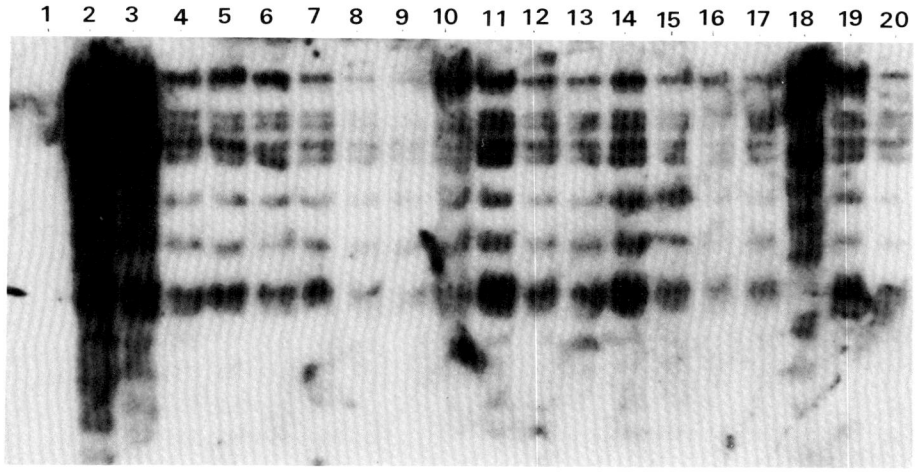

Fig. 2. Detection of human *alu* sequences in primary tumors and metastases induced in nude mice by injection of NIH 3T3 cells transfected with AS tumor DNA. DNAs (10 µg each) from the indicated tumors and metastases were digested with *Eco*RI and analyzed by Southern hybridization to ^{32}P-labeled, nick-translated *alu* probe (Palu.1, Oncor, Inc.). **Lane1:** NIH 3T3. **Lane 2:** AS-2T. **Lanes 3–7:** Individual lung colonies of AS-2M. **Lane 8:** AS-1T. **Lane 9:** AS-1M. **Lane 10:** AS-3T. **Lanes 11–16:** Individual lung colonies of AS-3M. **Lane 17:** AS-4T. **Lanes 18–20:** Individual lung colonies of AS-4M.

tumors and metastases induced by AS DNA contained human *alu* sequences (Fig. 2). Interestingly, all the primary tumors and metastases induced by AS DNA exhibited a common set of human repetitive sequences. In contrast, the two tumors induced by NIH 3T3 cells transfected with human placental DNA contained very little or no human sequences (data not shown).

In order to determine whether the primary tumors and metastases contained specific oncogenes, their DNAs were analyzed for the presence of human Ha- and

Ki-*ras* genes by Southern analysis. None of the primary tumors and metastases induced by AS DNA contained the human Ki-*ras* gene (data not shown). The hybridization pattern observed with the Ki-*ras* probe in primary tumors and metastases was similar to that of untransfected NIH 3T3 cells. However, when duplicate blots were hybridized with the Ha-*ras* probe, all the primary tumors and metastases induced by AS DNA exhibited additional bands besides the mouse endogenous Ha-*ras* sequences (Fig. 3). In contrast, the two tumors induced by transfection with human placental DNA did not contain the human Ki- or the Ha-*ras* gene (data not shown). These data, together with the observation that the two tumors induced by human placental DNA transfectants contained very little or no human *alu* sequences, suggests that these two tumors were induced by spontaneous transformation.

Interestingly, DNA from AS tumor contained amplified copies of the Ha-*ras* gene compared with the Ha-*ras* gene present in human placental DNA. Similarly, the Ha-*ras* gene in all the primary tumors and metastases, with the exception of AS-1T, was further amplified compared with the Ha-*ras* present in AS tumor. In addition, *Bam*HI fragments homologous to the Ha-*ras* gene present in most primary tumors and metastases were different from the 6.6-kilobase (kb) fragment found in AS tumor DNA and in human placental DNA. Whereas DNAs from AS-1T, AS-1M, and AS-4M contained only the 6.6-kb *Bam*HI fragment of the Ha-*ras* gene, DNAs from AS-2T, AS-2M, and AS-3M contained, in addition to the 6.6-kb fragment, a novel 9.4-kb *Bam*HI fragment homologous to the Ha-*ras* gene. On the other hand, DNAs from AS-3T and AS-4T contained only the 9.4-kb and not the 6.6-kb *Bam*HI fragment of the Ha-*ras* gene. The newly acquired 9.4-kb *Bam*HI fragment of the Ha-*ras* gene present in some tumors and metastases could be attributable to the loss of a restriction site on integration of the donor DNA into the recipient cell DNA. In addition, these

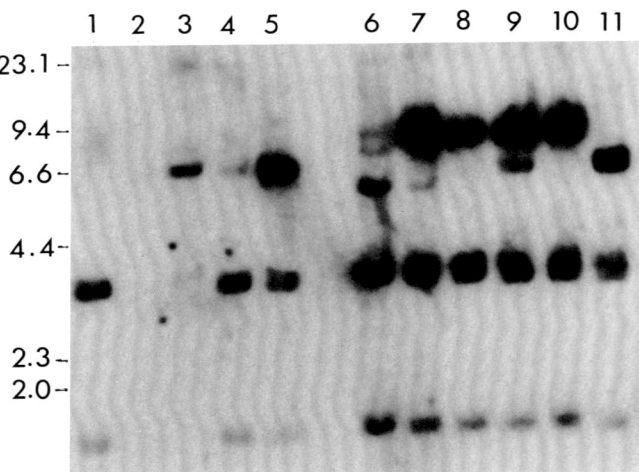

Fig. 3. Detection of Ha-*ras* sequences in primary tumors and metastases induced in nude mice by injection of NIH 3T3 cells transfected with AS DNA. Various DNAs (10 μg each) were digested with *Bam*HI and analyzed by Southern blot hybridization to ^{32}P-labeled, nick-translated Ha-*ras* probe (*Pras*.1, Oncor, Inc.) under conditions of high stringency. **Lane 1:** NIH 3T3. **Lane 2:** Human placenta. **Lane 3:** AS tumor. **Lane 4:** AS-1T. **Lane 5:** AS-1M. **Lane 6:** AS-2T. **Lane 7:** AS-2M. **Lane 8:** AS-3T. **Lane 9:** AS-3M. **Lane 10:** AS-4T. **Lane 11:** AS-4M. Numbers on the left are *Hind*III-digested lambda phage DNA molecular weight markers.

results also demonstrate the heterogeneous nature of the transfected cells. Since these tumors were induced in mice by injection of pooled G418-resistant colonies, it is likely that they were made up of a heterogeneous population of cells.

Genomic DNAs from a representative primary tumor (AS-3T) and a metastasis (AS-2M) was used again in a second round of transfection. Both AS-3T and AS-2M secondary transfectants not only induced tumors in nude mice at the site of injection but also metastasized spontaneously to the lungs (Table II). The lung colonies induced by the secondary transfectants were similar in number (2–14) and size to those induced by the primary transfectants.

DNAs from secondary tumors and metastases were analyzed for the presence of human *alu* and Ha-*ras* sequences. All the secondary tumors and lung metastases tested contained a common set of human *alu* sequences (Fig. 4). In most cases, there were only one or two discrete bands, which suggests that these sequences may be tightly linked to the Ha-*ras* oncogene. Southern blot analysis of DNAs from secondary

TABLE II. Tumorigenicity of Secondary Transfectants*

Donor DNA	Group	Tumor diameter (mm) on week—					Metastasis	Tumor Designation
		1	2	3	4	5		
AS-3T	1	0	0	0	4.0	9.5	Yes	AS-3T-1T, AS-3T-1M
	2	0	0	3.0	6.0	11.0	Yes	AS-3T-2T, AS-3T-2M
AS-2M	3	0	0	4.0	8.0	17.0	Yes	AS-2M-3T, AS-2M-3M
	4	0	0	6.0	10.5	19.0	Yes	AS-2M-4T, AS-2M-4M
Human placenta	5	0	0	0	0	0	—	
	6	0	0	0	0	0	—	—
None	7	0	0	0	0	0	—	—
	8	0	0	0	0	0	—	—

*Each group represents a pool of G418-resistant colonies and each line a nude mouse injected with 5×10^6 cells from two plates.

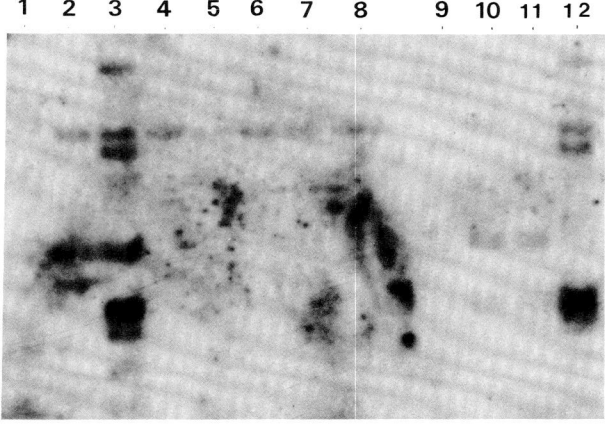

Fig. 4. Presence of human *alu* sequences in secondary tumors and metastases induced in nude mice by injection of NIH 3T3 cells transfected with DNAs from AS-3T tumor as AS-2M metastasis. Various DNAs were analyzed for human repeat sequences as described in Materials and Methods. **Lane 1:** NIH 3T3. **Lane 2:** AS-3T-1T. **Lane 3:** AS-3T-2T. **Lanes 4–8:** Individual lung metastases of AS-3T-1M. **Lane 9:** AS-2M-3T. **Lanes 10, 11:** Individual lung colonies of AS-2M-3M. **Lane 12:** AS-2M-4T.

tumors and metastases with an Ha-*ras* probe revealed that all of them contained the unique, highly amplified 9.4-kb *Bam*HI fragment similar to those found in AS-3T tumor and AS-2M metastasis (Fig. 5).

DISCUSSION

Until recently, DNA transfection studies aimed at identifying oncogenes were limited to using the NIH 3T3 "focus assay." Very often the genes from tumors that had focus-forming activity were found to be members of the *ras* family of oncogenes. In an attempt to detect new transforming genes, Blair et al [9] and Fasano et al [10] developed an NIH 3T3 "tumorigenicity assay," in which transfected NIH 3T3 cells are injected into athymic nude mice. Using this assay, we simultaneously transferred tumorigenic and metastatic phenotypes by transfection of NIH 3T3 cells with genomic DNA from a human squamous cell carcinoma (AS). Both the tumors and metastases induced in nude mice by injection of transfected cells contained the human Ha-*ras* oncogene.

We were surprised to find that s.c. injection of NIH 3T3 cells cotransfected with DNAs from AS tumor and pSV2-*neo* not only induced tumors at the site of injection but also metastasized spontaneously to the lungs in 100% of mice injected. The tumorigenic and metastatic phenotypes again cotransferred in a second round of DNA transfection. Southern blot hybridization with *ras* probes revealed that a majority of the tumors and metastases induced by AS DNA contained highly amplified Ha-*ras* oncogene. Interestingly, DNA from AS tumor also contained high copy numbers of the Ha-*ras* gene compared with that present in human placental DNA. Therefore, we conclude that further amplification of the Ha-*ras* gene in tumors and metastases induced by AS DNA might have occurred during or after gene transfer. Such

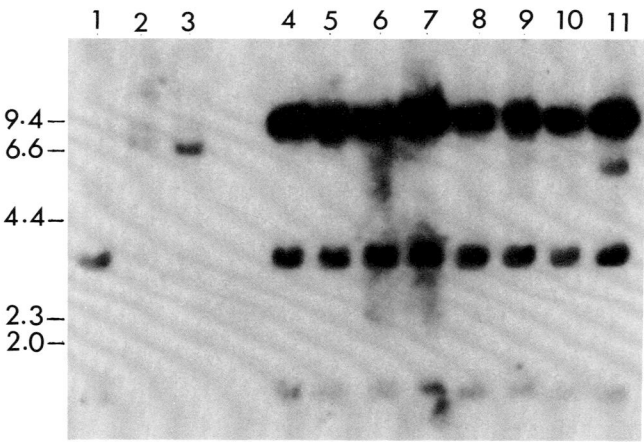

Fig. 5. Presence of Ha-*ras* sequences in secondary tumors and metastases induced in nude mice by injection of NIH 3T3 cells transfected with DNAs from AS-3T tumor and AS-2M metastasis. DNAs from indicated tumors and metastases were analyzed for Ha-*ras* sequences as described in Materials and Methods. **Lane 1:** NIH 3T3. **Lane 2:** Human placenta. **Lane 3:** AS tumor. **Lane 4:** AS-3T-1T. **Lanes 5, 6:** Individual lung colonies of AS-3T-1M. **Lane 7:** AS-3T-2T. **Lane 8:** AS-2M-3T. **Lanes 9, 10:** Individual lung colonies of AS-2M-3M. **Lane 11:** AS-2M-4T. Numbers on the left are *Hind*III-digested lambda phage DNA molecular weight markers.

amplification and rearrangement of genes are known to occur during DNA transfection [10,37,38].

DNAs from most tumors and metastases induced by primary and secondary transfectants contained amplified copies of the Ha-*ras* gene. In addition, DNAs from a majority of primary tumors and metastases and all secondary tumors and metastases induced by AS tumor DNA contained a unique 9.4-kb *Bam*HI fragment of the amplified Ha-*ras* gene. This suggests that this amplified 9.4-kb *Bam*HI fragment of the Ha-*ras* gene was responsible for induction of both tumorigenic and metastatic phenotypes in NIH 3T3 cells transfected with DNA from AS tumor. However, we do not know at present whether the amplified Ha-*ras* gene in AS tumor and in tumors and metastases induced by AS DNA contains structural mutations. Previous studies have shown that introduction of activated c-Ha-*ras*-1 gene into NIH 3T3 [39–43] and early-passage rat fibroblast [42,44,45] cells results in induction of both tumorigenic and metastatic phenotypes. In contrast, NIH 3T3 cells transformed by elevated levels of the Ha-*ras* proto-oncogene were tumorigenic but not metastatic [42]. Based on these and our studies, we can speculate that the Ha-*ras* gene in AS DNA and in tumors and metastases induced by AS DNA may, in addition to being amplified, contain structural alterations.

Other strategies for studying the molecular basis of metastasis have included introduction of either cloned activated *ras* gene [42,46,47] or genomic DNA from metastatic cells [40] into tumorigenic but nonmetastatic cells, and assessment of the ability of transfected cells to metastasize in syngeneic immunocompetent hosts. Using this approach, Vousden et al [46] and Collard et al [47] demonstrated that activated human c-Ha-*ras*-1 oncogene conferred metastatic potential when introduced into nonmetastatic but tumorigenic cells by DNA-mediated gene transfer. In contrast, Muschel et al [42] found that transfection of tumorigenic, but nonmetastatic murine C127 cells with activated c-Ha-*ras* gene did not confer metastatic potential, even though the C127 transformants expressed increased levels of the Ha-*ras* protein. On the other hand, Bernstein and Weinberg [40] reported that the metastatic phenotype induced by transfection of *ras*-transformed, nonmetastatic tumor cells with genomic DNA from a human metastatic tumor was associated with an unidentified gene. In another study, Gallick et al [48] found that human metastatic colon tumors expressed decreased levels of $p21^{ras}$ protein compared with the levels expressed in primary tumors. Thus, these contradictory findings imply that both *ras* and non-*ras* genes may be involved in the regulation of the metastatic phenotype. Although our data strongly suggest that the amplified Ha-*ras* oncogene is associated with the metastatic phenotype in NIH 3T3 cells transfected with AS tumor DNA, the involvement of other non-*ras* genes, if any, in the regulation of the metastatic phenotype remains to be determined.

ACKNOWLEDGMENTS

We wish to thank Lisa Daniels for excellent technical assistance, Dr. Corazon Bucana for assistance in photography, Dr. I. J. Fidler for support of this work, and Helen Farr for typing the manuscript. This work was supported by a grant from the M. K. Ash Foundation.

REFERENCES

1. Shih C, Shilo B, Goldfarb M, Dannenberg A, Weinberg R: Proc Natl Acad Sci USA 76:5714–5718, 1979.

2. Murray MJ, Shilo BZ, Shih C, Cowing D, Hsu HW, Weinberg RA: Cell 25:355–361, 1981.
3. Perucho M, Goldfarb M, Shimizu K, Lama C, Fogh J, Wigler M: Cell 27:467–476, 1981.
4. Balmain A, Pragnell IB: Nature 303:72–74, 1983.
5. Krontiris TG, Cooper GM: Proc Natl Acad Sci USA 78:1181–1184, 1984.
6. Balmain A, Ramsden M, Bowden GT, Smith J: Nature 307:658–660, 1984.
7. Sukumar S, Notario V, Martin-Zanca D, Barbacid M: Nature 306:658–661, 1983.
8. Sukumar S, Pulciani S, Doniger J, DiPaolo JA, Evans CH, Zbar B, Barbacid M: Science 223:1197–1199, 1984.
9. Blair DG, Cooper CS, Oskarsson MK, Eader LA, Vande Woude GF: Science 281:1122–1125, 1982.
10. Fasano O, Birnbaum D, Edlund L, Fogh J, Wigler M: Mol Cell Biol 4:1695–1705, 1984.
11. Cooper CS, Park M, Blair DG, Tainsky MA, Huebner K, Croce CM, Vande Woude GF: Nature 311:29–33, 1984.
12. Schechter AL, Stern DF, Vaidyanathan L, Decker SJ, Drebin JA, Greene MI, Weinberg RA: Nature 312:513–516, 1984.
13. Spector DH, Varmus HE, Bishop JM: Proc Natl Acad Sci USA 75:4102–4106, 1978.
14. Muller R, Slamon DJ, Tremblay JM, Kline MJ, Verma IM: Nature 299:640–644, 1982.
15. DeFeo D, Gonda MA, Young HA, Chang EH, Lowy DR, Scolnick EM, Ellis RW: Proc Natl Acad Sci USA 78:3328–3332, 1981.
16. Dalla Favera R, Wong-Staal F, Gallo RC: Nature 299:61–63, 1982.
17. Tabin CJ, Bradley SM, Bargmann CI, Weinberg RA, Papageorge AG, Scolnick EM, Dhar R, Lowy DR, Chang EH: Nature 300:143–149, 1982.
18. Reddy EP, Reynolds RK, Santos E, Barbacid M: Nature 300:149–152, 1982.
19. Capon DJ, Seeberg PH, McGrath JP, Hayflick JS, Edman U, Levinson AD, Goddel DV: Nature 304:507–513, 1983.
20. Pulciani S, Santos E, Lauver AV, Long LK, Robbins KC, Barbacid M: Proc Natl Acad Sci USA 79:2845–2849, 1982.
21. Der C, Krontiris T, Cooper G: Proc Natl Acad Sci USA 79:3637–3640, 1982.
22. Parada LF, Tabin CJ, Shih C, Weinberg RA: Nature 297:474–478, 1982.
23. Santos E, Tronick SR, Aaronson SA, Pulciani S, Barbacid M: Nature 298:343–347, 1982.
24. Shimizu K, Goldfarb M, Suard Y, Perucho M, Li Y, Kamata T, Feramisco J, Starnezer E, Fogh J, Wigler M: Proc Natl Acad Sci USA 80:2112–2116, 1983.
25. Hall A, Marshall GJ, Spur NK, Weiss RA: Nature 303:396–400, 1983.
26. Taparowsky E, Suard Y, Fasano O, Shimizu K, Goldfarb M, Wigler M: Nature 300:762–765, 1982.
27. Taparowsky E, Shimizu K, Goldfarb M, Wigler M: Cell 581–586, 1983.
28. Yuasa Y, Srivastava SK, Dunn CY, Rhim JS, Reddy EP, Aaronson SA: Nature 303:775–779, 1983.
29. Zarbl H, Sukumar S, Arthur AV, Martin-Zanca D, Barbacid M: Nature 315:382–385, 1985.
30. Quintanilla M, Brown K, Ramsden M, Balmain A: Nature 322:78–80, 1986.
31. Blum HF: "Carcinogenesis by Ultraviolet Light." New Jersey: Princeton, 1978.
32. Scotto J, Fears TR: Natl Cancer Inst Monogr 50:169–177, 1978.
33. Wigler M, Pellicer A, Silverstein S, Axel R: Cell 14:725–731, 1978.
34. Maniatis T, Fritsch EF, Sambrook J: "Molecular Cloning, A Laboratory Manual." Cold Spring Harbor, NY: Cold Spring Harbor Laboratory, 1982.
35. Southern PJ, Berg PA: J Mol Appl Genet 1:327–341, 1982.
36. Southern EM: J Mol Biol 98:503–517, 1975.
37. Pellicer A, Wigler M, Axel R, Silverstein S: Cell 14:133–141, 1981.
38. Goldfarb M, Shimizu K, Perucho M, Wigler M: Nature 296:404–409, 1982.
39. Thorgeirsson UP, Turpeenniemi-Hujanen T, Williams JE, Westin EH, Heilman CA, Talmadge JE, Liotta LA: Mol Cell Biol 5:259–262, 1985.
40. Bernstein SC, Weinberg RA: Proc Natl Acad Sci USA 82:1726–1730, 1985.
41. Greig RG, Koestler TP, Trainer DL, Corwin SP, Miles L, Kline T, Sweet R, Yokoyama S, Poste G: Proc Natl Acad Sci USA 82:3698–3701, 1985.
42. Muschel RJ, Williams JE, Lowy DR, Liotta LA: Am J Pathol 121:1–8, 1985.
43. Bradley MO, Kraynak AR, Storer RD, Gibbs JB: Proc Natl Acad Sci USA 83:5277–5281, 1986.
44. Pozzatti R, Muschel R, Williams J, Padmanabhan R, Howard B, Liotta L, Khoury G: Science 232:223–227, 1986.
45. Van Roy FM, Messiaen L, Liebant G, Gao J, Dragonetti CH, Fiers WC, Mareel MM: Cancer Res 46:4787–4795, 1986.
46. Vousden KH, Eccles SA, Purvies H, Marshall CJ: Int J Cancer 37:425–433, 1986.
47. Collard JG, Schijren JF, Roos E: Cancer Res 47:754–759, 1987.
48. Gallick GE, Kurzrock R, Kloetzer WS, Arlinghaus RB, Gutterman JU: Proc Natl Acad Sci USA 82:1795–1799, 1985.

Cytogenetic Diversity in Primary Human Tumors

Sandra R. Wolman, Patricia M. Camuto, and Mary Ann Perle

Department of Pathology, NYU School of Medicine, New York, New York 10016

Cytogenetic patterns from primary short-term culture of breast cancer, renal carcinoma, and tumors of the central nervous system are presented to illustrate the range of karyotypic diversity of human solid tumors as well as their biologic differences in culture systems that support their growth. These studies have illustrated several major issues. 1) Results vary with the tissue of origin: primary cultures from breast are almost uniformly diploid, while renal tumors are near-diploid, mosaic, and show clonal aberrations; and CNS tumors are heterogeneous: some diploid, some near-diploid and some highly aneuploid. 2) Results after short-term culture are selective, representing subpopulations from the heterogeneous cells that are detected on direct analysis of fresh tumors by cytogenetics or flow cytometry (FCM). It is not yet clear whether prognosis depends on the dominant population of the primary tumor or alternatively should be influenced by detection of small aneuploid subpopulations. 3) Evidence from all three tumor types supports the interpretation that cytogenetically normal diploid cells constitute part of some tumor populations, and may be better adapted to routine growth in culture than aneuploid subpopulations from the same primary tumors. These cells may also compose a major portion of the viable population of tumors in vivo and, therefore, could represent a useful model for studies of tumorigenesis and therapeutic regimens.

Key words: renal carcinomas, cytogenetic heterogeneity, flow cytometry, CNS tumors, breast tumors

Human tumors display a wide range of karyotypic diversity. Many tumors are characterized by extensive numerical and structural chromosome aberrations. Some, however, show minimal deviation from the normal karyotype, and a few tumors appear to be largely represented by normal diploid cells. In the leukemias and lymphomas, chromosome aberrations are relatively uniform throughout a tumor cell population. In contrast, many human solid tumors display great intratumoral cytogenetic heterogeneity. Moreover, tumors of the same morphologic subtype may display a wide range of karyotypic deviations.

Recent studies in the leukemias and lymphomas have demonstrated relatively uniform and probably causal relationships between certain chromosome rearrange-

Received May 15, 1987; accepted June 16, 1987.

© 1988 Alan R. Liss, Inc.

ments and specific tumors. One of the best examples of such a relationship is the 8; 14 translocation (or t(2;8) or 8;22) found in cells of Hodgkin's lymphoma. At the molecular level these translocations result in transposition of the myc oncogene into a region adjacent to a functioning immunoglobulin locus. In lymphoid cell lineages, the functional result of the transposition is oncogene activation, which presumably is responsible for acquisition of tumor-relevant properties. These and other similar relationships between chromosome rearrangements and specific tumors are discussed by Dr. Carlo Croce [1]. Their demonstration is facilitated when tumors have a near-diploid chromosome constitution.

Similarly, the diploid and near-diploid populations of cells from primary solid human tumors could represent a desirable model for the study of early events in tumorigenesis and for rational approaches to therapy. The cellular models used for experimental approaches to tumor therapy often utilize well-established tumor cell cultures. Such cultures, frequently derived from advanced stages of tumor in vivo, often undergo further evolution in culture [2]. Thus, the cultured cells may differ greatly from the original primary tumor against which therapy should be targeted.

We will present examples from primary human tumors which illustrate different spectra of cytogenetic patterns in short-term culture, intrinsic biologic differences in their ability to adapt to growth in culture, and differing responses to selective culture systems. Some selective factors are probably responsible for the reduced karyotypic diversity seen in short-term tumor cultures in comparison to that found by direct cytogenetic analysis of the fresh tissues. These differences are amply demonstrated in studies of breast cancer [3-5]. Several important sources of variability for the DNA content and karyotypic patterns of human tumors are shown in Figure 1. The source of tumor reflects the state of tumor progression to some extent. Metastases, whether solid, in marrow, or from effusion fluids, represent more advanced stages of tumor development than the primary lesion. Needle aspirates, in contrast to the solid primary tumor mass, are likely to include cells with less adhesive and presumably less differentiated characteristics. For example, in an epithelial tumor, intercellular bridges, a sign of differentiation, are likely to result in adherent cell masses. From any of the sources in Figure 1, the fresh tumor is likely to consist of a mixed population of cells of differing viability, and of both tumor and non-tumor origin. Both the transport medium and the first processing of the tumor by disaggregation methods may select differentially between cells of greater and lesser viability. If the cells are not analyzed

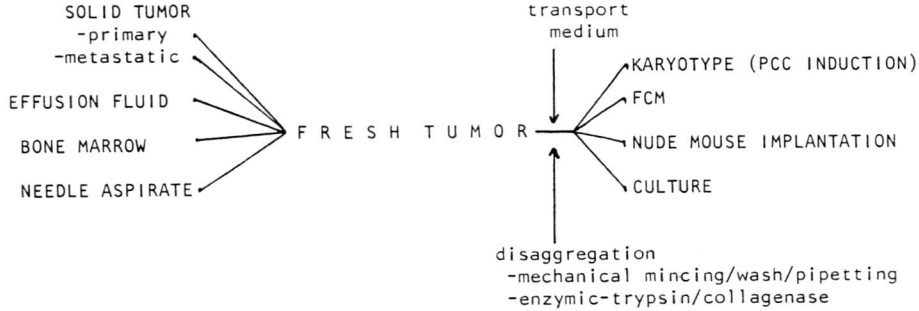

Fig. 1. Sources of fresh tumor are shown at left and processing techniques on the right. Premature chromosome condensation (PCC) is a method that permits visualization of chromosomes from interphase cells [18].

directly, either for karyotype or for DNA content by flow cytometry, then further selection among existing subpopulations will occur unobserved, as the tumor is processed either for tissue culture or for nude mouse implantation prior to study of DNA or karyotype. (Another modification which can be introduced is the induction through premature chromosome condensation of karyotypes from cells that were not dividing spontaneously within the tumor).

Culture of the tumor cell population prior to karyotypic study introduces a large number of new variables, many of which are intentionally selective or preferential for tumor cells. Table I lists a number of procedures that are commonly used either to deter the growth of normal cells or to enhance the concentration of tumor cells prior to culture. Table II presents modifications of the physical aspects of substrate, medium, or environment—all of which are potentially selective for specific subsets within a tumor cell population.

BREAST CANCER

With these considerations as background, we will present results from primary cultures of three types of human solid tumors. The first set of data are derived from

TABLE I. Pretreatment of Cells Prior to Culture

Purposes
    To deter fibroblast, monocyte or other normal cell contamination
    To enhance concentration of tumor cells
Methods
    Differential adhesion or response to trypsin
    Passage in soft agar
    Isolation by cloning (rings or wells)
    Disaggregation; selection for single cells vs clumps
    Ficoll or Percoll gradients
    Elimination of special populations
        Phagocytes by Fe uptake and magnets
        Reaction with antibody-coated surfaces

TABLE II. Selection of Cell Type by Culture Conditions

Monolayer vs suspension growth
Feeder layer
    Cell source
    Method of inactivation
Substrate modification
    Laminin
    Fibronectin
    Collagen
    Polylysine
    Extracellular matrix
3-D growth
    Agar or collagen gel
Medium and environment
    % oxygen
    % serum
    Conditioning of media by cultured cells
    Supplements; growth factors, hormones, etc.

breast cancers. Remarkably little cytogenetic data have been obtained from direct studies of human tumors or from cell cultures [6]. A recent review revealed fewer than 20 cases analyzed directly by banded methods and not all could be completely analyzed. Direct analyses of advanced breast cancer, mainly in the form of effusion fluids, also are few in number. Cell lines, almost all derived from effusion fluids, have shown cytogenetic instability and heterogeneity with unpredictable emergence of new clonal karyotypes. Lines that are widely used as models for therapeutic strategies, such as MCF-7, show great variability and marked karyotypic differences between cells grown in vivo and in vitro [2]. Until recently human breast tissue and tumors have been extraordinarily difficult to propagate in culture. Even now the growth of normal or tumor-derived breast epithelium is dependent on supplementation of culture media by hormones, growth factors, and other poorly defined additives, such as conditioned media from other cell culture sources. The cells we studied were grown by Dr. Helene Smith and co-workers [7,8] from fresh solid tumor after prolonged enzymic disaggregation, followed by removal of the single cell suspension and culture of the adherent cell masses termed "organoids." The cell masses attach and begin to divide in a medium supplemented with hormones, insulin, cholera toxin, and growth factors derived from existing cell cultures. Even under these conditions they are capable of very limited growth in culture. The cells are epithelial in morphology, form secretory domes, show junctional complexes, and have mammary milk-fat globule antigens. Chromosome analyses of 15 tumor-derived primary cultures in either first or second passage has yielded predominantly diploid cells [5]. Chromosomal banding at levels of 550 or higher resolution has not revealed structural aberrations. No clonal aberrations have been detected in the primary cultures although occasional nonclonal structural or numerical aberrations have been found. Morphologic, antigenic and functional markers indicative of breast cell origin are cited above but indicators of malignant characteristics are less decisive. Of the latter, the most convincing is the demonstration of invasion of amniotic membrane in vitro, a property not shared by breast cells derived from non-malignant sources [9]. Other evidence suggesting that the diploid cells represent subpopulations of tumor in approximately two-thirds of primary breast cancers has been reviewed [10].

RENAL CARCINOMA

In contrast to the modifications necessary to culture breast cancer, some human tumors grow well in simple culture systems. A high proportion of renal cell carcinomas grow well on standard plastic surfaces with unmodified serum-supplemented media, after either mincing or collagenase dissociation of the fresh tumor material. The cultures have yielded chromosome harvests from over 2/3 of the samples received. Most of those which we were unable to culture were either extremely limited in sample volume or had reduced viability because of tumor infarction.

Within the first 2–3 weeks the cultured cells show a highly characteristic, relatively uniform morphology. They form a monolayer which is typically epithelial and pavement-like. Individual cells are commonly triangular in two-dimensional appearance, and have characteristic heavy granulation in the immediate perinuclear region. Electron microscopy of the fresh surgical specimen is similar to that of the cultured cells after 2–5 weeks. Cells from both sources share characteristics of extensive cytoplasmic vacuolization, circumferential papillation of the cytoplasmic border, and dense reticulated chromatin patterns in the one or two nucleoli of each nucleus. Thus, there is morphologic evidence that the cultured cells are tumor-derived. The cytogenetic analyses of these cultures, presented in Table III and IV, are divided into cultures from which harvests were obtained in 2 weeks or less, and those with prolonged culture prior to chromosome analysis. The results do not differ qualitatively, but the frequency of clonally aberrant chromosome populations was higher when harvests were obtained relatively early. Three patterns are evident. Two cultures showed exclusively aberrant cytogenetic patterns, while a few cultures contained exclusively normal diploid cells. Among those that were diploid, several cases may be inappropriate for inclusion in the study; for example, cases 4959 and 4749 were reclassified as an adenoma and as an oncocytoma, respectively. The remaining cases included both a normal diploid population and a clonally aberrant population. Cases with aberrant populations were generally marked by chromosome losses and gains. Of these, seven contained clones missing the Y chromosome and seven, some overlapping, showed trisomy for chromosome 7. In cases 5151 and 5512, the clonal aberrations were structural. In summary, 10 of the 19 cultures showed clonal chromosome aberrations. These cultures, therefore, showed not only a high

TABLE III. Cytogenetics of Cultured Renal Tumors With 1st Harvest ≤ 14 Days

Case no.	Harvest time (days)	No. metaphase cells analyzed	Karyotype
4632	9	29	47,X,−Y,+7,+10/50,X, −Y,+7,+10,+12,+16,+17
4667	8	6	46,XY
4674	12	18	46,XY/46,X,−Y,+7/ 43,XY,+7,+ others
4823	12	30	46,XY/45,X,−Y/ 46,X,−Y,+7/ 47,X,−Y,+7,+12
4942	13	14	46,XX/47,XX,+7
4959 (adenoma)	10	13	46,XX
5151	10	13	46,XY/46,XY,16q−
5188	10	25	46,XY/45,X,−Y
5300	14	28	46,XY/45,X,−Y/ 46,X,−Y,+7

TABLE IV. Cytogenetics of Cultured Renal Tumors With Successful Harvest After 14 Days

Case no.	Harvest time	No. metaphase cells analyzed	Karyotype
4635	2 months	9	45,X,−Y
4661	1 1/2 months	8	46,XY
4673	40 days	10	46,XX
4712	2 months	10	46,XX
4731	1 month +	24	46,XY
4749	33 and 38 days	11	46,XX
5111	21 days	18	46,XX
5199	19 days	36	46,XY
5310	20 days	26	46,XY/45,X,−Y/? 45,X,−Y,+7,−20
5512	22 days	18	46,XY/47,XY,+7/ 48,XY,+7,+7

proportion of karyotypic abnormality but also considerable specificity for particular chromosomally aberrant clones. Recent work suggests that with modifications such as addition of growth factors, we can retrieve higher frequencies of chromosomally aberrant cells, particularly those with structural alterations.

What is not clear is whether the diploid cells are truly representative of tumor subsets or result from contamination of cultures by normal cell populations. This question is under investigation using cytochemical markers, but markers that clearly, reliably, and uniformly distinguish stromal or normal kidney from tumor-derived cells are not yet available to us. Recent results of direct analysis and short-term cultures from other laboratories have emphasized frequent rearrangement of chromosome 3 [11-13], an observation of great interest because of the family in which inheritance of a balanced translocation between chromosomes 3 and 8 was closely associated with the appearance of renal tumors [14]. Direct harvest also appears to yield a higher frequency of aberrant karyotypes [15].

We have attempted to pursue further the question of intratumoral heterogeneity in renal carcinoma by flow cytometry. The results, shown in Table V, appear to support the cytogenetic results based on cell culture. Most of the karyotypic abnormalities diagnosed would not be detectable by whole cell flow cytometry. The limits of resolution of the instrumentation used (Ortho Cytofluorograph 504 interfaced with a model 2150 computer) preclude detection of differences from the normal karyotype of less than 5 chromosomes (unpublished observations). In two instances, cases 4673 and 4674, flow cytometry of the fresh tumors showed both diploid and aneuploid peaks. The aneuploid cells in both cases were not recovered from culture. In case 4673, the fixed paraffin-embedded tissues were also analyzed by flow cytometry. The flow diagrams shown in Figure 2 are taken from two sections, one of which was almost exclusively tumor while the other was half tumor and half normal kidney. Despite the large differences in sampling, the flow diagrams did not differ substantially in the sizes of their diploid and aneuploid peaks. These results indicate the strong probability that a diploid subpopulation existed within the tumor.

To summarize the data obtained thus far, we have been able to culture cells from renal cell carcinomas with relative ease. We have defined clonal karyotypic abnormalities in more than 50% of the tumors analyzed, with apparent specificity for trisomy 7 and for loss of the Y chromosome. Although similarities of morphology

TABLE V. Renal Tumor Study

Case no.	Karyotype	Flow cytometry
4632	47,X,−Y,+7,+10/ 50,X,−Y,+7,+10, +12,+16,+17	Diploid
4635	45,X,−Y	Diploid
4667	46,XY	Diploid
4673	46,XY	Diploid, aneuploid
4674	46,XY/46,X,−Y,+7	Diploid, aneuploid
4712	46,XX	Diploid
4749 (oncocytoma)	46,XX	Diploid
4823	46,XY/45,X,−Y/47,X,−Y,+7,+12	Diploid
5512	46,XY/47,XY,+7/48,XY,+7,7	Diploid

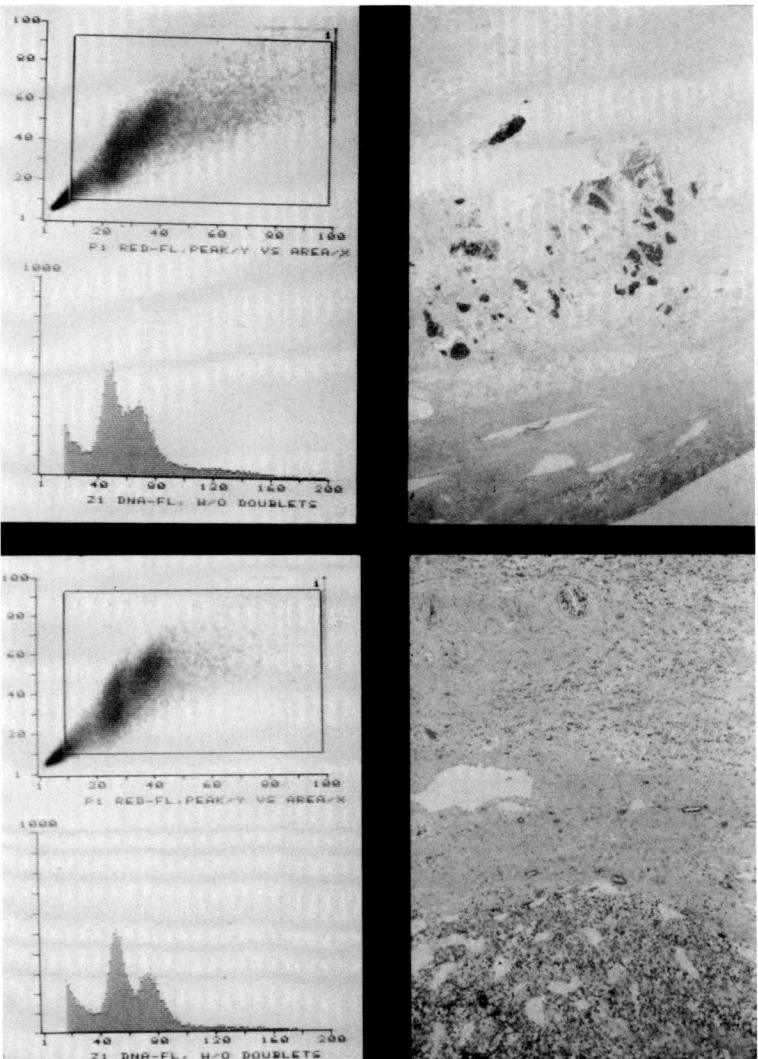

Fig. 2. On the left are the peak vs area scatter and flow histograms for two samples of the same renal carcinoma (case 4673). The paraffin blocks from which the flow samples were prepared are represented by the photomicrographs to the right of each. The histograms do not differ significantly, although the upper sample was more than 90% tumor, while the lower consisted of equal amounts of tumor and normal kidney.

suggest that the diploid cells in culture originate from tumor, we do not yet have clear proof that this is the case. In a few cases, it appears that aneuploid populations do not survive in this culture system.

CENTRAL NERVOUS SYSTEM TUMORS

Tumors of the central nervous system, in contrast to the previous two tumor types, have been cultured with considerable frequency by other investigators [16,17].

The most consistent aberrations reported in glial tumors have been loss of a sex chromosome or trisomy 7, although many karyotypically normal cells were also found. Structural rearrangements and extensive chromosome aberrations were far more common in highly malignant tumors. Since normal brain tissue is nondividing and since the supporting stromal cells of the central nervous system can only be cultured with great difficulty, problems of potential contamination with normal cell populations are more remote. Cellular morphology in culture is also highly characteristic and aids in identification of the growing populations. In culture there is almost invariably a mixed population, including bipolar cells that are characteristic of glial origin admixed with stellate and pavement cells. We have successfully cultured 28 of 29 samples received. Of these, only 11 cytogenetic results are available at present. Table VI shows that some of these tumors have grown as pure diploid populations; others have shown loss of the second sex chromosome; some are a mixture of diploid and aneupolid cells. For example, case 5464 is aneuploid for a population that has lost the second sex chromosome while case 5674 is aneuploid for a population which is highly abnormal with multiple translocations. In case 5786 we have found only karyotypically abnormal cells in culture; one clone is pseudodiploid, while the other is markedly aneuploid. Thus, in this system where contamination by normal cells is unlikely, the results thus far, similar to those for renal carcinoma, include a number of cases that are diploid or show loss of a sex chromosome. The overall success rate of growth in culture is high in defined or modified culture media (additives such as zinc, etc).

TABLE VI. Cytogenetics of Cultured CNS Tumors

Case no.	Tumor diagnosis	Karyotype
5464	Medulloblastoma	46,XY/45,X,−Y
5521	Glioblastoma Gr.IV	46,XX
5536	Astrocytoma Gr. III	46,XX
5556	Oligo-dendroglioma/ependymoma	46,XY
5583	Glioma, astrocytoma Gr. IV	46,X,−X
5674	Glioblastoma, astrocytoma Gr. IV	46,XY/abnormal clone with multiple aberrations
5786	Regrowth medulloblastoma (?)	46,X,?Y,+multiple aberrations/55,X,?Y,+ multiple X aberrations
5889	Low-grade astrocytoma (?)	46,XX
5901	Pineablastoma	46,XX
5965	Hemangioblastoma	46,XX
6070	Medulloblastoma	46,XY

CONCLUSIONS

These studies of different primary human tumors illustrate several major problems. First, results appear to vary depending upon the tissue of origin. Simple unspecialized culture systems will not support the growth of cells from primary breast cancers or indeed cells from normal breasts, while they will support the growth of a large fraction of tumors of renal origin and almost 100% of tumors from the central nervous system. Moreover, primary cultures from breast are composed almost uniformly of normal diploid cells, while those of renal and CNS tumors include diploid and near-diploid cells. Both appear to contain mosaic populations and both show clonal aberrations in near-diploid cells. Unmodified and nonspecialized culture media do not appear to support highly aneuploid populations from renal tumors. Special media are necessary for the growth of cells from breast cancers and improve success in the culture of cells from CNS tumors. There is additional evidence that short-term culture conditions are highly selective in that the heterogeneous or multiclonal populations that historically have been detected using direct cytogenetic techniques have not been found in our cell cultures from breast and renal tumors.

Flow studies on the same tumors in a few cases suggest that subpopulations of renal tumors are not growing in culture. Evidence from all tumor types suggests that cytogenetically normal diploid cells constitute part of some tumor populations. The evidence is stronger for cultures derived from breast and central nervous system tumors, while further work is necessary to support that interpretation for the renal carcinoma cultures. It is clear that diploid and near-diploid cells from all three types of tumor appear better adapted to routine growth in culture than do aneuploid subpopulations from the same primary tumors.

In some respects we are very much like the blind men attempting to describe an elephant with our tools limited to investigation of one part or another of the entire beast. It is important to remember that for many or most primary solid tumors of man, the tumor has encompassed 7/8 of its entire life span prior to clinical detection. Considerable evolution and development of diversity can have occurred during this period and our studies of solid tumors in culture suggest that this is indeed the case. It is likely in some human tumors that at least one subset of the tumor cell population is karyotypically diploid. These cells, less altered than the remainder of the tumor cell population, are less vulnerable to therapeutic attack and, therefore, better fitted to carry on and survive as the tumor stem line. If some tumor populations are indeed cytogenetically normal, what significance can we attribute to the clonal karyotypic abnormalities that appear to be specific to solid tumor subtypes? We suggest that the primary and important events in tumor initiation and progression most often occur at the level of the gene rather than the chromosome, but that these consistent and apparently specific chromosome aberrations may serve as signposts for genes that are critically oncogenic for particular cell lineages or stages of differentation. Since the pathways for significant genetic alteration may depend on the unique functioning portions of specialized cell types, it is reasonable to expect that the clonal cytogenetic aberrations that characterize specific tumor types will differ. It is also reasonable to expect that evolution within a primary tumor or its metastases will be associated with new biological attributes which may in turn depend upon chromosomal rearrangement, loss, or reduplication. Thus it is reasonable to expect considerable cytogenetic diversity within individual tumors as well among different tumors. These differences must be explored and described for individual tumor types before they can be exploited for tumor therapeutic efforts.

ACKNOWLEDGMENTS

We are indebted to Niola Jezukaitis for manuscript preparation.

REFERENCES

1. Croce CM: Cancer Res 46:6019, 1986.

2. Seibert K, Shafie SM, Triche TJ, Whang-Peng JJ, O'Brien SJ, Toney JH, Huff KK, Lippman ME: Cancer Res 43:2223,1983.
3. Rodgers CS, Hill SM, Hulten MA: Cancer Genet Cytogenet 13:95,1984.
4. Hill SM, Rodgers CS, Hulten MA: Cancer Genet Cytogenet 24:45,1987.
5. Wolman SR, Smith HS, Stampfer M, Hackett AJ: Cancer Genet Cytogenet 16:49,1985.
6. Wolman SR: In Medina D, Kidwell W, Heppner G, Anderson E (eds): "Cellular and Molecular Biology of Experimental Mammary Cancer." New York: Plenum Press, 1987 (in press).
7. Smith HS, Lan S, Ceriani R, Hackett AJ, Stampfer MR: Cancer Res 41:4637, 1981.
8. Smith HS, Wolman SR, Hackett AJ: Biochim Biophys Acta 738:103,1984.
9. Smith HS, Liotta LA, Hancock MC, Wolman SR, Hackett AJ: Proc Nat Acad Sci USA 82:1805,1985.
10. Smith HS, Wolman SR, Auer G, Hackett AJ: In Rich MA, Hager JC, Taylor-Papadimitriou J (eds): "Breast Cancer: On the Frontiers of Discovery." Boston: M Nijhoff,1986,pp 75–89.
11. Teyssier JR, Henry I, Dozier C, Ferre D, Adnet JJ, Pluot M: J Natl Cancer Inst 77:1187,1986.
12. Yoshida MA, Ohyashiki K, Ochi H, Gibas Z, Pontes JW, Prout GR, Huben R, Sandberg AA: Cancer Res 46:2139,1986.
13. Berger CS, Sandberg AA, Todd IAD, Pennington RD, Haddad FS, Hecht BK, Hecht F: Cancer Genet Cytogenet 23:1,1986.
14. Cohen AJ, Li PF, Berg S, Marchetto DJ, Tsai S, Jacobs SC, Brown RS: N Engl J Med 301:592,1979.
15. Ferti-Passantonopoulou A, Panani A, Raptis S: Cancer Genet Cytogenet 11:227,1984.
16. Shapiro JR: Semin Oncol 13:4,1986.
17. Bigner SH, Mark J, Bullard DE, Mahaley MS, Bigner DD: Cancer Genet Cytogenet 22:121,1986.
18. Hittleman WN: In Rao PN, Johnson RT, Sperling K (eds): "Premature Chromosome Condensation: Applications in Basic, Clinical, and Mutation Research." New York: Academic Press, 1982, pp 309.

Heparanases and Tumor Metastasis

Motowo Nakajima, Tatsuro Irimura, and Garth L. Nicolson

Department of Tumor Biology, The University of Texas M.D. Anderson Hospital and Tumor Institute, Houston, Texas 77030

The successful penetration of endothelial basement membranes is an important process in the formation of hematogenous tumor metastases. Heparan sulfate (HS) proteoglycan is a major constituent of endothelial basement membranes, and we have found that HS-degradative activities of metastatic B16 melanoma sublines correlate with their lung-colonizing potentials. The melanoma HS-degrading enzyme is a unique endo-β-D-glucuronidase (heparanase) that cleaves HS at specific intrachain sites and is detectable in a variety of cultured human malignant melanomas. The treatment of B16 melanoma cells with heparanase inhibitors that have few other biological activities, such as N-acetylated N-desulfated heparin, results in significant reductions in the numbers of experimental lung metastases in syngeneic mice, indicating that heparanase plays an important role in melanoma metastasis. HS-degrading endoglycosidases are not tumor-specific and have been found in several normal tissues and cells. There are at least three types of endo-β-D-glucuronidases based on their substrate specificities. Melanoma heparanase, an $M_r \sim 96,000$ enzyme with specificity for β-D-glucuronosyl-N-acetylglucosaminyl linkages in HS, is different from platelet and mastocytoma endoglucuronidases. Elevated levels of heparanase have been detected in sera from metastatic tumor-bearing animals and malignant melanoma patients, and a correlation exists between serum heparanase activity and extent of metastases. The results suggest that heparanase is potentially a useful marker for tumor metastasis.

Key words: endo-β-D-glucuronidase, heparan sulfate, melanoma, heparin, serum enzyme, basement membrane

Most cancer mortality is the result of metastasis of tumors to regional and distant sites. Metastasis formation occurs via a sequential and complex series of unique interactions between tumor cells and normal host cells and tissues. For example, during the process of metastasis formation migrating tumor cells are confronted by natural tissue barriers, such as connective stroma and basement membranes. The ability of malignant cells to penetrate these barriers is thought to depend on the presence of tumor and/or host enzymes capable of degrading stromal and basement membrane components—mainly collagenous and noncollagenous glycoproteins and proteoglycans. Recent progress on degradative enzymes secreted by invasive

Received May 14, 1987; accepted July 16, 1987.

© 1988 Alan R. Liss, Inc.

and metastatic tumors has been reviewed by Nicolson [1], Nicolson and Poste [2], Jones and De Clerck [3], Mullins and Rohrlick [4], and Pauli et al [5]; and by Terranova et al [6], Liotta et al [7], and Wooley [8] (collagenases); by Sloane and Honn [9] (cysteine proteinases); by Danø et al [10] (plasminogen activators); and by Bernacki et al [11] (exo- and endoglycosidases).

Basement membranes are continuous sheets of extracellular matrix that separate parenchymal cells from underlying interstitial connective tissue. They have characteristic permeabilities and play a role in maintaining normal tissue architecture [12,13]. Enzymatic degradation of basement membrane components by metastatic tumor cells has been observed by using intact basement membranes, their isolated components, or the extracellular matrices produced by endothelial or endodermal cells [14–22]. The activities of several cell-associated enzymes are thought to be involved in the destruction of basement membranes and their activities correlate with metastatic potential in several types of malignant cells [14,15,17,21–25] (Fig. 1). Here we focus on tumor endoglycosidases capable of degrading heparan sulfate (HS) proteoglycans and discuss their possible use as markers of tumor metastasis.

MOUSE B16 MELANOMA HEPARANASE

Due to their unique physical and chemical properties the HS proteoglycans are important structural elements of basement membranes [26,27]. For example, HS proteoglycan promotes basal lamina matrix assembly by enhancing the interactions of

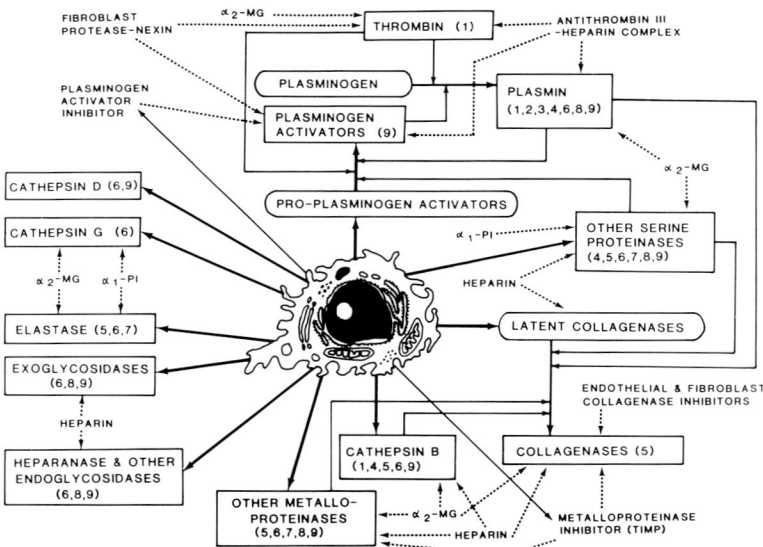

Fig. 1. Tumor-associated degradative enzymes and plasma proteinases: their possible roles in metastatic processes and their regulation by inhibitors derived from tumor and normal cells. The bold solid lines represent the release of enzymes or activation of proenzymes. The broken lines represent possible inhibitory mechanisms. The numbers represent the possible roles of degradative enzymes: (1) platelet aggregation, (2) fibrinolysis, (3) lamininolysis, (4) fibronectinolysis, (5) collagenolysis, (6) proteoglycanolysis, (7) elastinolysis, (8) host cell lysis, (9) other activities. Abbreviations: α_1PI, α_1-proteinase inhibitor; α_2-MG, α_2-macroglobulin.

collagenous and noncollagenous protein components while protecting them against proteolytic attack [28,29]. Thus, the destruction of the HS proteoglycan barrier could be important in basement membrane invasion by tumor cells.

The interactions between malignant cells and vascular endothelium have been studied by using monolayers of cultured vascular endothelial cells that synthesize an extracellular matrix resembling a basement membrane [15-17]. With this model, Kramer et al [16] found that metastatic B16 melanoma cells degrade matrix glycoproteins such as fibronectin and sulfated glycosaminoglycans, but predominantly HS. Since HS was released in solution as fragments approximately one-third their original size, it was proposed that metastatic tumor cells have an HS endoglycosidase [16]. We have examined the relationship between metastatic properties and the ability of the five B16 melanoma sublines of various implantation and invasion characteristics to enzymatically degrade subendothelial extracellular matrix and have found that highly invasive and metastatic B16 sublines degrade sulfated glycosaminoglycans faster than did sublines of lower metastatic potential [17].

Using purified lung HS, intact B16 cells (or their cell extracts) with a high potential for lung colonization degrade HS at higher rates than B16 cells with a poor potential for lung colonization [17]. We then examined the abilities of B16 cells to degrade HS from various origins and other purified glycosaminoglycans such as heparin, chondroitin 4-sulfate, chondroitin 6-sulfate, dermatan sulfate, keratan sulfate and hyaluronic acid [18,30,31]. HS purified from basement-membrane producing EHS sarcoma [18] and PYS-2 carcinoma [30], lung, kidney, and extracellular matrices of bovine aortic endothelial [18], and corneal endothelial cells [31] was degraded into HS fragments of characteristic molecular weight, in contrast to other glycosaminoglycans listed above, which were essentially undegraded [18]. Interestingly, heparin but not other glycosaminoglycans inhibited HS degradation [18]. The time dependence of HS degradation into particular molecular weight fragments indicated that melanoma heparanase cleaves HS at specific intrachain sites.

In order to determine the heparanase-specific HS cleavage points, the newly formed reducing termini of HS fragments were investigated. From this analysis the HS-degrading enzyme was identified as an endo-β-D-glucuronidase that cleaves β-D-glucuronosyl-N-acetylglucosaminyl linkages of the HS molecule [18]. To distinguish the melanoma HS-degrading endoglucuronidase from HS-specific elimination enzymes, such as heparitinase (EC 4.2.2.8) from *Flavobacterium heparinum*, we proposed that the melanoma enzyme should be called a heparanase (Fig. 2) [18].

HEPARAN-SULFATE-DEGRADING ENDOGLYCOSIDASES IN NORMAL AND TUMOR CELLS

The enzymatic degradation of HS proteoglycan by tumor cells has now been observed by several laboratories [19,22,24,32-34]. Vlodavsky et al [24] found that highly metastatic ESb T-lymphoma cells degrade HS proteoglycans present in the subendothelial matrix into low-molecular-weight HS fragments at faster rates than the less-invasive Eb subline. Becker et al [22] reported the degradation of HS proteoglycans in bovine corneal endothelial cell extracellular matrix by metastatic variants of rat rhabdomyosarcoma cells and a correlation between their enzyme activity and spontaneous metastatic potential was established. Ricoveri and Cappelletti [32] noted that cell extracts or intact metastatic mouse fibrosarcoma and B16 melanoma degraded

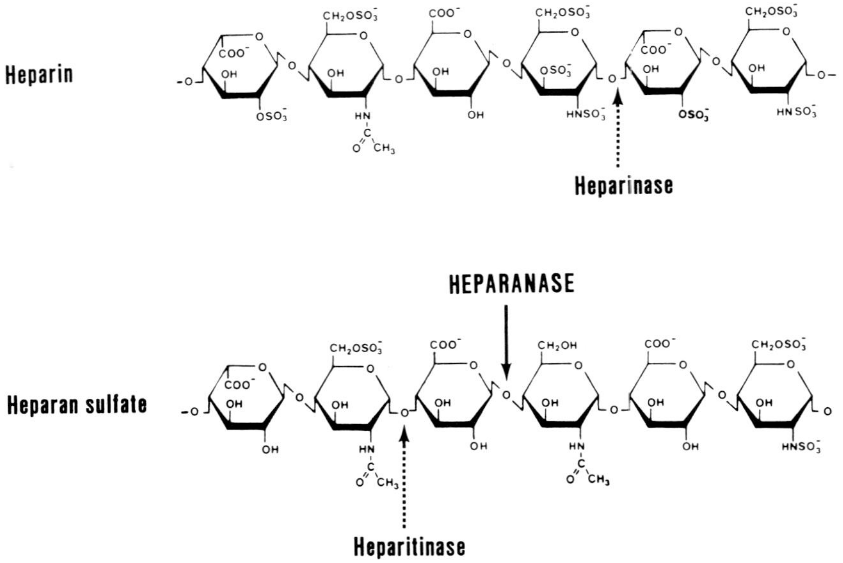

Fig. 2. Specificities of melanoma heparanase (endo-β-D-glucuronidase) and Fravobacter eliminases such as heparinase (EC 4.2.2.7) and heparitinase (EC 4.2.2.8).

HS faster than did their nonmetastatic counterparts. The optimum pH for HS degradation by HS endoglycosidases of mouse fibrosarcoma and B16 melanoma cells was about 5.6, but significant activity is still present at physiological pH [17,18,32].

To perform rapid microquantitative assays of large sample numbers of heparanase, we recently developed a solid-phase HS substrate by crosslinking of partially N-desulfated and N-[^{14}C or ^{3}H]acetylated HS onto agarose beads via one covalent linkage [35]. With this solid-phase substrate, several malignant human melanoma cell lines and normal cells such as fibroblasts and endothelial cells were assayed for HS-degrading activity [35,36]. All of the 15 human melanoma cells tested had HS-degradative activity, and some possessed activities comparable to that of mouse B16-F10 melanoma cells [36]. However, normal mouse skin fibroblasts and aortic endothelial cells showed very low activities [35] (Table I). These results suggest that melanoma cells generally possess heparanase and that this enzyme may perform an important role in human melanoma metastasis.

As stated above, HS-degrading endoglycosidase activity (Table II) is not unique to metastatic tumor cells, and the following normal tissues and cells have been found to possess HS-degrading endoglycosidases: liver [37,38], spleen [39], skin fibroblasts [40], placenta [41], platelets [42–45], T-lymphocytes [46,47], and inflammatory macrophages [47,48]. Enzymes present in rat liver, human skin fibroblasts, human placenta, and human platelets have also been identified as endoglucuronidases [38,40,41,43,44]. In some cases these normal cell enzymes have been shown to be different from tumor enzymes. For example, a platelet endo-β-D-glucuronidase different from melanoma heparanase have been purified by Oosta et al [44]. This normal cell enzyme is capable of degrading both HS and heparin and has an M_r of 134,000. In contrast, heparin is a potent inhibitor of melanoma heparanase [18].

TABLE I. Heparan Sulfate (HS) Degradation Activity in Mouse and Human Malignant Melanoma Cells [35,36]

Cell line	HS degradation activity[a]	
	Mean cpm ± SD	Ratio[b]
Mouse		
B16-F1	341 ± 32	1.00
B16-F10	510 ± 34	1.50
B16-BL6	758 ± 58	2.22
B16-B15b	716 ± 71	2.10
Human		
SK-MEL-19	379 ± 40	1.11
SK-MEL-23	397 ± 29	1.16
SK-MEL-93 (D×1)	625 ± 36	1.83
SK-MEL-93 (D×3)	381 ± 25	1.12
SK-MEL-93 (D×6)	703 ± 19	2.06
Hs 294T	381 ± 44	1.12
Hs 852T	202 ± 16	0.59
Hs 939	619 ± 44	1.82
T294	366 ± 15	1.07
M40	787 ± 75	2.31
RON	457 ± 27	1.34
BMCL	118 ± 31	0.35
A375 parent	392 ± 38	1.15
A375 Met Mix	659 ± 22	1.93
A375 M6	612 ± 48	1.79
Mouse skin fibroblasts	58 ± 17	0.17
Bovine aortic endothelia cells	42 ± 18	0.12

[a]Heparanase assay was carried out by the incubation of a Triton X-100 cell extract (2.4×10^5 cells) with PNDS-N[^{14}C]Ac-HS immobilized on agarose beads (4,500 cpm) at 37°C for 12 hr. The amount of radioactivity released in the presence of heat-inactivated enzymes (52 ± 12 cpm) was subtracted from the raw data (n = 3).
[b]Activity relative to the activity of B16-F1 (1.00).

We have purified melanoma heparanases from mouse B16-F10, human A375 Met, and Hs939 melanoma cells by using heparin-Sepharose, concanavalin A–Sepharose, and N-acetylated N-desulfated heparin-Sepharose affinity column chromatography. The human and mouse melanoma heparanases are of M_r ~96,000, as determined by SDS–polyacrylamide gel electrophoresis, and their pI is 5.2. At neutral pH such heparanases are highly active, while they are totally inactive at pH less than 5 and above 8.

The results of the studies on enzyme substrate specificities [18,37,38,45] suggest that there are at least three different types of mammalian cell endo-β-D-glucuronidases. Melanoma and liver glucuronidases appear to degrade HS but not heparin [18,37,38]. The human platelet enzyme depolymerizes both HS and heparin and cleaves the β-glucuronidic linkage in the antithrombin-binding octasaccharide of heparin molecules [45]. Another endoglucuronidase from mouse mastocytoma catalyzes the depolymerization of macromolecular heparin proteoglycans into fragments similar in size to commercial heparin [49,50]. The mastocytoma enzyme has little or no activity against HS and does not cleave the antithrombin-binding regions of the heparin [45,49].

TABLE II. HS-Degrading Endoglycosidases in Mammalian Cells

Normal cells	
Rat liver cells	Höök et al [37]
	Kjellén et al [38]
Rat spleen cells	Höök et al [39]
Human skin fibroblasts	Klein et al [40]
Human placenta	Klein and von Figura [41]
Human platelets	Wasteson et al [42]
	Oldberg et al [43]
	Oosta et al [44]
	Thunberg et al [45]
Rat activated T-lymphocytes	Naparstek et al [46]
Murine-activated T-lymphocytes	Savion et al [47]
Murine inflammatory macrophages	Savion et al [47]
Rat resident, alveolar, intratumoral, and inflammatory macrophages	Nakajima et al [48]
Tumor cells	
Murine melanoma cells	Kramer et al [16]
	Nakajima et al [17,18]
	Vlodavsky et al [19]
	Ricoveri and Cappelletti [32]
Murine T-lymphoma cells	Vlodavsky et al [24]
	Bar-Ner et al [34]
Human melanoma cells	Nakajima et al [35,36]
Rat rhabdomyosarcoma cells	Becker et al [22]
Murine fibrosarcoma cells	Ricoveri and Cappelletti [32]
Human colon carcinoma cells	Iozzo [33]
Rat mammary adenocarcinoma cells	Nakajima et al (unpublished)

HEPARANASE INHIBITORS

To confirm the biological significance of heparanases in metastatic processes, inhibitors against these enzymes have been used. Heparin is a potent inhibitor of heparanase; however, it has a variety of other biological activities, including anticoagulation [51,52] (Fig. 1). In certain experimental tumor systems heparin protects against metastases [53–55], while in others enhancement of tumor cell dissemination occurs [56–58]. The inhibitory effects of heparin on metastasis are thought to be mainly a consequence of the inhibition of blood coagulation and platelet aggregation that are known to facilitate implantation of tumor cells in organ capillaries. Most heparins are actually mixtures of polysaccharides that have intrinsic heterogeneity and molecular diversity; thus it is difficult to determine the role of particular structures in their complex biological activities.

We have attempted to ascertain the structural requirement for heparanase inhibition and find potent heparanase inhibitors that lack anticoagulation activity by chemically modifying heparin molecules [59]. Heparin modifications such as desulfation, deacetylation, sulfation, acetylation, and carboxyl-reduction were performed, and among several modified heparins, N-acetylated N-desulfated heparin, N-resulfated N- and O-desulfated heparin, and carboxyl-reduced heparin were found to maintain their heparanase inhibitory activity (Table III). These substrates also inhibited the degradation of mouse lung endothelial cell extracellular matrix by B16 melanoma cells. Treatment of B16-BL6 melanoma cells with the heparanase inhibitors resulted in significant reductions in the numbers of experimental melanoma lung

TABLE III. Effects of Heparin Derivatives on Heparanase Activity and Blood-Borne Lung Colonization of B16-BL6 Melanoma Cells in Mice [59]

Treatment	Heparanse inhibition[a]	Lung colonies[b]	
		No.	Median
None	0	0, 1, 26, 48, 75, 163, 193, 200+, 200+	75
Heparin	100.7	0, 0, 0, 0, 0, 1, 1, 2, 12	0
N-acetylated N-desulfated heparin	88.5	0, 1, 2, 3, 5, 5, 25, 37, 200+	5
N-resulfated N-, O-desulfated heparin	40.3	0, 0, 2, 5, 8, 13, 20, 90, 200+	8
Carboxyl-reduced heparin	53.2	7, 13, 42, 49, 51, 55, 58, 89, 120	51

[a]Heparanase activity was measured by incubating B16-BL6 melanoma cell lysates equivalent to 10^6 cells with a suspension of [^{3}H]HS-agarose beads and 1.25 mg/ml heparanase inhibitor at 37°C for 24 hr.
[b]The cells were incubated with chemically modified heparins (500 µg/ml) at 4°C for 2 hr before intravenous injection of 5×10^4 cells/0.1 ml into C57BL/6 mice. Experimental blood-borne metastasis to lung and other organs was determined after 20 days.

metastases in syngeneic mice (Table III) [59], supporting our hypothesis that heparanase plays an important role in melanoma metastasis. It is known that surgery, chemotherapy, and radiotherapy may enhance tumor cell dissemination. Therefore, antimetastasis treatments employing degradative enzyme inhibitors such as heparanase inhibitors may be useful in combination with other therapies to prevent further tumor spread.

SERUM ENZYME LEVELS AND TUMOR METASTASIS

The expression of certain serum proteins, such as carcinoembryonic antigen [60], α-fetoprotein [61], and placentalike alkaline phosphatase [62], is associated with some human cancers, and their immunologic detection has been used diagnostically for neoplastic disease. High levels of glycosyltransferases, such as sialyl- and galactosyltransferases, have been found in the sera of animals bearing spontaneously metastasizing tumors [63–65]. There is no clear functional relationship, however, between elevated serum levels of such components and metastatic disease.

Since tissue-degrading enzymes are secreted in high amounts from invasive tumor cells, the levels of such enzymes in body fluids could be useful as diagnostic markers of tumor invasion and metastasis. In fact, high levels of β-N-acetylglucosaminidase and β-glucuronidase were found in the sera of animals and patients with various types of tumors [11]. The release of these exoglycosidases from lysosomes has been related to the ability of Lewis lung carcinoma cells to form lung metastases [66], and changes in dipeptidase and acid proteinase activities in blood plasma of mice were associated with the presence of ascites tumors [67]. Pietras et al [68] investigated hydrolytic enzyme activities in sera of 121 women with invasive cancer and found that cathepsin B1–like activity in sera before therapy was an average of 45 times greater than that of normal controls, and cathepsin B1–like activity increased

TABLE IV. HS-Degrading Activities in the Sera From Rats Subcutaneously Injected With Highly Metastatic 13762NF Mammary Adenocarcinoma Cells [70]

Days after injection of cells (or DPBS)	HS-degrading activity in the sera, U/ml[a] (control rats injected with DPBS)	
0	0.12	(0.12)
9	0.10	(0.10)
16	0.46	(0.11)
23	0.96	(0.12)
30	2.01	(0.12)

No. of metastases[b]	(No. of rats)	HS-degrading activity in the sera, U/ml[a]
Lung		
0	(8)	0.47
1–10	(3)	0.44
>250	(10)	1.91
Lymph nodes		
0	(4)	0.10
1–2	(5)	0.49
>4	(12)	1.77

[a]HS-degrading activity was measured by incubation of ^{3}H-labeled solid-phase heparanase substrates with the serum diluted tenfold with 0.1 M sodium acetate, 0.15 M sodium chloride, pH 6.0. One unit of activity refers to the amounts of enzyme that liberates 1 μg of HS per minute.
[b]Rats were killed at various periods after subcutaneous injection of 1×10^6 MTLn3 (T44).5 cells in 0.1 ml of Dulbecco's phosphate-buffered saline (DPBS) and the numbers of metastases and serum enzyme activities were measured.

progressively during the transition from preinvasive to invasive cervical carcinoma. Ishihara et al [69] found increased neutral proteinase activity in the sera of rats bearing AH109A ascites hepatoma cells. The partially purified serum protease fraction contained both serine and cysteine proteinase activities and degraded pepsin-treated chains of basement membrane type IV collagen [69].

We have found that HS-degrading endoglycosidase is released from metastatic tumor cells, and this enzyme can circulate in the body fluids of tumor-bearing animals. We have assessed the sera from rats bearing mammary adenocarcinomas of differing metastatic potentials for this enzyme [70]. HS-degradative activity in sera diluted tenfold increased with time after subcutaneous injection of highly metastatic MTLn3 mammary adenocarcinoma cells in female F344 rats (Table IV). In contrast, sera from rats bearing mammary adenocarcinoma of low metastatic potential, such as clone MTC, possessed low levels of enzyme, even 30 days after tumor cell injection. In contrast to MTLn3 cells, clone MTC cells remained localized at the injection site and did not metastasize to regional lymph nodes or distant sites. Enzyme activities in the sera of rats bearing subcutaneous MTLn3 tumors correlated with extent of metastases. Rats with large numbers of metastases in the lung and/or lymph nodes had much higher activities of HS-degradative enzymes in their sera than rats with few or no metastases (Table IV). These results suggest that the activity of heparanase in

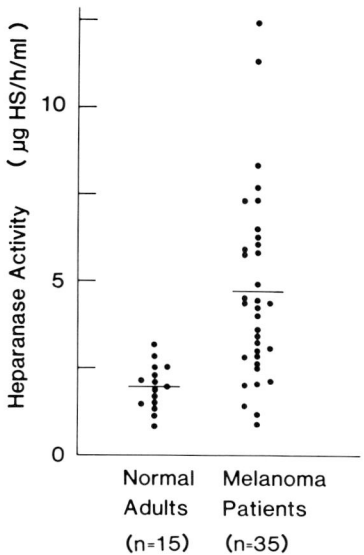

Fig. 3. Heparan sulfate degrading activity in sera of normal adults and malignant melanoma patients. The enzyme activity was measured by using solid-phase assay substrates (Table I).

serum is related to the occurrence of metastases to lung and lymph nodes. Thus, HS-degradative enzymes may be useful serum markers of tumor metastasis.

Since human malignant melanoma tissues have high heparanase activities and the heparanase is released from melanoma cells, we tested sera from malignant melanoma patients and normal adults for heparanase (Fig. 3). The average serum heparanase activities of melanoma patients (n=35) and normal adults (n=15) were 3.72 and 1.98 U/ml serum, respectively ($P < .05$). The sera from the patients having metastases in lymph nodes, liver, lung, and brain showed more than four times the level of heparanase activity than normal controls ($P < .001$). The source of HS-degradative activity in the normal adult serum includes platelets and other blood cells, because heparin-degrading activity was also detected. Therefore, the difference in serum heparanase may be much greater in patients with metastatic disease than we have estimated. A more specific enzyme assay for tumor-associated heparanaase should lead to more accurate analyses of clinical samples.

CONCLUSION

The development of sensitive methods to diagnose and predict metastasis and to monitor the therapy of metastases is an important goal. Studies on the role of basement-membrane degrading enzymes in tumor metastasis led to our hypothesis that such tumor enzymes may be useful markers for tumor metastasis and also possible targets to block the process of metastasis. Although basement-membrane degradative enzymes are not unique to malignant tumor cells; elevated levels of these enzymes in serum have been found to be associated with many types of metastatic tumors, and certain enzyme inhibitors were shown to have antimetastatic effects. Future research on metastasis-associated-degradative enzymes should allow the development of new approaches to diagnose and monitor tumor metastases, and this could lead to the synthesis of unique inhibitors of metastatic disease.

ACKNOWLEDGMENTS

This work was supported by National Institutes of Health grants RO1-CA41524 to M. Nakjima, R35-CA44352 to G.L. Nicolson, and RO1-CA39319 to T. Irimura and by a grant from the National Foundation for Cancer Research and the Meadows Foundation to G.L. Nicolson.

REFERENCES

1. Nicolson GL: Biochim Biophys Acta 695:113, 1982.
2. Nicolson GL, Poste G: Int Rev Exp Pathol 25:77, 1983.
3. Jones PA, De Clerck YA: Cancer Metastasis Rev 1:289, 1982.
4. Mullins DE, Rohrlich ST: Biochim Biophys Acta 695:177, 1983.
5. Pauli BU, Schwartz DE, Thonar EJ-M. Kuettner KE: Cancer Metastasis Rev 2:129, 1983.
6. Terranova VP, Hujanen ES, Martin GR: J Natl Cancer Inst 77:311, 1986.
7. Liotta LA, Thorgeirsson UP, Garbisa S: Cancer Metastasis Rev 1:277, 1982.
8. Wooley DE: Cancer Metastasis Rev 3:361, 1984.
9. Sloane BF, Honn KV: Cancer Metastasis Rev 3:249, 1984.
10. Danø K, Andreasen PA, Grondahl-Hansen J. Kristense P, Nielsen LS, Skriver L: Adv Cancer Res 44:139, 1985.
11. Bernacki RJ, Niedbala MJ, Korytnyk W: Cancer Metastasis Rev 4:81, 1985.
12. Vracko R: Am J Pathol 77:313, 1974.
13. Kefalides NA, Alper R, Clark CC: Int Rev Cytol 61:167, 1979.
14. Liotta LA, Abe S, Robey PG, Martin GR: Proc Natl Acad Sci USA 76:2268, 1979.
15. Nicolson GL: J Histochem Cytochem 30:214, 1982.
16. Kramer RH, Vogel KG, Nicolson GL: J Biol Chem 257:2678, 1982.
17. Nakajima M, Irimura T, Di Ferrante D, Di Ferrante N, Nicolson GL: Science 220:611, 1983.
18. Nakajima M, Irimura T, Di Ferrante N, Nicolson GL: J Biol Chem 259:2283, 1984.
19. Vlodavsky I, Ariav Y, Atzmon R, Fuks Z: Exp Cell Res 140:145, 1982.
20. Kramer RH, Vogel KG: J Natl Cancer Inst 72:889, 1984.
21. Starkey JR, Hosick HL, Stanford DR, Liggitt HD: Cancer Res 44:1585, 1984.
22. Becker M, Moczar M, Poupon MF, Moczar E: J Natl Cancer Inst 77:417, 1986.
23. Liotta LA, Tryggvason K, Garbisa S, Hart I, Foltz CM, Shafie S: Nature (Lond) 284:67, 1980.
24. Vlodavsky I, Fuks Z, Bar-Ner M, Ariav Y, Schirrmacher V: Cancer Res 43:2704, 1983.
25. Sloane BF, Dunn JR, Honn KV: Science (Wash) 212:1151, 1981.
26. Parthasarathy N, Spiro RG: J Biol Chem 256:507, 1981.
27. Kanwar YS, Linker A, Farquhar MG: J Cell Biol 86:688, 1980.
28. Hascal VC: In Ginsburg V (ed): "Biology of Carbohydrates." New York: John Wiley and Sons, 1981, pp 1–49.
29. Chiarugi VP: Anticancer Res 2:275, 1982.
30. Irimura T, Nakajima M, Di Ferrante N, Nicolson GL: Anal Biochem 130:461, 1983.
31. Wang Z-W, Irimura T, Nakajima M, Belloni PN, Nicolson GL: Eur J Biochem 153:125, 1985.
32. Ricoveri W, Cappelletti R: Cancer Res 46:3855, 1986.
33. Iozzo RV: J Biol Chem 262:1888, 1987.
34. Bar-Ner M, Kramer MD, Schirrmacher V, Ishai-Michaeli R, Fuks Z, Vlodavsky I: Int J Cancer 35:483, 1985.
35. Nakajima M, Irimura T, Nicolson GL: Anal Biochem 157:162, 1986.
36. Nakajima M, Irimura T. Nicolson GL: Cancer Lett 31:277, 1986.
37. Höök M, Wasteson Å, Oldberg Å: Biochem Biophys Res Commun 67:1422, 1975.
38. Kjellén L, Pertoft H, Oldberg Å, Höök M: J Biol Chem 260:8416, 1985.
39. Höök M, Pettersson I, Ögren S: Thromb Res 10:857, 1977.
40. Klein U, Kresse H, von Figura K: Biochem Biophys Res Commun 69:158, 1976.
41. Klein U, von Figura K: Biochem Biophys Res Commun 73:569, 1976.
42. Wasteson Å, Glimelius B, Busch C, Westermark B, Heldin C-H, Norling B: Thromb Res 11:309, 1977.
43. Oldberg ÅA, Heldin C-H, Wasteson Å, Busch C, Höök M: Biochemistry 19:5755, 1980.

44. Oosta GM, Favreau LV, Beeler DL, Rosenberg RD: J Biol Chem 257:11249, 1982.
45. Thunberg L, Bräckström G, Wasteson Å, Robinson HC, Ögren S, Lindahl U: J Biol Chem 257:10278, 1982.
46. Naparstek Y, Cohen IR, Fuks Z, Vlodavsky I: Nature 310:241, 1984.
47. Savion N, Vlodavsky I, Fuks Z: J Cell Physiol 118:169, 1984.
48. Nakajima M, North S, Irimura T, Nicolson GL: J Cell Biol 101:215a, 1985.
49. Ögren S, Lindahl U: J Biol Chem 250:2690, 1976.
50. Robinson HC, Horner AA, Höök M, Ögren S, Lindahl U: J Biol Chem 253:6687, 1978.
51. Jaques LB: Pharmacol Rev 31:99, 1980.
52. Casu B: Adv Carbohydr Chem Biochem 43:51, 1985.
53. Hagmar B, Norrby K: Int J Cancer 5:72, 1970.
54. Tsubura E, Yamashita T, Kobayashi M, Higuchi Y, Isobe J: Gann Monogr Cancer Res 20:147, 1977.
55. Hilgard P: In Nicolson GL, Milas L (eds): "Cancer Invasion and Metastasis: Biologic and Therapeutic Aspects." New York: Raven Press, 1984, pp 353-360.
56. Maat B: Br J Cancer 37:369, 1978.
57. Hagmar B, Boeryd B: Pathol Eur 4:274, 1969.
58. Chan SY, Pollard M: J Natl Cancer Inst 64:1121, 1980.
59. Irimura T, Nakajima M, Nicolson GL: Biochemistry 25:5322, 1986.
60. Gold, P, Freedman SO: J Exp Med 121:439, 1965.
61. Abelev GI: Adv Cancer Res 14:295, 1971.
62. Kellen JA, Bush RS, Malkin A: Cancer REs 36:269, 1976.
63. Chatterjee SK: Eur J Cancer 15:1351, 1979.
64. Bernacki RJ, Kim U: Science 195:577, 1977.
65. Kondo Y, Sato K, Ueyama Y, Ohsawa N: Cancer Res 41:2912, 1981.
66. Dobrossy L, Pavelic ZP, Vaughan M, Porter N, Bernacki RJ: Cancer Res 40:3281, 1980.
67. Ottoson R, Sylvén B: Arch Biochem Biophys 87:41, 1960.
68. Pietras RJ, Szego CM, Mangan CE, Seeler BJ, Burtnett MM: Gynecol Oncol 7:1, 1979.
69. Ishihara A, Nabeshima K, Koono M: Invasion Metastasis 6:225, 1986.
70. Nakajima M, Welch DR, Irimura T, Nicolson GL: Prog Clin Biol Res 212:113, 1986.

Mechanism of Induction of Class I Major Histocompatibility Antigen Expression by Murine Leukemia Virus

Douglas V. Faller, Lise D. Wilson, and David C. Flyer

Division of Pediatric Oncology, Dana Farber Cancer Institute and Department of Pediatrics, Harvard Medical School and Childrens Hospital Medical Center, Boston, Massachusetts 02115 (D.V.F., L.D.W.), Department of Microbiology, Milton S. Hershey Medical Center, Hershey, Pennsylvania 17033 (D.C.F.)

Alterations in expression of major histocompatibility complex (MHC) antigens on tumor cells clearly correlate with the tumorgenicity and metastatic potential of those cells. These changes in the biological behavior of the tumor cells are presumably secondary to resulting changes in their susceptibility to immune recognition and destruction. Murine leukemia viruses (MuLV) exert regulatory effects on class I genes of the MHC locus. MuLV infection results in substantial increases in cell surface expression of all three class I MHC antigens. These viral effects on MHC antigen expression profoundly influence immune-mediated interaction with the infected cells, as assessed by cytotoxic T lymphocyte recognition and killing. Control of class I MHC and beta-2 microglobulin genes by MuLV takes place via a *trans*-acting molecular mechanism. MuLV controls expression of widely separated endogenous cellular MHC genes, transfected xenogeneic class I MHC genes, and unintegrated chimeric genes consisting of fragments of class I MHC genes linked to a bacterial reporter gene. These findings indicate that MuLV exerts its effects on MHC expression via a *trans* mechanism. The MuLV-responsive sequences on the MHC genes appear to lie within 1.2 kilobases upstream of the initiation codon for those genes.

Key words: immune surveillance, *trans* activation, retroviruses, class I MHC antigens, leukemia viruses

The level of cellular immune response against tumors appears to be a major factor in determining tumor growth and metastatic behavior [1–6]. Any process which alters immune recognition may therefore alter the response of the organism to the tumor, either facilitating the interaction of the tumor with the immune system or permitting the escape of these transformed cells from immune destruction. The class I major histocompatibility complex (MHC) antigens are polymorphic cell surface glycoproteins that function as targets, directing the attack of cytotoxic T lymphocytes

Received May 4, 1987; revised and accepted August 5, 1987.

© 1988 Alan R. Liss, Inc.

(CTL) against virally transformed cells. CTL function and recognition of target cells require associated recognition between foreign antigens and self-MHC components [6–8]. In the case of lymphomas induced by murine leukemia viruses, these foreign antigens can be either virally encoded proteins or nonviral tumor-specific antigens induced in the course of tumorgenesis [9,10]. The level of expression of MHC class I proteins on virus-infected cells has been correlated with the degree of effectiveness with which they are recognized by CTL [11,12]. On some tumors, the new or enhanced expression of specific class I MHC antigens is associated with increased potential for invasion and metastasis [13]. It is, therefore, reasonable to expect that viruses with the capability of altering class I MHC expression in the cells they infect may be influencing their own survival and the survival of the cells they transform.

Previously, this laboratory has reported that mouse cells express significantly increased surface levels of murine class I MHC H-2K, H-2D, and H-2L proteins after infection with the Moloney murine leukemia virus (M-MuLV) [11]. The infected cells are efficiently lysed by M-MuLV-specific CTL and also by allospecific CTL, a reflection of their increased level of H-2 antigens. Coinfection of cells with M-MuLV and the replication-defective, acutely transforming Moloney murine sarcoma virus (M-MSV) eliminates the H-2 enhancement as well as decreasing the immunosensitivity of the infected cells.

This report describes our efforts to define the mechanism by which the murine leukemia viruses induce class I MHC expression. Our findings indicate that as a result of MuLV infection, cells increase their synthesis of MHC class I mRNA, as well as beta-2 microglobulin mRNA. Analysis of MuLV-infected cells transfected with MHC class I genes suggests that the viral regulation of H-2 transcription occurs in *trans*. We also show that sequences upstream of at least one murine class I gene are responsive to this *trans* regulation and will direct increased production of an attached bacterial reporter gene in M-MuLV-infected cells.

MATERIALS AND METHODS

Viruses

Moloney murine leukemia virus clone 1 [14] was obtained from Drs. C. Tabin and R. Weinberg. In some experiments the source of the virus was a producer cell line of BALB/c-3T3 cells transfected with an infectious proviral clone of Moloney MuLV designated pMoV-9 [15], or with an infectious proviral clone of an amphotropic MuLV, strain 4070, kindly provided by Dr. A. Oliff.

Cells

BALB/c-3T3 fibroblasts and NIH-3T3 fibroblasts were obtained through the American Type Culture Collection (Rockville, MD). LB10SV, a fibroblast cell line derived from C57BL/10 mice, was described previously [9]. Infected and uninfected fibroblasts were cultured in Dulbecco's modified Eagle's medium (GIBCO Laboratories, Grand Island, NY) supplemented with 10% heat-inactivated fetal calf serum (FCS) and 2 mM L-glutamine.

Monoclonal Antibodies

Hybridoma cell lines producing monoclonal antibodies specific for H-2K^d (31.3.45), H-2D^d (34.2.12), H-2L^d (28.14.8), and H-2K^b (B8-24-3) were provided by Dr. David Sachs. Monoclonal antibody specific for HLA-A2 was obtained from hybridoma PA2.5 (American Type Culture Collection, Rockville, MD). Cell-free supernatants from hybridoma-conditioned medium were used undiluted for cell surface antigen labeling. An antisera raised in rabbits against purified H-2^k, which cross-reacts with all murine H-2 proteins, was the generous gift of Dr. S. Herrmann, and was used as a 1:25 dilution for cell staining.

Concanavalin A (Con A) Supernatant

Spleen cells from Lewis rats (Charles River Laboratories, Wilmington, MA) were cultured in the presence of 5 μg/ml Con A (Pharmacia Fine Chemicals, Uppsala, Sweden) for 24 h. The cell-free supernatant was partially purified by ammonium sulfate precipitation as described [11,16].

Generation of CTL

Allospecific CTL (anti-H-2^b) were generated in 5-day, one-way mixed lymphocyte cultures. BALB/c spleen cells (5×10^6) were cultured with an equal number of gamma-irradiated (2,500 rads) C57BL/6 spleen cells in 16-mm Linbro plates (Flow Laboratories, Inc., McClean, VA), in 2 ml of RPMI 1640 (GIBCO), supplemented with 100 U/ml penicillin/streptomycin, 2 mM L-glutamine, 10 mM HEPES, 5×10^{-5} M 2-mercaptoethanol, and 10% FCS. Anti-H-2^d allospecific CTL were generated in an analogous way, except that irradiated BALB/c spleen cells were used as stimulators and C57BL/6 spleen cells were used as the responding population.

^{51}Cr-Release Assay

^{51}Cr-release assays were carried out in duplicate in 96-well V-bottomed microtiter plates. Varying numbers of immune lymphocytes were added to 10^4 ^{51}Cr-labeled target cells in 0.2 ml wells and were incubated for 4 h. After incubation, the cells were pelleted, and 50% of the well supernatant was removed and was counted in a gamma counter (Packard Instrument Co., Grove, IL). Percent specific ^{51}Cr release was calculated as follows:

$$\frac{(^{51}\text{Cr release with immune lymphocytes}) - (\text{spontaneous }^{51}\text{Cr release})}{(\text{Maximum }^{51}\text{Cr released with 3\% Triton}) - (\text{spontaneous }^{51}\text{Cr release})} \times 100$$

Immunofluorescent Labeling and Analysis

Live cells were incubated with hybridoma culture supernatants followed by Fluorescein-conjugated, affinity-purified F(ab')$_2$ fragment of sheep antimouse IgG (Cooper Biomedical, Malvern, PA), as described [11]. After fixation in 2% paraformaldehyde, labeled cells were analyzed by an Epics V fluorescence-activated cell sorter (Coulter Electronics, Inc., Hialeah, FL). As a control, some cell populations were exposed to recombinant murine interferon gamma (Genentech, South San Francisco, CA), at a concentration of 100 U/ml for 48 h prior to staining.

Northern Blot Analysis of Total Cellular RNA

Total cellular RNA was extracted from cells using a modification of the guanidine hydrochloride extraction technique described by Strohman et al. [17]. Briefly, after three serial ethanol precipitations in the presence of 6 M guanidine/100 mM potassium acetate, the nucleic acids were extracted with a phenol/chloroform mixture and ethanol precipitated. Twenty micrograms of RNA were loaded per lane on a 1.2% agarose gel containing formaldehyde and ethidium bromide [18]. Following electrophoresis, transfer to nitrocellulose was carried out using standard techniques. After baking in vacuo, prehybridization of the filters was performed in $5 \times$ SSC (0.75 M NaCl, 75 mM trisodium citrate, pH 7.0) and 50% formamide at 42°C. Hybridization was carried out under the same conditions, in the presence of 10% dextran sulphate and 2×10^6 cpm of radiolabeled probe/ml of hybridization fluid. The blots were washed under stringent conditions (68°C, $0.2 \times$ SSC) and autoradiography was carried out using intensifying screens at -70°C. Densitometric scanning (Helena Laboratories, Beaumont, TX) was performed to quantitate relative amounts of hybridization.

The probe used to detect H-2 class I sequences was a 2.5-kilobase (kb) Bam HI fragment from a plasmid clone containing the H-2D^b genomic clone (kindly provided by Drs. H. Allen and R. Flavell). This fragment contains the strongly conserved exons 4-8 and the 3' untranslated sequences and hybridizes to all murine class I mRNA species. The probe for beta-2 microglobulin was previously described [11]. Probes were labeled to a specific activity of $>10^8$ cpm/μg, using the random oligo primer method [19]. In order to normalize for the amount of RNA in each lane, blots were stripped of probe following autoradiography and rehybridized with an actin cDNA probe [20].

DNA-Mediated Gene Transfer

The Human Leukocyte Antigen-A2 (HLA-A2) gene, subcloned into the Eco RI site of pBR328 [21], was kindly provided by Drs. A. Biro and J. Strominger. This DNA was coprecipitated with the selectable marker pMSV-*neo* (10, and see below) or pSV2-*neo* [22] and salmon sperm DNA as carrier. Transfection and isolation of clones was carried out as previously described [10]. Clones were selected for cell surface expression of HLA-A2 by immunofluorescent staining and analyzed by fluorescence-activated cell sorting.

CAT Vector Constructions

The subclone of the genomic H-2K^b gene in pBR327 [23] was digested with the restricted enzymes Hind III and Nru I to generate a 2.1-kb fragment. After isolation, the fragment was blunt-ended with the large fragment of *Escherichia coli* DNA polymerase I and ligated to Hind III oligonucleotide linkers. The linkered fragment was then ligated into the Hind III site of the chlorampenicol acetyl transferase (CAT) vector, pSVO-CAT [24]. Transformation of competent *E. coli* HB101 resulted in Amp^R colonies which were screened by the minilysate technique [25] for insertion and correct orientation of the H-2K^b promoter sequences relative to the bacterial CAT gene (pKbHN-CAT, see Fig. 4). The construction pKbPN-CAT was generated by isolating the 1.2-kb Pvu II-Nru I fragment of the H-2K^b gene, ligating it to Hind III linkers and cloning it into pSVO-CAT as above (see Fig. 4). All enzymes and linkers were obtained from New England Biolabs (Beverly, MA) and were used according to the supplier's recommendations.

Assay for Transient CAT Expression

All CAT plasmids were isolated by lysozyme-SDS lysis and cesium chloride-ethidium bromide equilibrium gradient centrifugation. Cells were plated at 10^6/100-

mm tissue culture dish approximately 18 hr before transfection. Calcium phosphate precipitates containing 10 μg of the CAT vector and 20 μg salmon sperm carrier DNA were prepared, and transfections were carried out as described previously [10]. The CAT vector pSV2-CAT [24], provided by Drs. R. Mulligan and J. Nye, was used as a positive control for CAT expression in each of the cell lines tested. Forty-eight hours after transfection, the cell monolayers were washed with and scraped into ice-cold phosphate-buffered saline. The pelleted cells were resuspended in 100 μl of 0.25 M Tris-HCl, pH 7.8, and cell extracts were prepared by freezing and thawing the resuspended cells three times. Cellular debris was removed by centrifugation in a microfuge for 5 min at 4°C. The extracts were then measured for protein content and assayed for CAT activity as described by Gorman et al. [24]. Controls including purified CAT enzyme (.001 unit/assay; Pharmacia, Piscataway, NJ), instead of cell extract, were also run as standards for acetylation states of the chloramphenicol.

RESULTS

Infection of murine fibroblasts with M-MuLV results in enhancement of cell surface expression of MHC antigens. By using monoclonal antibodies specific for each of the three murine class I MHC proteins on BALB/c cells (H-2K^d, H-2D^d, and H-2L^d) it was demonstrated that the levels of all three antigens are upregulated on the surface of chronically infected BALB/c-3T3 cells (Fig. 1). The magnitude of the increase is up to tenfold for H-2K and somewhat less for H-2D and H-2L. The temporal course of this increase in class I antigen expression parallels the relatively slow spread of viral infection through newly infected cells (as monitored by expression of viral glycoprotein and positive immunofluorescence using a fluorescein isothiocyanate (FITC)-conjugated anti-viral glycoprotein monoclonal antibody). However, some increase in class I MHC expression can be demonstrated as soon as

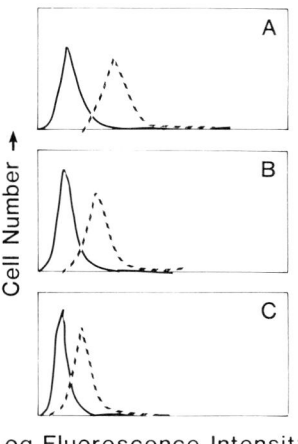

Fig. 1. Effect of murine leukemia virus infection of BALB/c-3T3 fibroblasts on cell surface class I MHC antigen expression. Binding of monoclonal antibodies specific for H-2K^d(**A**), H-2D^d(**B**), and H-2L^d(**C**) was measured by flow cytofluorometry after reacting infected or uninfected BALB/c cells with anti-H-2 monoclonal antibodies, followed by FITC-conjugated goat anti-mouse IgG. Uninfected BALB/c-3T3,(———); M-MuLV-infected BALB/c3T3, (— — — —).

48 hr after exposure of the cells to virus-containing media (data not shown). Similarly, MuLV-infection of NIH-3T3 cells causes an increase in cell surface expression of class I MHC antigen (Fig. 2A). Because NIH-3T3 cells are not from a defined inbred and MHC-phenotyped mouse strain, a pan-reactive antimurine class I rabbit serum was initially used to detect all class I-related molecules on the surface of these cells. Figure 2B demonstrates enhanced reactivity of NIH-3T3 cells with this serum following treatment with interferon gamma. Subsequently, we found that a monoclonal antibody specific for H-2D^b would detect class I molecules induced on NIH-3T3 cells by MuLV infection (data not shown).

Another way of assessing levels of immunologically active MHC antigens on the surface of cells is by analysis of their reactivity with allospecific T lymphocytes. The susceptibility of MuLV-infected BALB/c cells to lysis by anti-H-2^d-specific CTL paralleled their increase in H-2^d expression as determined by antibody staining, in that MuLV infection resulted in a greater than fourfold enhancement in lysis by allospecific CTL (Table I). Relative susceptibility to allospecific lysis is determined by the need for a fourfold increase in the effector-to-target-cell ratio for equivalent killing of the uninfected versus the MuLV-infected BALB/c cells. Infection of BALB/c cells with another murine retrovirus, amphotropic MuLV, also resulted in increased lysis by alloreactive CTL. Similarly, MuLV-infected NIH-3T3 cells demonstrated an

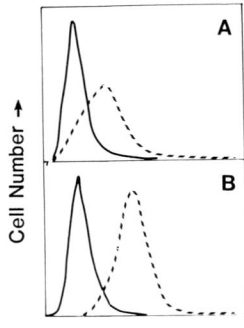

Fig. 2. Effect of murine leukemia virus infection of NIH-3T3 cells on cell surface class I MHC antigen expression. Binding of a rabbit antiserum which is pan-reactive with all murine H-2 antigens was measured by flow cytofluorometry after reacting uninfected, M-MuLV-infected, or interferon gamma-treated cells with the serum at a 1:25 dilution, followed by FITC-conjugated sheep anti-rabbit IgG. Uninfected NIH-3T3, (———). M-MuLV-infected NIH-3T3 (A) or interferon gamma-treated NIH-3T3 (B) (– – – – – –).

TABLE I. Lysis of MuLV-Infected BALB/c-3T3 Cells by Allogeneic CTL

Cell line	Virus[a]	% Cytotoxicity[b]		
		12:1[c]	25:1	50:1
BALB/c	—	33.0	43.1	57.1
BALB/c	M-MuLV	54.9	69.2	76.5
BALB/c	A-MuLV	46.3	59.3	78.3

[a]Cells were uninfected or infected with Moloney MuLV (M-MuLV) or with amphotropic MuLV (A-MuLV).
[b]Percent specific ^{51}Cr release.
[c]Effector-to-target cell ratios.

increase in their susceptibility to killing by anti-H-2^b-specific alloreactive CTL (Table II). In fact, they were lysed more efficiently than the usual H-2^b target cell line LB10SV. This finding, combined with the monoclonal antibody reactivity described above, suggests that the MHC phenotype of the NIH-3T3 cell line may contain some H-2^b-reactive elements.

To determine the molecular level at which induction of MHC by MuLV was occurring, analysis of class I-specific mRNA species in uninfected and infected BALB/c cells was carried out. The molecular probe used to detect MHC transcripts was selected on the basis of its ability to hybridize with all three types of murine class I transcripts (D, K, and L) and to cross-react to a molecular region highly conserved in all class I genes. BALB/c cells infected with M-MuLV express 4–6-fold more class I-specific transcripts than do uninfected cells (Fig. 3A). Normalization for the level of actin transcripts in infected versus uninfected cells (Fig. 3C) did not affect this ratio. Beta-2 microglobulin is a nonpolymorphic protein which associates with class I MHC polypeptides and is (in most cases) necessary for cell surface expression of MHC antigens [26]. The gene encoding beta-2 microglobulin does not lie within the MHC locus, yet the expression of beta-2 transcripts often parallels changes in the

TABLE II. Lysis of Moloney MuLV-Infected NIH-3T3 Cells by Allogeneic CTL

Cell line	% Cytotoxicity[a]			
	6:1[b]	12:1	25:1	50:1
LB10SV	13.4	29.6	38.1	52.3
NIH-3T3	7.7	8.8	14.0	18.0
M-MuLV-infected NIH-3T3	18.6	35.6	51.8	72.6

[a]Percent specific ^{51}Cr release.
[b]Effector-to-target cell ratios.

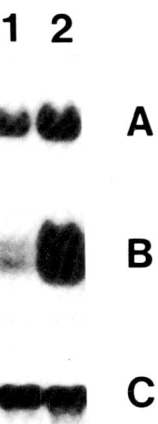

Fig. 3. Levels of class I MHC, beta-2 microglobulin, or beta-actin transcripts in BALB/c-3T3 cells, in the presence or absence of M-MuLV. Equal amounts of total cellular RNA extracted from BALB/c-3T3 cells (**lane 1**) or from M-MuLV-infected BALB/c-3T3 cells (**lane 2**) were separated on a 1.2% agarose gel, transferred to nitrocellulose, and hybridized sequentially to radiolabeled probes specific for H-2 (**A**), beta-2 microglobulin (**B**), and beta-actin (**C**) transcripts. Results of 15-hr autoradiographic exposure are shown here.

expression of class I transcripts [27]. Multiple analyses of mRNA species in infected or uninfected fibroblasts using a probe specific for murine beta-2 microglobulin revealed an average fivefold increase in the steady-state levels of both the 0.7- and 0.9-kb beta-2 microglobulin transcripts (Fig. 3B).

The finding that levels of all three class I MHC molecules and the genetically unlinked beta-2 microglobulin were elevated in M-MuLV-infected cells, and that this was reflected in an increase in the respective mRNA levels, suggested that MuLV was acting in a *trans* fashion to induce MHC and MHC-related genes. Such a *trans* mode of action should be capable of enhancement of other MHC genes which have been artificially introduced into the cell and stably integrated at loci distinct from the MHC region. To test this hypothesis, NIH-3T3 cells were transfected with the xenogeneic (human) class I MHC gene encoding HLA-A2. The resulting G418-resistant cell lines were sorted by fluoresence-activated flow cytometry and a population expressing HLA-A2 antigen on the cell surface was selected. Treatment of these transfected cells with interferon gamma resulted in an increased level of HLA-A2 expression (Fig. 4B). This heterogeneous population was then infected with M-MuLV and the cell surface levels of HLA-A2 compared to that of uninfected cells. Figure 4A demonstrates enhancement of HLA-A2 expression in the infected population.

Similarly, *trans* activation of MHC genes by MuLV should take place even in the absence of genomic integration, i.e., during transient expression of newly transfected genes. To amplify the fairly weak signal obtained during such transient gene expression assays, the 5' upstream region of the $H-2K^b$ gene was attached to the prokaryotic reporter gene CAT, which encodes the bacterial enzyme chloramphenicol acetyl transferase. The initial chimeric gene construction (called pKbHN-CAT, Fig. 5) included 2.1 kb of upstream sequence, terminated at an Nru I site 19 base pairs (bp) upstream of the ATG codon of the exon encoding the $H-2K^b$ leader peptide, and thus contained the essential sequences for effective promoter activity (i.e., TATA box, CCAAT box, and CAP site). Upon transfection of this recombinant gene into

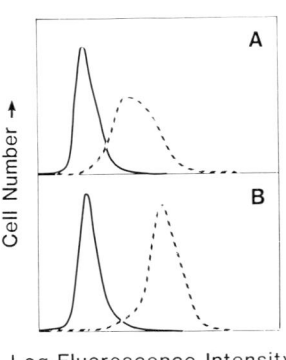

Fig. 4. Effect of murine leukemia virus infection of NIH-3T3 cells transfected with the HLA-A2 gene on the expression of HLA-A2. NIH-3T3 cells were transfected with the HLA-A2 gene and cell lines which stably expressed the A2 antigen were selected. Binding of a monoclonal antibody specific for HLA-A2 was measured by flow cytofluorometry after reacting uninfected, M-MuLV-infected, or interferon gamma-treated A2-transfected cells with the antibody, followed by FITC-conjugated goat anti-mouse IgG. Uninfected A2-transfected cells, (———). A2-transfected cells after infection with M-MuLV (**A**); or after treatment with interferon gamma (**B**), (- - - -).

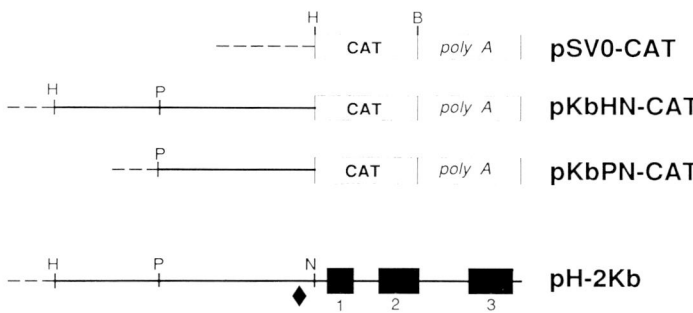

Fig. 5. Construction of pKbHN-CAT and pKbPN-CAT. The restriction map of the 5' portion of the H-2K^b gene showing the location of the promoter (♦) and exons 1-3 (■) has been adapted from Allen et al. [23]. H = Hind III; B = Bam HI; P = Pvu II; N = Nru I. The Nru I site is located 19 bp upstream from the ATG of the H-2K^b exon 1 (leader sequence). The 2.1 kb Hind III-Nru I fragment, and the 1.2 kb Pvu II-Nru I fragment, both from the H-2K^b 5' region (heavy lines), were ligated to Hind III oligonucleotide linkers and cloned into the Hind III site of the pSVO-CAT vector. Plasmid sequences are indicated by the broken lines. The E. coli Tn 9 chloramphenicol acetyl transferase gene (CAT) and the simian virus 40 (SV40) fragment containing the poly A addition site (poly A) are indicated.

uninfected, or M-MuLV-infected, BALB/c-3T3 cells and assay of cytoplasmic CAT activity at 48 hr, we found a consistent 4–5-fold increase in enzyme activity in the cells containing the leukemia virus (Fig. 6A). Normalization of this data to results obtained when the control plasmid, pSV2-CAT, was introduced into the same cell lines did not alter this ratio and negligible CAT activity was detected when the promoterless plasmid pSVO-CAT was introduced into either cell line. The relative increase in CAT expression in M-MuLV-infected cells compared to uninfected cells did not vary with time of incubation or with the amount of extract used in the incubation (data not shown).

The finding that a chimeric gene containing just the upstream elements of a class I MHC gene was controlled by M-MuLV in a fashion similar in direction and magnitude to the viral control of endogenous class I MHC genes allowed us to begin mapping those K^b control sequences which are responsive to murine leukemia virus. A second vector containing only 1.2 kb of K^b upstream sequence, and designated pKbPN-CAT (Fig. 5), was constructed and tested for activity in the same cell lines as the pKbHN-CAT vector. The difference in CAT expression driven by pKbPN-CAT in M-MuLV-infected versus uninfected cells was on average 2.5-fold (Fig. 6B). These results suggested that the MuLV effect on class I MHC expression may be mediated through an interaction somewhere within the 2.1 kb of DNA upstream from the coding sequence for the class I proteins. Shortening that sequence to 1.2 kb decreases the magnitude of the observed effect but does not eliminate it.

DISCUSSION

Abnormal regulation of MHC genes has been observed in tumors generated in a number of diverse ways, including chemically transformed cells, radiation-induced tumor cells, and spontaneously occurring leukemia cells in high-incidence mouse strains [reviewed in 28]. Attempts have been made to correlate changes in MHC expression with the metastatic or tumorgenic potential of the transformed cell [reviewed in 29]. We have shown here, and in previous studies [11], that cells in culture

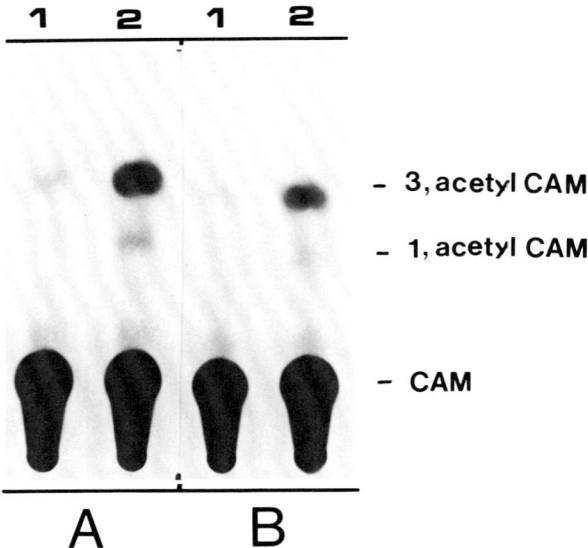

Fig. 6. Effect of leukemia virus infection on the level of CAT expression directed by pKbHN-CAT or pKbPN-CAT. Uninfected (**lane 1**), or M-MuLV-infected (**lane 2**), BALB/c-3T3 cells were transfected with calcium phosphate precipitates including 10 μg of pKbHN-CAT (**A**) or pKbPN-CAT (**B**). Cell extracts were prepared 48 hr post-transfection and assayed by incubating 500 μg of extract with 1 μCi ^{14}C-chloramphenicol for 2 hr at 37°C. The reaction products were separated by thin-layer chromatography (TLC). The autoradiograph of the TLC plate is shown with the positions of the unacetylated chloramphenicol (CAM) and acetylated reaction products (1-acetyl CAM and 3-acetyl CAM) indicated. Spots were cut from the plate and counted by liquid scintillation counting to determine the percent conversion of chloramphenicol to its acetylated derivatives. Percent chloramphenicol conversion for pKbHN-CAT-transfected, uninfected cell extracts was 0.15 ± 0.02, and for M-MuLV-infected cell extracts was 0.68 ± 0.05. Percent conversion for pKbPN-CAT-transfected, uninfected cell extracts was 0.16 ± 0.03, and for M-MuLV-infected cell extracts it was 0.37 ± 0.04.

increase their surface expression of class I MHC proteins shortly after infection with MuLV. It is highly unlikely that the increase is due to de novo expression of previously unexpressed class I genes, or to recombinational events leading to the formation of novel class I-like proteins, because increased levels of all three of the BALB/c class I antigens (H-2K, -L, and -D) are detected with H-2K^d-, H-2D^d-, and H-2L^d-specific monoclonal antibodies. Additional evidence that MuLV infection alters the expression of normal class I proteins is provided by our findings, using class I-specific CTL, that the immunological function of these antigens parallels their cell surface levels as assessed by monoclonal antibodies.

We show here an increase in the steady-state levels of both H-2 and beta-2 microglobulin mRNA species in MuLV-infected cells, and, in other studies, have demonstrated a parallel increase in transcription of these genes, as assessed by nuclear run-off assay [30]. Therefore, the increased level of H-2 protein in MuLV-infected cells is most likely the result of an increase in the rate of transcription of the H-2, as well as the beta-2 microglobulin, genes. Having observed parallel regulation of three class I genes which are widely separated within the mouse MHC locus, as well as the gene encoding beta-2 microglobulin, which is genetically unlinked to MHC and lies on a separate chromosome, it was of interest to determine whether MuLV infection would satisfy other criteria for a *trans*-acting mechanism of transcriptional activation. Accordingly, we have shown here that MuLV infection of a heterogeneous population of cells transfected with a human class I MHC gene (HLA-A2) results in enhanced expression of that A2 antigen. The incorporation of exogenous genes into the cellular genome after DNA-mediated gene transfer is known to be a random process [31]. It is therefore improbable that this induction of MHC antigen expression is the result of a *cis*-acting effect of the integrated provirus on transcription of each of the endogenous class I genes, the beta-2 microglobulin genes, and each of the randomly integrated HLA-A2 genes which were introduced by transfection.

A *trans*-activating effect by MuLV should also be capable of enhancing transcription of unintegrated class I genes or chimeric genes consisting of class I upstream elements linked to a reporter gene in a transient expression assay. Hybrid K^b-CAT constructions were utilized to test for such an activity and to provide some information relating to the genomic control sequences which respond to this regulatory activity. The temporal constraints on transient expression assays allow for minimal, if any, association of the transfected CAT vectors with the cellular genome, and most of the CAT mRNA is derived, therefore, from transcription of the vectors as extrachromosomal elements. The expression of CAT directed from at least 1.2 kb of H-$2K^b$ upstream sequences, when transfected into M-MuLV-infected cells, mimicked the MuLV-induced up-regulation of expression of the whole H-$2K^b$ gene.

Molecular mechanisms other than *trans*-regulation have been proposed to explain the effects of certain retroviruses on H-2 protein expression. Merulo et al. [32] have obtained evidence for altered methylation and structural rearrangements of the MHC complex in Radiation Leukemia Virus (RadLV)-induced tumors, presumably because of proximal integration of the viral genome. Like MuLV, RadLV induces class I MHC expression soon after infection; however, RadLV tumors that arise after a long latent period express little or no H-2 antigen [33].

Interferons are capable of inducing class I MHC expression on mesenchymal cells, and endogenous cellular interferon beta can be elaborated by cells in response to infection with some viruses. Although the response of cells to interferon gamma and to M-MuLV infection is similar [11], we have ruled out interferon as the mediator of MuLV induction of MHC in other studies [30]. We demonstrated that M-MuLV-infected cells do not produce detectable levels of interferon, or any other H-2-enhancing soluble factor, express no detectable mRNA species for interferon beta, and exhibit no interferon-induced antiviral state. In addition, we have previously found that interferon treatment of M-MuLV-infected cells has an additive effect on the H-2 level, suggesting that the site of action of interferon differs from that of the virus. Friedman and Stark have identified a consensus sequence upstream of the protein-coding regions of certain interferon-regulated genes [34]. This interferon response sequence lies approximately -137 to -165 bp upstream relative to the cap site in H-$2K^b$ [27]. Thus the interferon target sequence, as well as the presumably distinct target sequence(s) for MuLV control, are within the 1.2 kb of upstream H-$2K^b$ DNA contained in our chimeric CAT constructions. Fine mapping of these control regions is under way, to determine if they are truly discrete.

The murine sarcoma viruses have evolved a mechanism for keeping MHC expression in the cells they infect to a level suboptimal for recognition and killing by virus-specific or tumor-specific cytotoxic T lymphocytes [11]. Why the leukemia viruses would encode an activity designed to enhance the levels of these same proteins

would satisfy other criteria for a *trans*-acting mechanism of transcriptional activation. Accordingly, we have shown here that MuLV infection of a heterogeneous population of cells transfected with a human class I MHC gene (HLA-A2) results in enhanced expression of that A2 antigen. The incorporation of exogenous genes into the cellular genome after DNA-mediated gene transfer is known to be a random process [31]. It is therefore improbable that this induction of MHC antigen expression is the result of a *cis*-acting effect of the integrated provirus on transcription of each of the endogenous class I genes, the beta-2 microglobulin genes, and each of the randomly integrated HLA-A2 genes which were introduced by transfection.

A *trans*-activating effect by MuLV should also be capable of enhancing transcription of unintegrated class I genes or chimeric genes consisting of class I upstream elements linked to a reporter gene in a transient expression assay. Hybrid K^b-CAT constructions were utilized to test for such an activity and to provide some information relating to the genomic control sequences which respond to this regulatory activity. The temporal constraints on transient expression assays allow for minimal, if any, association of the transfected CAT vectors with the cellular genome, and most of the CAT mRNA is derived, therefore, from transcription of the vectors as extrachromosomal elements. The expression of CAT directed from at least 1.2 kb of H-$2K^b$ upstream sequences, when transfected into M-MuLV-infected cells, mimicked the MuLV-induced up-regulation of expression of the whole H-$2K^b$ gene.

Molecular mechanisms other than *trans*-regulation have been proposed to explain the effects of certain retroviruses on H-2 protein expression. Merulo et al. [32] have obtained evidence for altered methylation and structural rearrangements of the MHC complex in Radiation Leukemia Virus (RadLV)-induced tumors, presumably because of proximal integration of the viral genome. Like MuLV, RadLV induces class I MHC expression soon after infection; however, RadLV tumors that arise after a long latent period express little or no H-2 antigen [33].

Interferons are capable of inducing class I MHC expression on mesenchymal cells, and endogenous cellular interferon beta can be elaborated by cells in response to infection with some viruses. Although the response of cells to interferon gamma and to M-MuLV infection is similar [11], we have ruled out interferon as the mediator of MuLV induction of MHC in other studies [30]. We demonstrated that M-MuLV-infected cells do not produce detectable levels of interferon, or any other H-2-enhancing soluble factor, express no detectable mRNA species for interferon beta, and exhibit no interferon-induced antiviral state. In addition, we have previously found that interferon treatment of M-MuLV-infected cells has an additive effect on the H-2 level, suggesting that the site of action of interferon differs from that of the virus. Friedman and Stark have identified a consensus sequence upstream of the protein-coding regions of certain interferon-regulated genes [34]. This interferon response sequence lies approximately -137 to -165 bp upstream relative to the cap site in H-$2K^b$ [27]. Thus the interferon target sequence, as well as the presumably distinct target sequence(s) for MuLV control, are within the 1.2 kb of upstream H-$2K^b$ DNA contained in our chimeric CAT constructions. Fine mapping of these control regions is under way, to determine if they are truly discrete.

The murine sarcoma viruses have evolved a mechanism for keeping MHC expression in the cells they infect to a level suboptimal for recognition and killing by virus-specific or tumor-specific cytotoxic T lymphocytes [11]. Why the leukemia viruses would encode an activity designed to enhance the levels of these same proteins is not as immediately understandable. Other investigators have demonstrated an association between enhanced or activated expression of certain class I MHC antigens on solid tumors and increased potential for metastasis and invasion [13; and see 28 and 29 for review]. It was postulated that the association of tumor antigens and these enhanced class I antigens might activate a suppressor lymphocyte network, thus inhibiting the immune destruction of the tumor. Alternative hypotheses are possible to provide a teleologic explanation for MHC enhancement by the leukemia viruses. MuLV, and other murine retroviruses such as RadLV, promote the induction of thymic leukemias only after a long latent period through a complex multistep process, involving the generation of novel recombinant retroviruses [35]. After infection by these thymotropic retroviruses, and during the preleukemic phase, high levels of class I MHC antigens and viral gene products are detected on the majority of cells in the thymus [36,33]. It has been proposed that the increased levels of these cell surface proteins may help to bring about the chronic immunostimulation which appears necessary during this stage for eventual leukemogenesis, either to provide the recombinant leukemogenic viruses with a proliferating target cell population [37,38], or perhaps to enhance autostimulation of MuLV-infected, MuLV-specific T lymphocytes, producing a premalignant lymphoid hyperplasia [39]. Thus, the ability of MuLV to enhance H-2 expression in its target cells may be intrinsic to its ability to eventually generate lymphoid neoplasia.

ACKNOWLEDGMENTS

These studies were supported by a research grant from the American Cancer Society and grants CA37169 and CA40585 from the National Institute of Health. L.D.W. was supported by a USPHS Fellowship. D.V.F. is the recipient of an American Cancer Society Senior Faculty Award.

REFERENCES

1. Schmidt W, Festenstein H: Immunogenetics 16:257–265, 1982.
2. Festenstein H, Schmidt W: Immunol Rev 60:85–100, 1981.
3. De Baetselier P, Katzav S, Gorelik E, Feldman M, Segal S: Nature 288:179–182, 1980.
4. Gooding LR: J Immunol 129:1306–1310, 1982.
5. Imamura M, Martin WJ: J Immunol 129:877–883, 1982.
6. Hui K, Grosveld F, Festenstein H: Nature 311:750–752, 1984.
7. Hanna N, Burton RC: J Immunol 127:1754–1760, 1981.
8. Braciale TJ, Andrew ME, Braciale VL: J Exp Med 153:1371–1379, 1981
9. Flyer DC, Burakoff SJ, Faller DV: J Immunol 137:3968–3972, 1986.
10. Flyer DC, Burakoff SJ, Faller DV: Nature 305:815–817, 1983.
11. Flyer DC, Burakoff SJ, Faller DV: J Immunol 135:2287–2292, 1985.
12. Plata F, Tilkin AF, Levy JP, Lilly F: J Exp Med 154:1795–1810, 1981.
13. Katsav S, Segal S, Feldman M: Int J Cancer 33:407–413, 1984.
14. Fan H, Paskind M: J Virol 14:421–429, 1974.
15. Chumakov I, Stuhlmann H, Harbers K, Jaenisch RJ: J Virol 42:1088–1098, 1982.
16. Mier JW, Gallo RG: Proc Natl Acad Sci USA 77:6134–6138, 1980.
17. Strohman RC, Moss PS, Micou-Eastwood J, Spector D, Przybyla A, Paterson B: Cell 10:265–273, 1977.
18. Goldberg DA: Proc Natl Acad Sci USA 77:5794–5799, 1980.
19. Feinberg AP, Vogelstein B: Anal Biochem 132:6–13, 1983.
20. Cleveland DW, Lopata MA, McDonald RJ, Cowan NJ, Rutter WJ, Kirschner MW: Cell 20:95–105, 1980.

21. Barbosa JA, Mentzer SJ, Minowada G, Strominger JL, Burakoff SJ, Biro PA: Proc Natl Acad Sci USA 81:7549–7554, 1984.
22. Southern PJ, Berg P: J Mol Appl Genet 1:327–341, 1982.
23. Allen H, Wraith D, Pala P, Askonas B, Flavell RA: Nature 309:279–281, 1984.
24. Gorman CM, Moffat LF, Howard BH: Mol Cell Biol 2:1044–1051, 1982.
25. Birnboim HC, Doly J: Nucleic Acids Res 7:1513–1523, 1979.
26. Hood L, Steinmetz M, Malissen B: Annu Rev Immunol 1:529–568, 1983.
27. Kimura A, Israel A, LeBail O, Kourilsky P: Cell 44:261–272, 1986.
28. Goodenow RS, Vogel JM, Linsk RL: Science 230:777–783, 1985.
29. Festenstein H, Garrido F: Science 322:502–503, 1986.
30. Wilson LD, Flyer DC, Faller DV: Mol Cell Biol 7:2406–2415, 1987.
31. Kucherlapati RS: ASM News 50:49–53, 1984.
32. Merulo D, Kornreich R, Rossomando A, Boral A, Silver JL, Buxbaum J, Weiss EH, Devlin JJ, Mellor AL, Flavell RA, Pellicer A: Proc Natl Acad Sci USA 83:4504–4508, 1986.
33. Merulo D, Nimelstein SH, Jones PP, Lieberman M, McDevitt HO: J Exp Med 147:470–487, 1978.
34. Friedman RL, Stark GR: Nature 314:637–639, 1985.
35. Teich N, Wyke J, Mak T, Bernstein A, Hardy W: In Weiss R, Teich N, Varmus H, Coffin J (eds): "RNA Tumor Viruses." New York: Cold Spring Harbor Laboratory, pp 785–998, 1984.
36. Chazon R, Naron-Chera N: Cell Immunol 23:356–375, 1976.
37. McGrath MS, Weissman IL: Cell 17:65–75, 1979.
38. Lee JC, Ihle JN: Nature 289:407–409, 1981.
39. O'Neill HC, McGrath MS, Allison JP, Weissman IL: Cell 49:143–151, 1987.

Isolation and Visualization of Met-72-Positive, Metastatic Variants Present in B16 Melanoma Tumor Masses

Nanette P. Parratto and Arthur K. Kimura

Department of Pathology, University of Florida College of Medicine, Gainesville, Florida 32610

Metastatic variants of the B16 melanoma displaying high experimental metastatic potential have been shown to express high levels of a 72,000-dalton glycoprotein (Met-72) on their cell surface (Kimura AK, Xiang J: *J Nat Can Inst* 76:1247–1253, 1986). Monoclonal antibodies (MoAb) directed against the Met-72 determinant have been used in this study as immunohistochemical reagents on preparations of fresh B16 melanoma tumors and their metastases. These immunohistochemical analyses have utilized frozen sections, impression smears, and cytospin preparations of fresh tumors harvested at various time points during tumor growth, to view the presence and location of Met-72-positive metastatic variants within tumor masses. Biotinylated anti-Met-72 MoAbs were reacted with freshly dissociated tumor cells from a B16 melanoma ovarian metastasis. These cells were then reacted with fluorescein isothiocyanate (FITC)-streptavidin and analyzed by flow cytometry. A discrete population of positively staining cells was detected and isolated by cell sorting techniques. Met-72-positive cells were then cloned and reanalyzed after several weeks of *in vitro* expansion and found to have high experimental metastatic potential to ovaries. Frozen sections of subcutaneous tumors and their metastases were analyzed by immunoperoxidase techniques. A consistent finding in these studies has been that the few tumor cells which showed high intensity of Met-72 staining were positioned perivascularly and at the invading front of B16 melanoma tumors.

Key words: B16 melanoma, metastatic variants, met 72/83 antigen, immunohistochemistry, localization *in situ*

A number of experimental systems have documented clonal heterogeneity within primary tumors and their metastases [1–5]. Thus, although certain tumors may be

---

Abbreviations used: ABC = avidin-biotin-horseradish peroxidase complex; AEC = amino ethyl carbazole; cPEG = phosphate buffered saline + ethylenediamine-tetraacetic acid + glucose; FACS = fluorescence activated cell sorter; FBS = fetal bovine serum; FITC = fluorescein isothiocyanate; MoAb = monoclonal antibody (ies); NCS = newborn calf serum; pA = protein A; PBS = phosphate buffered saline; sA = streptavidin.

Received May 4, 1987; revised and accepted August 17, 1987.

© 1988 Alan R. Liss, Inc.

judged clonal with respect to a given phenotype or cell surface marker, clonal components of the tumor can differ markedly in their ability to form metastases, or in susceptibility to immune attack or drug therapy [2–5]. Tumor cells with high metastatic potential have often been referred to as metastatic variants.

Histopathologic evaluation of most solid tumors has been hindered by the lack of reagents capable of specifically identifying metastatic variants. Direct, *in situ* visualization of metastatic tumor cell variants would provide a valuable handle towards understanding the clonal evolution and interactions of tumor cells within primary tumors and their metastases. Recently, we identified via monoclonal antibody (MoAb), a 72-kilodalton (Kd) cell surface glycoprotein (Met-72) quantitatively associated with highly metastatic tumor cell variants of the B16 melanoma [1]. The experimental metastatic potential of over 30 B16 melanoma clones has been correlated to a quantitative surface expression of Met-72 [1,6,7]. In addition, anti-Met-72 MoAb used in conjunction with fluorescence-activated cell sorting (FACS) has recently been used directly to isolate metastatic variants from the heterogeneous parental B16-F1 tumor [8].

The present study was designed to isolate and histologically localize Met-72-positive, metastatic variants present in fresh B16 melanoma tumor masses. Perhaps the most striking finding to emerge from these studies was the unique, localized distribution of Met-72-positive cells within the tumor mass. Anti-Met-72 MoAb staining was only observed on tumor cells located perivascularly and along the invading front of the developing tumor. These experiments show that our MoAb previously used to characterize the expression of Met-72 *in vitro*, may also be useful for isolation and localization of highly metastatic variants *in situ* in primary and metastatic B16 melanoma.

MATERIALS AND METHODS

Mice

C57BL/6 mice were obtained from the Jackson Laboratory, (Bar Harbor, ME) and housed in the Tumor Biology Unit mouse colony, Department of Pathology. Female mice, aged 8–16 weeks, were used in these studies.

Monoclonal Antibodies

Anti-Met 72 MoAb were generated by syngeneic immunization of C57BL/6 mice with selected B16 melanoma clones. The specificity and characteristics of these MoAbs have been reported in detail [1]. Hybridoma cells secreting an isotype-identical, negative control MoAb used in this study (anti-sheep red blood cell, N- S.7, IgG3: kappa) were obtained from the American Type Culture Collection (Rockville, MD).

Murine Melanoma Cell Lines

The C57BL/6 melanoma, B16, and various *in vitro* and *in vivo* selected lines derived from it were obtained from the Division of Cancer Treatment Tumor Bank (E.G. and G. Mason Research Institute, 57 Union St., Worcester, MA) where they had been deposited by Dr. I.J. Fidler. Clones were derived by limiting dilution and micromanipulation [1] from both the parent line, B16-F1, and the *in vitro* selected, highly invasive metastatic form, B16-BL6 [9]. Stocks from early passages of these lines and clones were frozen at $-70°C$ and restarted every 8–12 weeks to limit the possibilities of functional and phenotypic drift. All cell lines and clones were maintained *in vitro* at 37°C in a humidified incubator containing 8% CO_2, by subculturing every 4 days. Monolayers of cells were detached from the petri dishes (Costar #3100, Cambridge, MA) by a 3-min room-temperature incubation with 0.5 mM EDTA in Ca^{++}- and Mg^{++}- free phosphate buffered saline (PBS) supplemented with 0.1% glucose (cPEG) [10]. For routine passage, cells were washed and replated at a concentration of 5×10^5/10 cm dish in 10 ml media.

The parent melanoma line, B16-F1, was maintained in Cellgro MEM (Sybron, Washington D.C.) supplemented with 10% fetal bovine serum (FBS), penicillin (100 U/ml), and streptomycin (100 µg/ml), 1 mM pyruvate, 2 mM glutamine, and 0.225% $NaHCO_3$. The highly invasive metastatic clone, BL6-10, was maintained in Eagles' Hanks' amino acid supplemented medium (EHAA, GIBCO, Grand Island, NY) [11] containing 10% newborn calf serum (NCS), penicillin, and streptomycin. A recently derived, poorly metastatic C5BL/6 melanoma, *JB/RH*, was provided by Dr. Jane Berklehammer (AMC Cancer Research Center, Denver, CO) [12,13] for comparison in our studies. These cells were maintained and passaged *in vitro* in EHAA + 10% NCS.

Biotinylation of MoAb and Flow Cytometric Analysis

IgG was purified from culture supernatants or ascites fluid by affinity fractionation through protein A-Sepharose 4B (Pharmacia, Piscataway, NJ) [14] and checked for purity by SDS polyacrylamide gel electrophoresis [15]. Affinity-purified IgG (1 mg/ml) was dialyzed against 0.1 M $NaHCO_3$ (pH 8.2) and then reacted with 2 mM NHS-LC-biotin (Pierce Chemical, Rockford, IL) dissolved in dimethylformamide (Sigma, St. Louis, MO) at biotin ester:protein ratios of 1:2.5 to 1:10 (w/w) for 4 hr at room temperature, in the dark. The reaction was stopped by the addition of 1M NH_4Cl to a final concentration of 0.1 M in the reaction mixture. Unreacted biotin was then removed by exhaustive dialysis against PBS. Biotin-conjugated protein concentrations were determined by optical density at 280 nm [16]. Optimal biotin ester/protein ratios used for the conjugation of the various preparations were determined empirically by flow cytometric analysis on cell preparations [17]. Briefly, 2×10^6 melanoma cells were incubated with biotinylated antibody at 4°C for 30 min in the dark. After three washes in PBS with 5% agamma horse serum (GIBCO), either native or biotinylated MoAb was incubated with FITC-streptavidin (Zymed Laboratories, San Francisco, CA) or FITC-sheep antimouse Ig for nonbiotinylated preparations. After three washes, 2×10^4 cells were counted and analyzed by flow cytometry [8,17].

Measurement of Purified and Biotinylated MoAb Binding by Radioimmunoassay

MoAb binding to the various cell types was measured indirectly with ^{125}I protein A (pA) as described [18] or with ^{125}I streptavidin (sA) with biotinylated MoAb using a modification of the method of Philpott et al [19]. Briefly, 2×10^5 freshly harvested *in vitro* grown cells were incubated for 1 hr with various dilutions of purified native or biotinylated MoAb. The cells were then washed three times with PBS plus 5% agamma horse serum and incubated for an additional 1 hr with 2×10^5 cpm radiolabeled pA or sA. Radioactivity bound to the cells after three washings was assessed by gamma scintillation counting. Background binding in these assays was routinely less than 600 cpm. MoAb binding to the different cell types is expressed as a binding index [1], calculated from triplicate determinations as follows:

$$\text{Binding index} = \frac{\text{mean cpm bound with anti-Met-72 MoAb}}{\text{mean cpm bound with anti-sheep red blood cell MoAb}}$$

This normalizes individual differences in background binding and allows comparison between the different cell types.

Generation of Subcutaneous Primary Tumor Foci, Spontaneous Metastases and Lung Colonization Assay

Primary tumor masses were generated by s.c. injection of 2×10^6 cells/100 μl PBS, at the dorsal thoracolumbar spinous junction. Experimental metastases were generated by tail vein injection of 3×10^5 cells into age- and sex-matched C57BL/6 mice.

Spontaneous metastases were generated by subcutaneous inoculation of 2×10^6 cells followed in 10 days by tumor excision with necropsy 21 days later (31 days after primary subcutaneous injection). Tumors were excised at various points of tumor growth.

Immunocytochemistry of Cytospin and Impression Smear Preparations of B16 Melanoma

B16 melanoma tumors were brought to a single cell suspension by teasing tumor masses into approximately 1 mm^3 pieces which were then subjected to an 8–10-hr incubation in Eagle's media supplemented with 0.1% collagenase V (Sigma, 10 ml/g tumor weight) at 4°C [20]. Viable cells were separated on Ficoll Hypaque (Pharmacia, Sweden) and resuspended in PBS. Cells were incubated with 0.3% H_2O_2 in PBS plus 5% agamma horse serum for 30 min at 4°C and washed three times with PBS. The cells were then incubated with biotinylated MoAb for 30 min at 4°C in the dark and washed three times. The antibody-labeled cells were incubated with avidin-biotin-horseradish peroxidase complex ([ABC]) Vector Laboratories, Burlingame, CA) for 30 min at 4°C in the dark, and washed three times. Approximately 3×10^4 labeled cells were then cytocentrifuged onto subbed slides. Slides were fixed in acetone for 30 sec, washed in PBS, and the reaction developed with aminoethylcarbazole ([AEC] Sigma) in the presence of H_2O_2, washed and counterstained with hematoxylin [21].

Impression smears of excised tumors were made by gently touching tumors, prerinsed in ice-cold PBS, onto subbed slides. The slides were air dried, fixed in acetone for 10 min, rinsed in PBS, and dried. Slides were either processed by immunohistochemistry methodology (see below) or stored at −70°C for future use. Impression smears provide a rapid screening method for detection of antigen expression *in vivo* [22].

Immunohistochemistry of Cryostat Sections of Primary and Metastatic B16 Melanoma

Primary and metastatic tumor masses obtained after 5–21 days of growth were excised, snap frozen in isopentane, and liquid nitrogen and stored at −70°C until sectioned. Cryostat sections 4 μm thick were air dried, fixed in cold acetone for 10 min, and washed in PBS using a modification of the technique by Suter et al [23]. Endogenous peroxidase was blocked by reaction with 0.3% H_2O_2 in PBS plus 5% agamma horse serum for 30 min at room temperature. Biotinylated antibodies at predetermined optimal concentrations were layered onto sections and allowed to react for 60 min at room temperature in a dark humidified chamber. Slides were then washed in three changes of PBS and reacted with ABC reagent for 30 min at room temperature in a dark, humidified chamber, and the slides were then washed in three changes of PBS. The reaction was developed with AEC in the presence of H_2O_2. The slides were washed, counterstained with hematoxylin, and examined under oil immersion.

RESULTS

Biotinylated Anti-Med-72 MoAb Specificity

Affinity purified anti-Met-72 or control MoAb were reacted with the biotin ester at varying weight/weight ratios. Flow cytometric analysis of biotinylated MoAb binding to B16 metastatic variants or sheep red blood cells was used to optimize conditions for biotin substitution. Three C57BL/6 melanoma lines of high and low experimental metastatic activities (Table I) were used as target cells in radioimmunoassay to insure that the process of biotinylation did not alter the specificity of anti-Met-72 MoAb. The ability of biotinylated anti-Met-72 MoAb to bind to murine melanomas of high metastatic potential is shown in Figure 1. Binding of biotinylated MoAb was measured indirectly after the addition of ^{125}I-streptavidin. The highly metastatic B16 melanoma clone, BL6-10, shows an approximately fivefold higher level of anti-Met-72 MoAb binding in RIA than to the poorly metastatic cell lines B16-F1 and *JB/RH*.

FACS Selection of Met-72-Positive Variants Isolated From a Fresh Experimental Ovarian Metastasis

Experimental metastases were generated by i.v. injection of B16-F1 melanoma cells as described. An ovarian metastasis was noted 21 days later, removed, and brought to a single-cell suspension for analysis of Met-72 expression by flow cytom-

TABLE I. Experimental Metastatic Potential of Three C57BL/6 Murine Melanomas*

Experiment	Cells	n[a]	Mean No. metastases pulmonary ± SE	Other sites of metastases
A	B16-F1	4	18 ± 3	Ovary, lymph node, liver
B	B16-F1	5	56 ± 16	Bone marrow
A	BL6-10	6	261 ± 96	Bone marrow, lymph node
B	BL6-10	14	160 ± 146	Ovary, bone marrow, lymph node, subcutis
A	JB/RH	6	0	
B	JB/RH	9	0	

*Experimental metastases were generated by tail-vein injection of 3×10^5 cells per 0.2 ml PBS.
[a]No. of age-matched female mice per group.

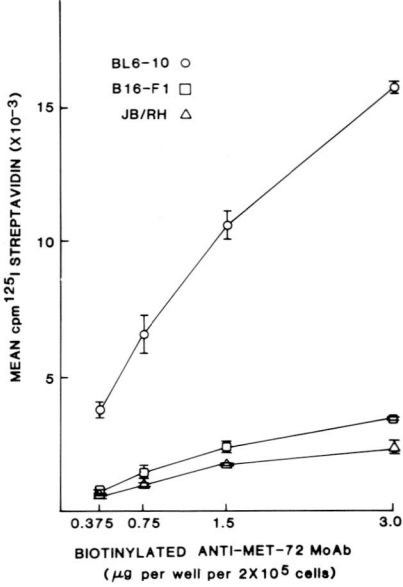

Fig. 1. Retention of binding specificity of anti-Met-72 MoAb after biotinylation. Various amounts of biotinylated anti-Met-72 MoAb were reacted with the highly metastatic B16 melanoma clone, BL6/10, the poorly metastatic B16 melanoma parent, B16-F1, and a recently derived, poorly metastatic C57BL/6 melanoma, *JB/RH*. The extent of specific binding was measured after the addition of ^{125}I-labeled streptavidin. Values are expressed as the mean of triplicate determinations of cpm bound ± SE.

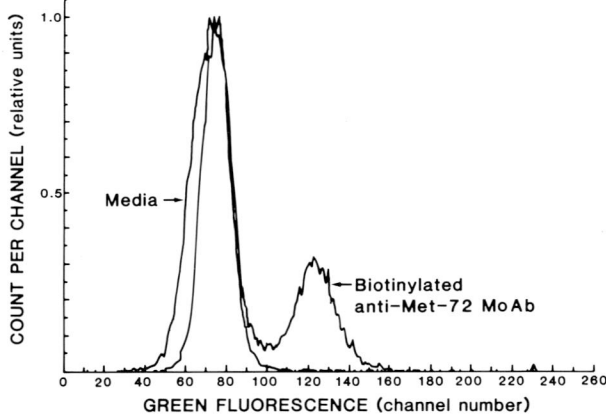

Fig. 2. Flow cytometric analysis of Met-72-positive metastatic variants within a fresh ovarian metastasis.

etry. Biotinylated anti-Met-72 MoAb and FITC-streptavidin treatment of these cells revealed two distinct populations within the freshly excised ovarian metastasis, one highly Met-72 positive (Fig. 2). Melanoma cells sorted from this population and maintained *in vitro* have retained a high binding profile to anti-Met-72 MoAb (data not shown). Cells obtained from the original ovarian metastasis (0-1) were cloned. One clone from the original ovarian metastasis was successively cycled by intravenous passage in the syngeneic host, three times (0-1.1, 0-1.2, 0-1.3), and each time organ selectivity and Met-72 expression of ovarian metastases were recorded. Repeated passage *in vivo* was seen to enhance organ selectivity for ovaries (53%, 56%, 87% of the mice having ovarian metastases) and to enrich for Met-72 expression (28, 36, 45 times background) (Fig. 3).

Immunocytology of Fresh Ovarian and Lung Metastases

B16 melanoma metastatic variants were isolated from fresh lung and ovarian experimental metastases by mechanical and enzymatic disaggregation. Single-cell suspensions were processed for immunocytology using anti-Met-72 MoAb. Cytospin preparations of an experimental ovarian metastasis showed positive immunoperoxidase staining (Fig. 4B). Impression smears of experimental and spontaneous lung metastases generated by injection of the poorly metastatic F1 parental B16 melanoma demonstrated similar levels of individual cellular binding to anti-Met-72 MoAb (Fig. 4D,F). Isotype identical MoAb (anti-sheep RBC, N-S.7) showed no staining in these assays (Fig. 4A,C,E).

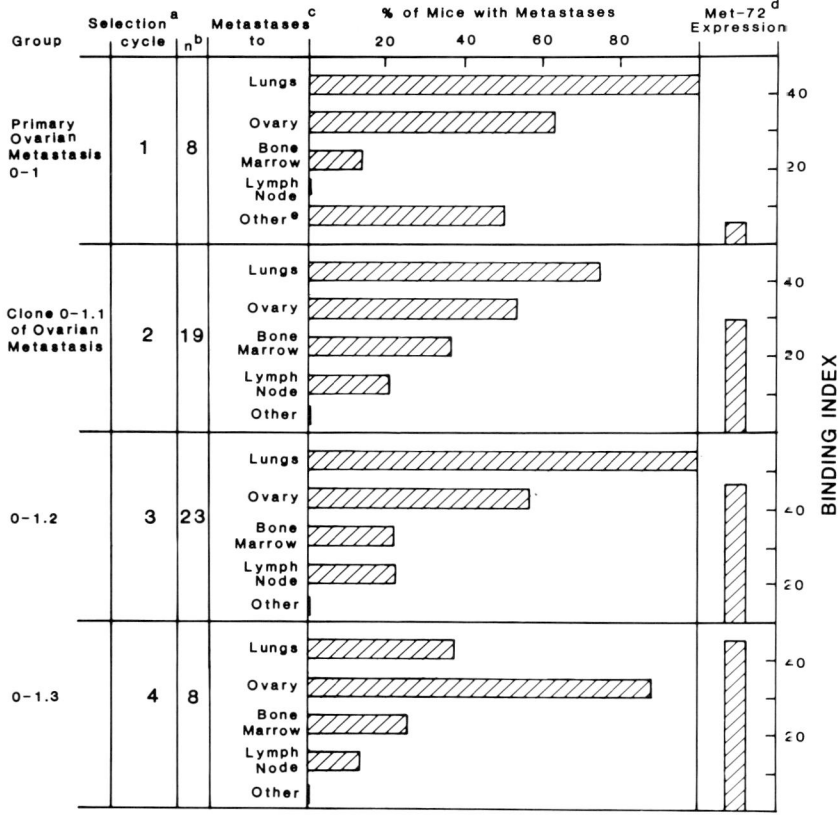

Fig. 3. Clones derived from experimental metastases to ovaries retain a high expression of Met-72 upon repeated cycling *in vivo*. **a:** In vivo cycle number for the selection of metastatic variants with ovary specificity. **b:** Number of mice per group. **c:** Organ site of metastasis. **d:** Binding of anti-Met-72 MoAb to ovarian metastatic variants as detected by RIA. Results are expressed as a binding index, which is calculated by dividing the mean cpm ^{125}I pA bound with anti-Met-72 MoAb divided by the mean cpm ^{125}I pA bound with N-S.7 MoAb (background binding). **e:** Other = kidney, mesentery.

Localized Distribution of Met-72-Positive Variants Within Progressing Subcutaneous Melanoma

Immunohistologic analyses of cryostat sections from subcutaneous B16-F1 melanomas were performed at various time points during tumor growth. Predeterminedoptimal concentrations of biotinylated MoAb were incubated with serial sections of snap-frozen tumor. Reactive sites were detected as red granules upon development with AEC. A common pattern of reactivity has been noted in all sections examined from tumors as early as 3 days to as late as 15 days of growth. A subcutaneous B16-F1 tumor excised after 7 days of growth was serially sectioned and stained with anti-Met-72 MoAb (Fig. 5). Background levels of peroxidase staining are shown in Figure 5A,B, using an isotype-identical biotinylated control MoAb, N-S.7. In contrast to the rather uniform staining of melanoma cells obtained from metastases (Fig. 4B,D,F), Met-72-positive cells seen in cryostat sections of primary tumors were observed only on advancing fronts and leading edges of the tumor mass (Fig. 5C,D,F), perivascular to extra-tumor vessels and intravascularly (Fig. 5E). No detectable binding was seen in the bulk of the tumor mass, which consisted of differentiated melanoma cells surrounding a necrotic, poorly vascularized, central core.

DISCUSSION

The existence of subpopulations of cells exhibiting a range of metastatic potential within heterogeneous tumors has been substantiated in a number of systems [2]. In the original studies leading to the present work, a strong correlation between the quantitative expression of a 72-Kd glycoprotein (Met-72) and experimental metastatic activity of over 30 *in vitro* growth B16 melanoma clones was demonstrated [1,6]. Flow cytometric analysis and cell sorting procedures using anti-Met-72 MoAb have directly shown that high levels of Met-72 expression are characteristic of cells with a high experimental metastatic potential [8]. Our current studies were designed to determine the potential utility of anti-Met-72 MoAb to visualize and localize Met-72-positive metastatic variants within progressively growing and metastatic B16 melanoma masses.

Results of the experiments reported here greatly expand our knowledge of Met-72 antigen expression and its correlation with metastatic potential *in vivo*. Localization of its expression in primary subcutaneous tumors is notably discrete, and not randomly distributed throughout the developing tumor mass.

Immunohistologic examination of progressively growing tumors excised at various times during subcutaneous growth shows a recurrent pattern of localization of Met-72-positive variants. In the present study we elected to study the staining and distribution of Met-72-positive, metastatic variants within the parent B16-F1 melanoma and metastases derived from it. Similar studies have been performed with our highly metastatic clone BL6-10, which was originally selected from the B16-F10 for increased invasiveness through bladder wall [9]. Subcutaneously derived tumors generated from both the parental B16-F1 and BL6-10 have been examined after 3, 7, 9, 12, and 15 days of growth. Met-72 expression was only observed on certain cells seen at the advancing front and perivascularly. These findings suggest that microenvironmental influences may function regionally to influence metastatic potential. The implication of this selective localization suggests that even if random somatic mutational events yield single metastatic variant cells within a solid tumor mass, their

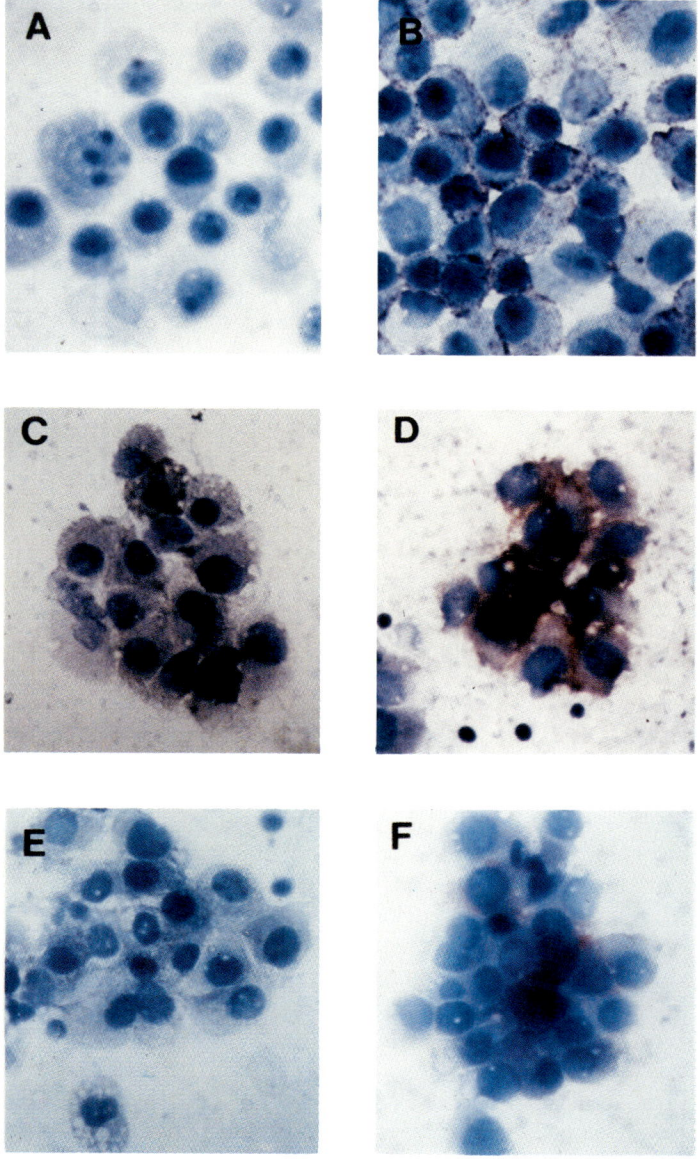

Fig. 4. Met-72-positive variants of B16 melanoma detected in cytospin and impression smear preparations of metastases. Cell suspensions from a fresh ovarian metastasis were stained using biotinylated control N-S.7 MoAb (**A**) or anti-Met-72 MoAb (**B**). Impression smears of experimental lung metastases (**C, D**) or spontaneous lung metastases (**E, F**) were stained using biotinylated N-S.7 MoAb (C,E) or anti-Met-72 MoAb (D,F). A–F, ×128.

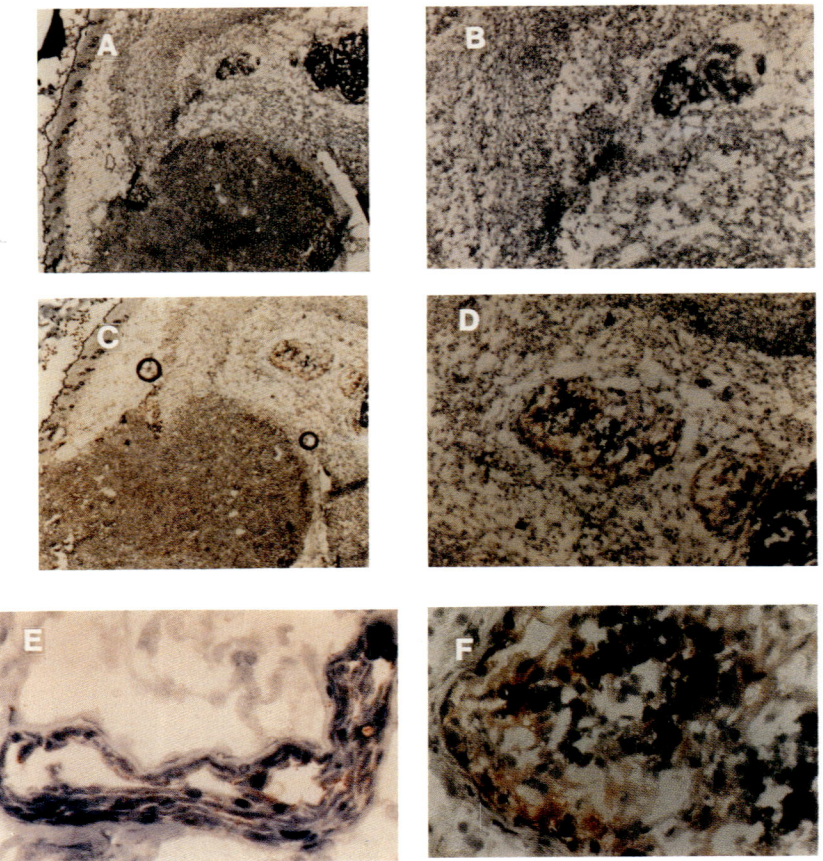

Fig. 5. Localization of Met-72-positive variants within developing B16 subcutaneous melanoma. Biotinylated N-S.7 MoAb bound to a cryostat section of a B16 F1 subcutaneous melanoma (**A**) ×10 and (**B**) ×25. Biotinylated anti-Met-72 MoAb bound to a section of the same B16 F1 subcutaneous melanoma ×10 (**C**), ×25 (**D**), ×100 (**E**), ×128 (**F**).

outgrowth into colonies may be directed by chemotactic or induction factors which are microenvironmentally determined. The fact that both the poorly metastatic B16-F1 and highly metastatic BL6-10 melanoma lines yield a similar distribution pattern after anti-Met-72 staining when grown subcutaneously suggests that considerable re-equilibration of the population occurs during growth as a primary tumor. Details of population re-equilibration and metastatic activity will be the subject of a separate communication (Parratto and Kimura, in preparation).

Our observations in the B16 melanoma model of metastasis are consistent with those of Gabbert et al [24]. They suggest that similar morphologic transitions at the invading front of rat malignant carcinoma may signify a localized process of tumor dedifferentiation. Tumor cell locomotion may be specifically enhanced in regions observed to have a loss of basement membrane and decreased numbers of desmosomes between tumor cells.

An important aspect of these studies focused on isolation and visualization of Met-72-positive variants within metastatic foci of B16 melanoma. The sophisticated capabilities of the fluorescence-activated cell sorter have provided evidence that Met-72 expression may be a common surface phenotype of B16 melanoma metastatic variants, irrespective of their organ colonization after i.v. inoculation. Experimentally induced ovarian metastases were directly shown to express Met-72, as has been reported for experimental lung metastases of the B16 melanoma [8]. As previously demonstrated with lung-colonizing melanoma cells [25], ovarian colonizing variants were selected by repeated *in vivo* cycling. These variants showed increased, stable levels of Met-72 expression (Fig. 3). Rapid cellular visualization of Met-72 was achieved by two immunocytologic methodologies: 1) cytospin preparations of experimental ovarian metastases, and 2) impression smears of experimental and spontaneous lung metastases. The ease of impression smear immunocytochemistry has permitted rapid characterization of the surface phenotype of cells dislodged from colonized lungs, which are technically refractory to cryostat sectioning. Primary melanomas and other well encapsulated masses do not present suitable specimens for impression smears.

The significant findings of these studies are that 1) Met-72-positive cells are consistently found only at two sites within B16 tumor masses, perivascularly, and at the advancing front and 2) cell surface expression of Met-72 may prove to be a generalized phenotype of B16 melanoma, metastatic variants irrespective of their organ selectivity. The ability to isolate metastatic variant cells from fresh tumor tissue may enable us to quantitate their presence and evaluate acquired qualitative differences during tumor progression and metastatic outgrowth.

ACKNOWLEDGMENTS

The technical assistance of Dr. Byron Croker, Cindy Bevis, Dr. Jianhua Xiang (NIH, Bethesda, MD) and Linda Lee-Ambrose is gratefully acknowledged. The skilled secretarial assistance of Mrs. Rose Mills is gratefully acknowledged. The generous gift of *JB/RH* cells from Dr. Jane Berkelhammer (AMC Cancer Research Center, Denver, CO) is gratefully acknowledged.

This work was supported in part by USPHS grants CA 09126 and CA 40351 from the National Cancer Institute, DHHS.

REFERENCES

1. Kimura AK, Xiang J: J Natl Cancer Inst 76:1247–1253, 1986.
2. Nicolson GL, Poste G: Curr Probl Cancer 7:4–83, 1982.
3. Nicolson GL, Poste G: Curr Probl Cancer 7:1–43, 1983.
4. Fidler IJ, Nicolson GL: Cancer Biol Rev 2:1–47, 1981.
5. Poste G: J Cell Biochem Suppl 11D:78, 1987.
6. Kimura AK, Mehta P, Xiang J, Lawson D, Dugger D, Kao KJ, Lee-Ambrose L: Clin Exp Metastasis in press, 1987.
7. Xiang J, Kimura AK: Clin Exp Metastasis 4:293–309, 1986.
8. Xiang J, Kimura AK: Clin Exp Metastasis in press, 1987.
9. Poste G, Doll J, Hart IR, Fidler IJ: Cancer Res 40:1636–1644, 1980.
10. Noonan K: Biochim Biophys Acta 551:22–43, 1979.
11. Click RE, Benck L, Alter BJ: Cell Immunol 3:264–276, 1972.
12. Berkelhammer J, Oxenhandler RW, Hook RR, Hennessy JM: Cancer Res 42:3157–3163, 1982.
13. Berkelhammer J, Luethens TN, Hook RR, Oxenhandler RW: Cancer Res 46:2923–2923, 1986.
14. Ey PL, Prowse SJ, Jenkin CR: Immunochemistry 15:429–436, 1978.

15. Laemmli UK: Nature 227:680–685, 1970.
16. Guesdon J-L, Ternynck T, Avrameas S: J Histochem Cytochem 27:1131–1139, 1979.
17. Braylan RC, Benson NA, Nourse V, Kruth HS: Cytometry 2:337–343, 1982.
18. Dorval G, Welsh KI, Wigzell H: J Immunol Methods 7:237–249, 1975.
19. Philpott GW, Kulczycki A, Grass EH, Parker CW: J Immunol 125:1201–1209, 1980.
20. Pretlow TP, Stinson AJ, Pretlow II TG, Glover GL: J Natl Cancer Inst 61:1431–1437, 1978.
21. Lam LT, English MC, Janckila AJ, Zeismer S, Li C-Y: Am J Clin Pathol 80:314–321, 1983.
22. Perry MD, Seigler HF, Johnston WW: J Natl Cancer Inst 77:1013–1021, 1986.
23. Suter L, Brocker EB, Bruggen J, Ruiter DJ, Sorg C: Cancer Immunol Immunother 16:53–58, 1983.
24. Gabbert H, Wagner R, Moll R, Gerharz C-D: Clin Exp Metastasis 3:257–279, 1985.
25. Fidler IJ, Nicolson GL: J Natl Cancer Inst 57:1199–1202, 1976.

Correlation of Immunomodulatory and Therapeutic Activities of Interferon and Interferon Inducers in Metastatic Disease

Paul L. Black, Hamblin Phillips, Henry R. Tribble, Robin Pennington, Mark Schneider, and James E. Talmadge

Preclinical Evaluation Laboratory, PRI, National Cancer Institute-Frederick Cancer Research Facility, Frederick, Maryland 21701

The mechanism of therapeutic activity of recombinant murine interferon-gamma (rMu IFN-γ) and the IFN inducer polyinosinic-polycytidylic acid solubilized with poly-L-lysine in carboxy methyl cellulose (pICLC) in treating metastatic disease was investigated by comparing effector cell augmentation with therapeutic activity in mice bearing experimental lung metastases (B16-BL6 melanoma). Effector cell functions in spleen, peripheral blood, and lung (the organ with tumor) were tested after 1 and 3 weeks of rMu IFN-γ or pICLC administration (intravenous, three times a week). In these studies, natural killer (NK), lymphokine-activated killer (LAK), cytolytic T lymphocytes (CTL) (against specific and nonspecific targets), and macrophage tumoricidal and tumoristatic activities were measured. rM IFN-γ and pICLC had therapeutic activity and immunomodulatory activity in most assays of immune function examined. Specific CTL activity of pulmonary parenchymal mononuclear cells (PPMC), but not in splenocytes or peripheral blood lymphocytes (PBL), during week 3 and not during week 1, correlated with the therapeutic activity of rMu IFN-γ and of pICLC. Macrophage tumoricidal activity in PPMC, but not in alveolar macrophages, also correlated with the therapeutic activity of rMu IFN-γ, but the opposite was true for the therapeutic activity of pICLC. NK

Abbreviations used: IFN; interferon; rMu IFN-γ, recombinant murine interferon-gamma; i.v., intravenous; tiw, three times a week; NK, natural killer; LAK, lymphokine-activated killer; CTL, cytolytic T lymphocytes; PPMC, pulmonary parenchymal mononuclear cells; BRM, biological response modifiers; PBL, peripheral blood lymphocytes; HBSS, Hanks' balanced salt solution; LPS, lipopolysaccharide; poly(I,C), polyinosinic-polycytidylic acid; poly(I,C)-LC or pICLC, poly(I,C) solubilized with poly-L-lysine in carboxymethyl cellulose.

Paul L. Black's present address is Virology Division, U.S. Army Medical Research Institute of Infectious Diseases, Ft. Detrick, Frederick, MD 21701.

Mark Schneider's and James E. Talmadge's present address is SmithKline and French Laboratories, King of Prussia, PA 19406.

Received June 3, 1987; accepted October 23, 1987.

Published 1988 by Alan R. Liss, Inc.

activity of PPMC, but not of splenocytes or PBL, during week 1 correlated with the therapeutic activity of pICLC; in contrast, NK activity at any site did not correlate with the therapeutic activity of rMu IFN-γ. LAK activity at any site did not correlate with the therapeutic activity of either agent.

Key words: treatment of metastases, interferon-gamma, double-stranded polyribonucleotides, mechanism of therapeutic activity, preclinical models, poly (I,C)-LC, cytolytic T lymphocyte (CTL), anti-tumor activity, tumor-specific

Interferons (IFN) consist of a family of glycoproteins whose synthesis and secretion are induced by viral infections and other stimuli. The IFNs induce an antiviral state in most cell types, and they inhibit the proliferation of many different types of tumor cells. Additionally, the IFNs have immunomodulatory activity, especially for the augmentation of macrophage tumoricidal activity and of natural killer (NK) cell cytotoxicity [1-7]. Although IFN-γ shares many properties with IFN-α and IFN-β, it has greater antiproliferative [8] and immunomodulatory [7,8] activities than IFN-α and IFN-β. Additionally, the cellular receptor for IFN-γ is distinct from the receptor for IFN-α and IFN-β [9].

The double-stranded polyribonucleotides such as polyinosinic-polycytidylic acid [poly(I,C)] stimulate the synthesis and secretion of IFNs [10-16]. Poly(I,C) also has potent immunomodulatory activity in a variety of assays of immune function, including antibody production [17,18], allograft rejection [19,20], protection against viral infection [15,21-25], and against transplantable tumor challenges [21,26-33], NK activity [6,20,34-39], and macrophage tumoricidal activity [39,40]. However, the effectiveness of poly(I,C) is limited in humans and primates by its susceptibility to the action of serum ribonucleases [41-43]. However, the complex of poly(I,C) admixed with poly-L-lysine and solubilized with carboxymethyl cellulose [poly(I,C)-LC] alleviates this problem [44,45].

Both recombinant murine interferon-gamma (rMu IFN-γ) [46] and poly (I,C)-LC [33,47,48] have consistently shown significant therapeutic activity in a variety of animal tumor models. However, demonstration of this preclinical therapeutic activity depends strictly on optimal dosage, schedule, route, and duration of administration [46-48]. Possibly as a result of these limitations, recombinant human (rH) IFN [49-62] and poly (I,C)-LC [63-69] have produced mixed results in clinical trials with a variety of cancer types. The use in clinical trials of excessively high doses of these biological response modifiers (BRMs), at or near the maximum tolerated dose, levels which exceeded the optimal therapeutic dose, may explain the discrepancy between the preclinical efficacy of these agents and their less impressive effects in clinical trials.

In the present studies, we investigated the immunomodulatory activity of rMu IFN-γ and of poly(I,C)-LC in tumor-bearing animals. Levels of NK, lymphokine-activated killer (LAK), cytolytic T lymphocyte (CTL), and macrophage tumoricidal and tumoristatic activities were assessed in cells from peripheral blood, spleen, and lungs (the organ with tumor), 1 and 3 weeks after the initiation of treatment, in mice bearing B16-BL6 experimental lung metastases. The therapeutic effects of rMu IFN-γ and of poly(I,C)-LC were correlated with their immunomodulatory activities in the various assay systems in an attempt to identify the immunomodulatory activities responsible for the therapeutic activity of these agents.

MATERIALS AND METHODS

Animals

Specific pathogen-free male C57BL/6 mice were obtained from the Animal Production Area of the NCI-Frederick Cancer Research Facility. Mice were 7–8 weeks old when they received tumor cells.

Tumors

The tumor cell lines used in these studies were B16-BL6 [70], a highly invasive variant derived from the B16 malignant melanoma of C57BL/6 origin, 3LL-M2 [71], a metastatic variant of the Lewis lung carcinoma line of C57BL/6 origin, YAC-1 [72], a lymphoma induced by Moloney virus in A/SN mice, and P815 [73], a mastocytoma induced by methylcholanthrene in DBA/2 mice. All cell lines were propagated by serial passage in vitro in complete Eagle's minimum essential medium with Earle's salts, supplemented with 5% fetal bovine serum, L-glutamine, sodium pyruvate, nonessential amino acids, and twofold vitamin solution. All cell lines were tested to ensure freedom from mycoplasma and murine viruses. All medium components were routinely tested for endotoxin contamination with a *Limulus* amebocyte lysate test, and only components with levels of endotoxin less than 0.125 EU/ml were used.

rMu IFN-γ

rMu IFN-γ, supplied through the courtesy of Dr. Michael Shepard (Genentech, South San Francisco, CA), had a specific activity of $\approx 2 \times 10^7$ U/mg. rMu IFN-γ was diluted in saline solution containing 0.5% normal mouse serum prior to injection. Poly(I,C)-LC was supplied through the courtesy of Dr. Hilton Levy (NIAID, NIH, NCI-FCRF, Frederick, MD) and was diluted with saline solution prior to injection.

Tumoricidal Assays

Single-cell suspensions of spleen cells were prepared by passing crushed spleens through a wire mesh sieve. Mononuclear cells from collagenase-dissociated pulmonary parenchyma, referred to as pulmonary parenchymal mononuclear cells (PPMC), were obtained by centrifugation on a Ficoll-Hypague density gradient. Blood, anticoagulated with EDTA, was obtained from the retroorbital sinus, and mononuclear cells were purified from whole blood by density gradient centrifugation on colloidal silica (Sepracell-MN, Sepratech, Oklahoma City, OK). The NK and LAK activities of single-cell suspensions of peripheral blood lymphocytes (PBL), splenocytes, and PPMC from each group were determined simultaneously. NK and LAK activities were routinely assessed in a 4-hr ^{51}Cr release assay, using YAC-1 cells as the targets for NK activity and P815 cells as targets for LAK activity, as previously described [74]. CTL activity of PBL, spleen cells, and PPMC was tested in an 18-hr [^{75}Se]methionine release assay [74]. B16-BL6 cells were used as specific targets in these assays, with syngeneic Lewis lung carcinoma cells (3LL-M2) serving as a specificity control. Macrophages, purified by 3 cycles of adherence at 37°C and washing, were obtained from lung lavage (alveolar macrophages) and from PPMC (pulmonary macrophages). Macrophage tumoricidal activity was determined in a 72-hr in vitro assay, with [^{125}I]UdR-labeled B16-BL6 cells as targets [74]. Macrophage tumoristatic activity was determined simultaneously in a 72-hr in vitro assay, in which reduction in [^{3}H]TdR uptake by B16-BL6 cells (terminally pulsed for the last 18 hr of culture) was measured. Macrophage tumoricidal and tumoristatic assays were performed in the presence and absence of added exogenous bacterial lipopolysaccharide (LPS), which functions as a second signal for macrophage activation [75,76], at a concentration of 5 ng/ml.

Experimental Design

Groups of 40 mice were inoculated intravenously (i.v.) with 40,000 viable B16-BL6 cells. After 24 hr, i.v. treatment with either rMu IFN-γ or poly(I,C)-LC was initiated. rMu IFN-γ doses ranging from 0.5–5 × 10^6 U/kg and poly(I,C)-LC doses ranging from 0.005 to 1.25 mg/kg were used, and treatment was maintained three times a week (tiw) for 4 weeks. One and three weeks after inoculation of tumor cells, 10 mice from each group were sacrificed, and we assessed NK, LAK, and CTL activities of splenocytes; NK, LAK, CTL, and macrophage tumoricidal and tumoristatic activities in PPMC; tumoricidal and tumoristatic activities of alveolar macrophages, and NK and CTL activities of PBL. To compare levels of lytic activity in different experimental conditions, levels of NK, LAK, and CTL activity were expressed as lytic units (LU)/10^{7}cells with 1 LU defined as the number of effector cells required to produce 20% specific release. Four weeks after tumor inoculation, ten mice from each group were sacrificed, and their lungs were removed, washed, and preserved in buffered formalin. The number of metastatic foci on the lungs was enumerated with the aid of a dissecting microscope. The remaining ten animals in each group were maintained until death to evaluate the effect of rMu IFN-γ or of poly(I,C)-LC on survival. Prolongation of survival and reduction in the number of pulmonary metastases were used as measures of the therapeutic efficacy of the treatment protocols. Each experiment was performed three times with similar results, and data from the three experiments were pooled.

Statistical Analyses

The survival of cohorts of mice receiving different treatment regimens is presented as Kaplan-Meier survival curves, and the statistical significance of these differences was analyzed with the Kruskal-Wallis test [77]. The statistical significance of the differences in the number of lung metastases was analyzed by the Mann-Whitney U-test [77]. The correlations of therapeutic efficacy, expressed as the median survival time or as the median number of lung metastases, with the various measures of effector cell function were analyzed by Pearson's correlation coefficient [77]. NK, LAK, and CTL activities were expressed as LU/10^7 cells. Macrophage tumoricidal activity was expressed as % specific release, and macrophage tumoristatic activity was expressed as % reduction in uptake of [^{3}H]TdR. For these analyses, therapeutic activity (median survival time or median number of lung metastases) at different doses of the BRMs was compared with immunomodulatory activity at the different BRM doses in a stepwise 2 × 2 correlation matrix. Simply put, demonstration of a correlation between the therapeutic and immunomodulatory activities of a BRM depends on there being a similar dose dependence for both activities.

RESULTS

Therapeutic Activity of rMu IFN-γ and of Poly(I,C)-LC

rMu IFN-γ doses of 1.5 and 2.5 × 10^6 U/kg significantly reduced the number of pulmonary metastases, compared to saline treatment [1.5 × 10^6 U/kg ($P = 0.0002$)

and 2.5×10^6 ($P = 0.0014$)], as shown in Table I. rMu IFN-γ doses of 0.5 and 5×10^6 U/kg had no significant therapeutic activity. Additionally, the two doses of rMu IFN-γ with therapeutic activity (1.5 and 2.5×10^6 U/kg) did not differ significantly from each other, but both doses had significantly greater therapeutic activity when compared to the 0.5 or 5×10^6 U/kg doses (Table I). When therapeutic activity was expressed as prolongation of survival, the therapeutic effects of rMu IFN-γ were observed at dosage levels identical with those for reduction in the number of long metastases, with therapeutic activity at doses of 1.5 and 2.5×10^6 U/kg and no therapeutic activity at doses of 0.5 and 5×10^6 U/kg (data not shown). Poly(I,C)-LC doses of 0.05, 0.5, and 1.25 mg/kg all significantly prolonged survival, compared to saline treatment, of animals bearing B16-BL6 experimental lung metastases [0.05 mg/kg ($P = 0.0016$), 0.5 mg/kg ($P = 0.0005$), and 1.25 mg/kg ($P = 0.0001$)], as shown in Figure 1. The lowest poly(I,C)-LC dose tested, 0.005 mg/kg, had no significant therapeutic activity compared with saline treatment, and this dose had significantly less therapeutic activity than the other three doses of poly(I,C)-LC (Fig. 1). The same three doses of poly(I,C)-LC had therapeutic activity, compared to saline treatment, when therapeutic activity was expressed as reduction in the number of pulmonary metastatic nodules (data not shown).

Effect of BRMs on NK and LAK Activities

The NK and LAK activities of splenocytes, PPMC, and PBL were examined 1 and 3 weeks after tumor inoculation. With rMu IFN-γ, no striking dose-response effects were seen because all the doses of rMu IFN-γ tested boosted the levels of NK activity (data not shown). Poly(I,C)-LC also boosted NK activity at most tested doses, but dose response effects could be seen during week 1 (Fig. 2). NK activity in PPMC peaked at a dose of 0.5 mg/kg of poly(I,C)-LC, and NK activity in splenocytes and PBL peaked at a dose of 0.05 mg/kg of poly(I,C)-LC. During week 3, poly(I,C)-LC did not augment NK activity in any site effectively (Fig. 2B). Little or no LAK activity was detected in any tested organ site, at any dose of either BRM, or at either time examined (data not shown).

Effect of BRMs on CTL Activity

The CTL activity of splenocytes, PPMC, and PBL was tested 1 and 3 weeks after tumor inoculation. Specific targets—B16-BL6 melanoma cells, the same cell type as the primary tumor—and nonspecific control targets—syngeneic Lewis lung

TABLE I. Therapeutic Activity of rMu IFN-γ on Experimental Lung Metastases†

| BRM | Dose (U/kg) | No. of metastases | | P values* | | | |
		Median	Range	vs. saline	vs. 0.5 $\times 10^6$	vs. 1.5 $\times 10^6$	vs. 2.5 $\times 10^6$
Saline		>300	18->300				
rMu IFN-γ	0.5×10^6	167	8->300	0.063			
rMu IFN-γ	1.5×10^6	15	3->300	0.0002	0.0003		
rMu IFN-γ	2.5×10^6	41	0->300	0.0014	0.04	0.095	
rMu IFN-γ	5×10^6	>300	58->300	0.31	0.014	0.0003	0.001

†Mice received i.v. inoculations of 40,000 B16-BL6 melanoma cells. rMu IFN-γ was administered i.v., tiw beginning 1 day later. After 4 weeks, mice were sacrificed, and the number of metastatic nodules on the lungs was enumerated with the aid of a dissecting microscope.
*Determined by Mann-Whitney U-test.

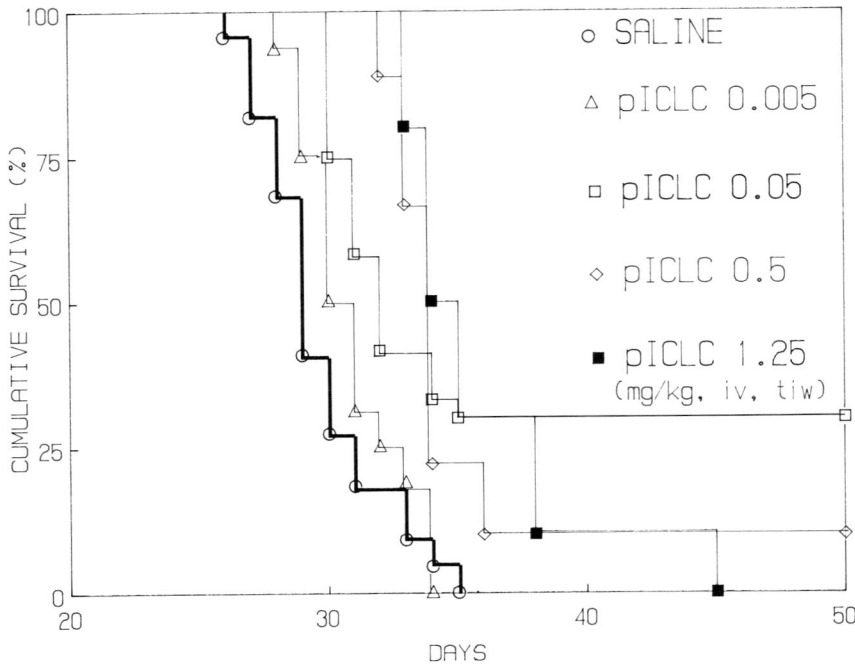

Fig. 1. Effect poly(I,C)-LC on survival of mice inoculated i.v. with 40,000 B16-BL6 melanoma cells. Treatment with poly(I,C)-LC (i.v., tiw) was initiated 1 day later. The statistical significance of the differences in survival was analyzed with the Kruskal-Wallis test. Results (P values) are presented in Table II.

TABLE II. Survival Data

Poly(I,C)-LC (mg/kg)	Median survival time (days)	Range	vs. saline	vs. 0.005 mg/kg	vs. 0.05 mg/kg	vs. 0.5 mg/kg
			\multicolumn{4}{c}{P values}			
0	29	26–35				
0.005	30	28–34	0.18			
0.05	32	30–>84	0.0016	0.048		
0.5	34	32–>84	0.0005	0.0022	0.32	
1.25	34	33–45	0.0001	0.0003	0.17	0.31

carcinoma (3LL-M2) cells—were tested. During week 1, lytic activity against B16-BL6 targets was seen in PBL from animals treated with all doses of rMu IFN-γ (Fig. 3A). PPMC displayed low levels of lytic activity against B16-BL6 targets at some doses of rMu IFN-γ, but splenocytes had little or no lytic activity against B16-BL6 targets (Fig. 3A). This activity does not represent specific CTL activity because PPMC had similar levels of lytic activity against the nonspecific control target, Lewis lung carcinoma (Fig. 3C), as against the specific target, B16-BL6 (Fig. 3A). In contrast, no lytic activity was seen against either target by effector cells from any organ of animals treated with poly(I,C)-LC during week 1 (data not shown). However during week 3, the pattern of lytic activity was quite different from that seen during week 1 for both poly(I,C)-LC and rMu IFN-γ. During week 3, lytic activity against

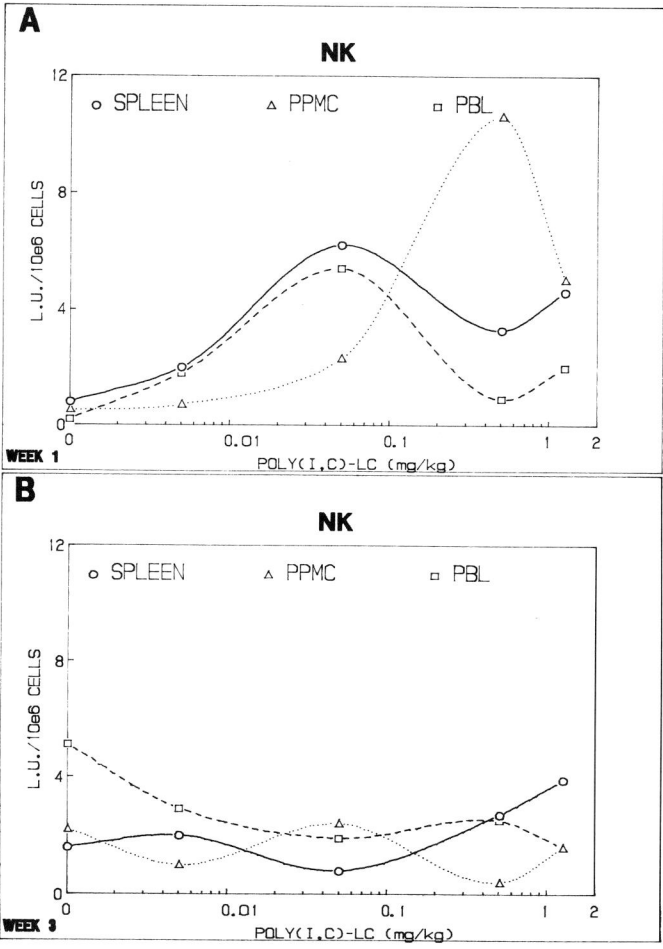

Fig. 2. Effect of i.v. poly(I,C)-LC on NK activity in mice bearing B16-BL6 experimental metastases. NK activity, expressed as lytic units/10^6 cells, was measured 1 **(A)** and 3 **(B)** weeks after tumor inoculation.

the specific target, B16-BL6, was observed only in PPMC, not in splenocytes or PBL (Figs. 3B, 4A). This lytic activity peaked at doses of 2.5×10^6 U/kg of rMu IFN-γ (Fig. 3B) and 0.5 mg/kg of poly(I,C)-LC (Fig. 4A), respectively. The lack of lytic activity by PPMC against the specificity control targets, Lewis lung carcinoma (Fig. 3D), during week 3, strongly suggests that this activity is mediated by specific CTL and was found only in the tumor-bearing organ, the lung. Furthermore, the PPMC did not mediate LAK activity during week 3 (data not shown). The identity of the effector cells in PPMC as CTL is further strengthened by the demonstration that treatment of PPMC with anti-Thy 1.2 plus complement, but not anti-asialo GM1 plus complement, ablated their ability to kill B16-BL6 target cells (Fig. 4A). With NK activity, the opposite effects were observed (Fig. 4B). These results confirm the T cell nature of the effector cells in PPMC and provide further support for their identity as specific CTL.

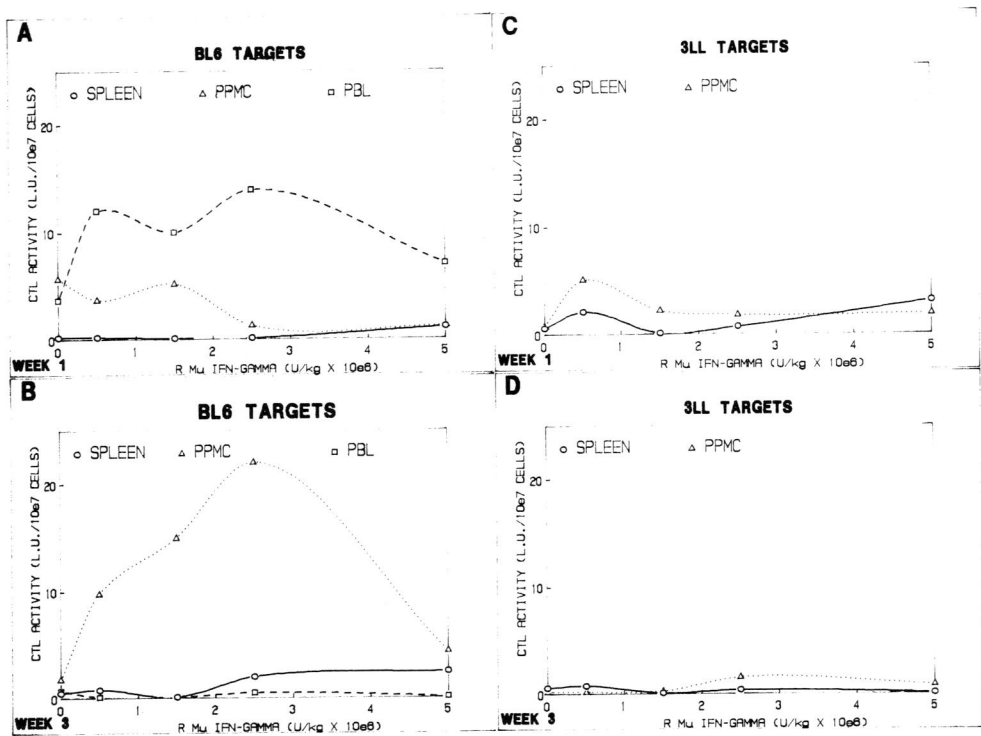

Fig. 3. Effect of i.v. rMu IFN-γ on CTL activity against specific (B16-BL6; **A,B**) and nonspecific (3LL; **C,D**) targets in mice bearing B16-BL6 experimental metastases. CTL activity, expressed as lytic units/10^7 cells, was measured 1(A,C) and 3(B,D) weeks after tumor inoculation.

Effect of BRMs on Macrophage-Mediated Cytotoxicity and Cytostasis

Macrophages were obtained from alveoli by lung lavage and from PPMC after 1 and 3 weeks of BRM treatment, and their tumoricidal and tumoristatic activities assessed. The results in Figure 5 demonstrate that rMu IFN-γ, administered i.v. tiw, augmented macrophage-mediated tumoricidal and tumoristatic activities. During week 1, rMu IFN-γ augmented tumoricidal activity in pulmonary macrophages with a peak at 1.5×10^6 U/kg (Fig. 5A). Also during week 1, rMu IFN-γ augmented macrophage tumoristatic activity, with a peak at 0.5×10^6 U/kg (Fig. 5C). During week 3, the tumoricidal (Fig. 5B) and tumoristatic (Fig. 5D) activities of pulmonary macrophages peaked at a dose of 2.5×10^6 U/kg. Alveolar macrophage activities did not show similar responses to rMu IFN-γ during week 3. In constrast, during week 1, poly(I,C)-LC boosted alveolar macrophage tumoricidal activity more effectively than pulmonary macrophage tumoricidal activity, with a peak at 0.5 mg/kg (Fig. 6A). There was some discrepancy between results from tumoricidal and tumoristasis assays because poly(I,C)-LC boosted the tumoristatic activity of pulmonary macrophages more effectively than that of alveolar macrophages, with a peak at 0.5 mg/kg (Fig. 6C). During week 3, however, macrophage tumoricidal and tumoristatic activities were not significantly boosted by poly(I,C)-LC (Fig. 6B,D).

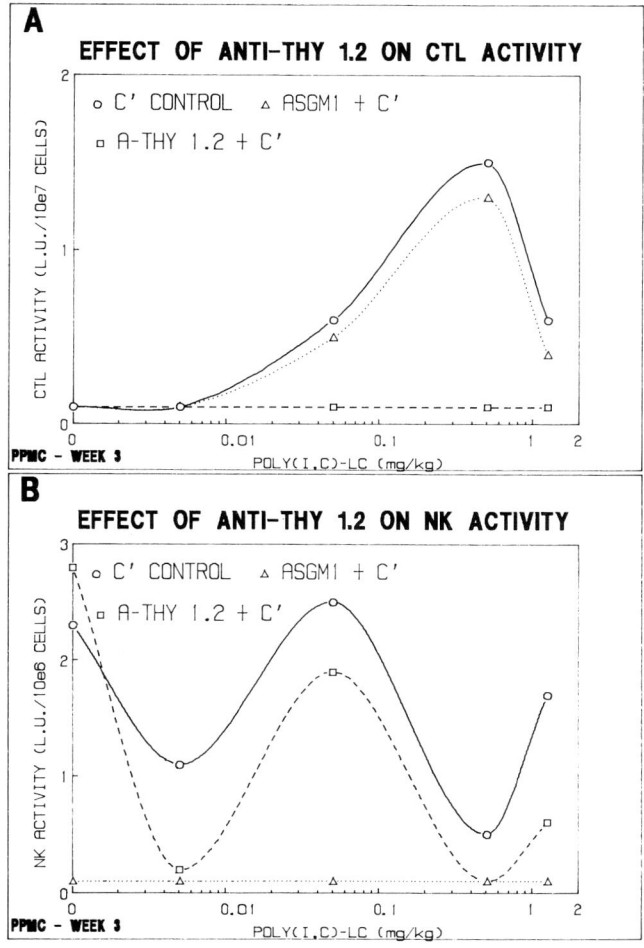

Fig. 4. Effect of antibody depletion with anti-Thy 1.2 (New England Nuclear, Boston, MA) or anti-asialo GM1 (Wako Chemical) on specific CTL (**A**) and NK (**B**) activity of PPMC from mice bearing experimental lung metastases, after 3 weeks of poly(I,C)-LC administration. Treatment with antibody plus complement (C') was performed as previously described [74]. B16-BL6 melanoma cells were the targets for specific CTL activity (A), and YAC-1 cells were the targets for NK activity (B).

Correlation of Therapeutic Activity With Effector Cell Function

In order to determine which effector cell functions were responsible for the therapeutic activity of rMu IFN-γ and of poly(I,C)-LC, the various effector cell functions in the different anatomical sites were correlated with therapeutic activity using Pearson's correlation coefficient [77]. This analysis revealed that the therapeutic activity of these BRMs correlated with augmented effector functions only in the organ with tumor, the lung, but not in the spleen or PBL (Tables III, IV). Specific CTL in PPMC at week 3 (with B16-BL6 as targets) correlated with the therapeutic activity of both rM IFN-γ ($P = 0.0088$, Table III) and of poly(I,C)-LC ($P = 0.037$, Table IV), but CTL activity in splenocytes or PBL at week 3 did not show a similar correlation. However, the CTL activity at any site tested during week 1 did not show a similar

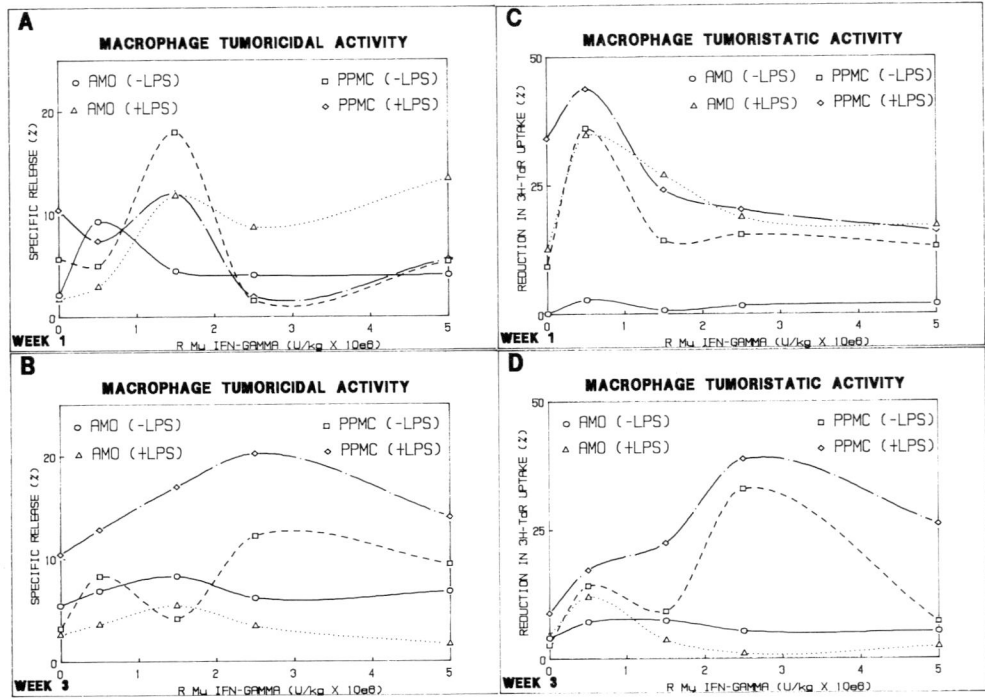

Fig. 5. Effect of i.v. rMu IFN-γ on macrophage tumoricidal (**A,B**) and tumoristatic (**C,D**) activities in mice bearing B16-BL6 experimental metastases. Macrophage tumoricidal activity, measured as specific release of [^{125}I]UdR from B16-BL6 targets in a 72-hr assay, and macrophage tumoricidal activity, expressed as reduction in [^{3}H]TdR uptake by B16-BL6 cells in a 72-hr assay, were measured 1(A,C) and 3(B,D) weeks after tumor inoculation.

correlation (Table III, IV) because no specific CTL activity was seen then (Fig. 3A,C). Macrophage tumoricidal and tumoristatic activities in PPMC but not in alveoli, also correlated with the therapeutic activity of rMu IFN-γ (Table III). With poly(I,C)-LC, the opposite was true, and its therapeutic activity correlated with alveolar macrophage tumoricidal activity but not with pulmonary macrophage tumoricidal activity (Table IV). The NK activity in PPMC, but not in splenocytes or PBL, correlated with the therapeutic activity of poly(I,C)-LC (Table IV) only during week 1, but not with the therapeutic activity of rMu IFN-γ (Table III). LAK activity in any tested site at either time did not correlate with therapeutic activity of either BRM (Tables III, IV).

DISCUSSION

Identifying agents with therapeutic activity against established metastatic disease, optimizing the administration protocols, and understanding the mechansim of their therapeutic activity are the primary goals of the preclinical studies of BRMs. Previous studies have demonstrated the importance of dosage, route, duration, and schedule of administration in optimizing the therapeutic activity of BRMs for the treatment of metastatic disease in preclinical models [46–48,74]. rMu IFN-γ and

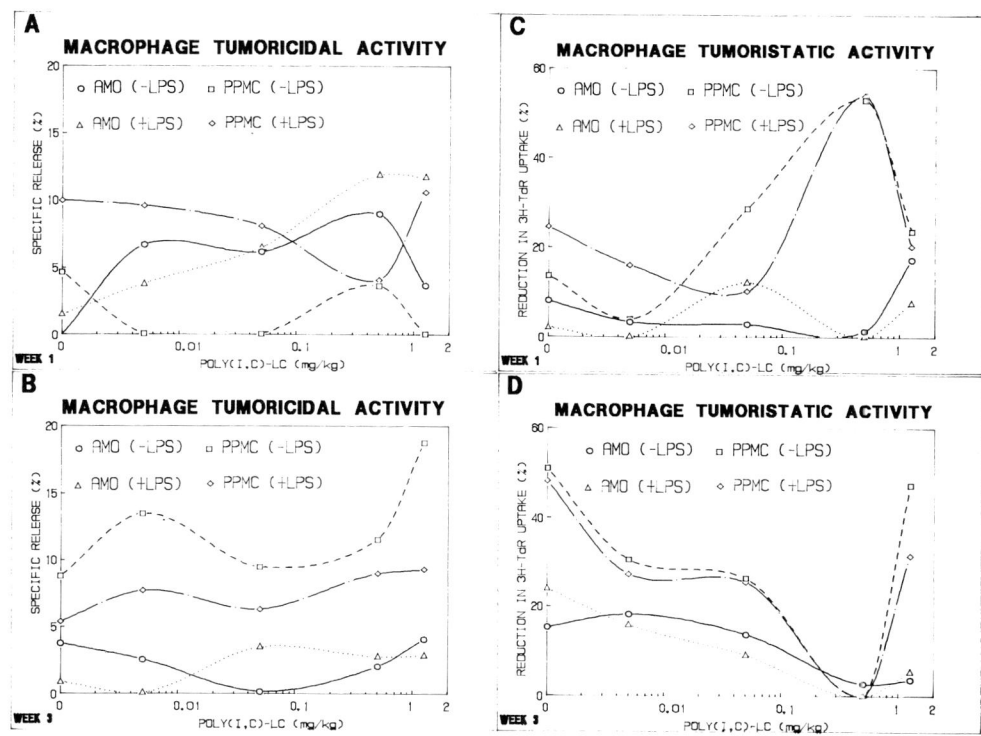

Fig. 6. Effect of i.v. poly(I,C)-LC on macrophage tumoricidal (**A,B**) and tumoristatic (**C,D**) activities in mice bearing B16-BL6 experimental metastases. Macrophage tumoricidal activity, measured as specific release of [^{125}I]UdR from B16-BL6 targets in a 72-hr assay, and macrophage tumoricidal activity, expressed as reduction in [^{3}H]TdR uptake by B16-BL6 cells in a 72-hr assay, were measured 1(A,C) and 3(B,D) weeks after tumor inoculation.

poly(I,C)-LC have consistently shown significant therapeutic activity in animal models of experimental and spontaneous metastases, but this therapeutic activity depends on utilization of optimal therapeutic protocols as discussed above. For example, i.v. administration of rMu IFN-γ produced greater therapeutic benefit compared with intraperitoneal or intramuscular administration [46], owing presumably to the higher, but less sustained serum levels of rMu IFN-γ obtained following i.v. administration compared with the other routes [46,78,79].

The results of the present studies are consistent with these concepts as therapeutic activity depended strongly on the dose of the BRM administered. Both rMu IFN-γ and poly(I,C)-LC also had immunomodulatory activity in most of the assay systems employed, with several exceptions. NK activity was not boosted, and may even have been depressed, after 3 weeks of poly(I,C)-LC (Fig. 2B) administration. This finding is consistent with other reports of NK hyporesponsiveness following repeated BRM administration [7,46,80–88]. LAK activity, measured by release of ^{51}Cr in a 4-hr assay with P815 cells as targets, was not boosted by treatment with either rMu IFN-γ or poly(I,C)-LC at any dosage level. In fact, LAK activity was not detected during these studies. Similarly, during week 3, rMu IFN-γ and poly(I,C)-LC did not augment CTL activity in splenocytes or PBL against either the specific or nonspecific target.

TABLE III. Correlation of Therapeutic Activity of rMu IFN-γ With Effector Cell Functions

	Effector cell function[a]							
	NK			LAK		CTL		
	Spleen	PPMC	PBL	Spleen	PPMC	Spleen	PPMC	PBL
Week 1	0.30[b]	0.18	0.15	0.44	0.60	0.10	0.51	0.58
Week 3	0.14	0.41	0.36	0.02	0.55	0.47	0.84 (0.0088)	0.41

	Macrophage activity							
	[^{125}I]UdR release				Reduction in [^{3}H]TdR uptake			
	AMO[c]		PPMC		AMO		PPMC	
	−LPS	+LPS	−LPS	+LPS	−LPS	+LPS	−LPS	+LPS
Week 1	0.41	0.24	0.17	0.37	0.26	0.35	0.74 (0.039)	0.82 (0.011)
Week 3	0.27	0.04	0.72 (0.036)	0.20	0.37	0.66	0.26	0.78 (0.023)

[a]Mice received i.v. inoculations of 40,000 B16-BL6 melanoma cells. rMu IFN-γ was administered i.v. beginning 1 day later. After 1 and 3 weeks, effector functions in various organs were tested. Effector cell functions were compared with median number of lung metastases using Pearson's correlation coefficient for medians.
[b]Correlation coefficients (P values for significant correlations).
[c]AMO, alveolar macrophages.

TABLE IV. Correlation of Therapeutic Activity of Poly(I,C)-LC With Effector Cell Functions

	Effector cell function[a]							
	NK			LAK		CTL		
	Spleen	PPMC	PBL	Spleen	PPMC	Spleen	PPMC	PBL
Week 1	0.62[b]	0.88 (0.049)	0.16	0.73	0.67	0.26	0.12	0.74
Week 3	0.61	0.45	0.77	0.58	0.79	0.02	0.90 (0.037)	0.15

	Macrophage activity							
	[^{125}I]UdR release				Reduction in [^{3}H]TdR uptake			
	AMO[c]		PPMC		AMO		PPMC	
	−LPS	+LPS	−LPS	+LPS	−LPS	+LPS	−LPS	+LPS
Week 1	0.62	0.99 (0.0006)	0.35	0.54	0.17	0.06	0.80	0.50
Week 3	0.12	0.69	0.50	0.82	0.92 (0.025)	0.96 (0.0079)	0.55	0.72

[a]Mice received i.v. inoculations of 40,000 B16-BL6 melanoma cells. Poly(I,C)-LC was administered i.v. beginning 1 day later. After 1 and 3 weeks, effector functions in various organs were tested. Effector cell functions were compared with median survival time using Pearson's correlation coefficient for medians.
[b]Correlation coefficients (P values for significant correlations).
[c]AMO, alveolar macrophages.

However, specific CTL activity against B16-BL6 in PPMC was augmented by both these agents in a dose-dependent manner, with peaks at 2.5×10^6 U/kg for rMu IFN-γ and at 0.5 mg/kg for poly(I,C)-LC. It should be emphasized that these effector cell populations in PPMC did not show any lytic activity against the nonspecific control target cells, syngeneic 3LL-M2 carcinoma. Furthermore, the effector cells in PPMC were sensitive to treatment with anti-Thy 1.2, but not anti-asialo GM1, plus complement. These results demonstrate that the effector cells responsible for the lytic activity against B16-BL6 targets in PPMC during week 3 are indeed specific CTL, as had been suggested by the target specificity of this lytic activity and by the absence of LAK cell activity. Furthermore, the restriction of specific CTL activity to one anatomic site, the lungs, may result from local antigen processing at the tumor site, local cytokine production, or chemotactic attraction of specific CTL to the tumor.

These studies also correlated the therapeutic and immunomodulatory effects of these BRMs in an effort to identify the mechanism of their therapeutic activity in treating metastatic disease. CTL in PPMC during week 3, but not during week 1, correlated with the therapeutic activity of both these BRMs, but CTL activity in splenocytes or PBL did not show a similar correlation. This difference in lytic activity between weeks 1 and 3 is predictable because about 10 to 14 days are required to produce a specific CTL response. Therefore, specific CTL activity would not have been expected during week 1. Macrophage antitumor activities also correlated with the therapeutic activity of these BRMs. However, the therapeutic activity of rMu IFN-γ correlated with macrophage activities in PPMC, while the therapeutic activity of poly(I,C)-LC correlated with alveolar macrophage activities. This difference may be associated with augmentation of the activities of different macrophage populations. The rMu IFN-γ may augment histiocytes (in situ tissue macrophages) while poly(I,C)-LC may augment monocytes whose activity appears as alveolar macrophages, but not histiocytes. This difference could represent a different mechanism of activation, with direct activation by rMu IFN-γ and indirect activation by poly(I,C)-LC, with the result that a mediator is diluted or inactive within parenchymal tissue.

Another discrepancy between the two BRMs' mechanisms of therapeutic activity occurred in NK activity. NK activity, at any site, at either time did not correlate with the therapeutic activity of rMu IFN-γ, but pulmonary NK activity during week 1, but not week 3, did correlate with the therapeutic activity of poly(I,C)-LC. It should be emphasized, however, that the lack of correlation of NK activity with the therapeutic activity of rMu IFN-γ is not necessarily due to a lack of NK augmentation because rMu IFN-γ boosted NK activity, but with a dose dependence different from that of rMu IFN-γ's therapeutic activity. For both these BRMs, pulmonary CTL activity during week 3 correlated with their therapeutic activity. Otherwise, effector functions only in the organ with tumor, the lung, showed correlations with therapeutic activity of either of these agents. These analyses revealed that both the particular effector function and the site sampled represent important factors in understanding the mechanism of therapeutic action of BRMs.

In summary, these studies support and extend the concept of optimal administration of BRMs for treating metastatic disease, and they provide information on the mechanism of therapeutic action of rMu IFN-γ and poly(I,C)-LC. In particular, monitoring immune functions in the tumor-bearing organ appears to be critical for identifying the mechanism of BRMs' therapeutic effects and for predicting such activity. Obviously it is not possibly routinely to obtain samples of tumor-bearing organs for immune monitoring of effector cell functions in patients during clinical trials of BRMs, and monitoring of effector functions in readily accessible sites such as peripheral blood may not accurately reflect the immunotherapeutic activity of BRMs. However in some situations, such as peritoneal effusions, this approach may be feasible and could prove highly informative.

ACKNOWLEDGMENTS

This research was sponsored by the DHHS, under contract No. NO1-23910 with Program Resources, Inc.

By acceptance of this article, the publisher or recipient acknowledges the right of the U.S. Government to retain a nonexclusive, royalty-free license in and to any copyright covering the article.

The contents of this publication do not necessarily reflect the views or policies of the Department of Health and Human Services, nor does mention of trade names, commercial products, or organizations imply endorsement by the U.S. Government.

REFERENCES

1. Fidler IJ, Raz A: Lymphokines 3:345, 1981.
2. Meltzer MS: Lymphokines 3:319, 1981.
3. Varesio L, Blasi E, Thurman GB, Talmadge JE, Wiltrout RH, Herberman RB: Cancer Res 44:4465, 1984.
4. Gidlund M, Orn A, Wigzell H, Senik A, Gresser I: Nature 273:759, 1978.
5. Schreiber RD, Hicks LJ, Celada A, Buchmeier NA, Gray PW: J Immunol 134:1609, 1985.
6. Djeu JY, Heinbaugh JA, Holden HT, Herberman RB: J Immunol 122:175, 1979.
7. Talmadge JE, Herberman RB, Chirigos MA, Maluish AE, Schneider MA, Adams JS, Phillips H, Thurman GB: J Immunol 135:2483, 1985.
8. Rubin BY, Gupta SL: Proc Natl Acad Sci USA 77:5928, 1980.
9. Branca AA, Baglioni C: Nature 294:768, 1981.
10. Hilleman MR: J Cell Physiol 71:43, 1968.
11. Ho M, Ke YH: Virology 40:693, 1970.
12. Beers RF, Braun W (ed): "Biological Effects of Polynucleotides." Berlin: Springer, 1971.
13. Buckler EC, Dubuy HG, Johnson ML, Baron S: Proc Soc Exp Biol Med 136:394, 1971.
14. Field AK, Tytell AA, Lampson GP, Hilleman MR: Proc Natl Acad Sci USA 58:1004, 1972.
15. Field AK, Tytell AA, Piperno E, Lampson GP, Nemes MM, Hilleman MR: Medicine 51:169, 1972.
16. Finter NB: In Finter NB (ed): "Interferons and Interferon Inducers." Amsterdam: Elsevier-North Holland, 1973.
17. Turner W, Chan SP, Chirigos MA: Proc Soc Exp Biol Med 133:334, 1970.
18. Harrington DL, Crabbs CL, Hilmas DE, Brown JR, Higbee CA, Cole FE, Levy HB: Infect Immun 24:60, 1979.
19. Cantor H, Asofsky R, Levy HB: J Immunol 104:1035, 1970.
20. Chirigos MA, Papademetriou V, Bartocci A, Read E, Levy HB: Int J Immunopharmacol 3:329, 1981.
21. Sarma PS, Shiu G, Meubauer R, Baron S, Huebner RJ: Proc Natl Acad Sci USA 62:1146, 1969.
22. Catalano LW, Baron S: Proc Soc Exp Biol Med 133:684, 1970.
23. Levy HB, London W, Piccoli DA, Baron S, Rice J: J Infect Dis 133:A256, 1976.
24. Olsen GA, Kern ER, Glasgow LA, Overall JC: Antimicrob Agents Chemother 10:668, 1976.
25. Hekman RACP, Prins MEF, Bosveld IJ, Trapman J: Int J Cancer 26:493, 1981.
26. Levy HB, Law LW, Rabson AS: Proc Natl Acad Sci USA 62:357, 1969.
27. Zeleznick CD, Bhuyan BK: Proc Soc Exp Biol Med 130:126, 1969.
28. Levy HB, Asofsky R, Riley R, Garapin A, Cantor H, Adamson R: Ann NY Acad Sci 173:640, 1970.

29. Kreider JW, Benjamin SA: J Natl Cancer Inst 49:1303, 1972.
30. Glasgow LA, Crane JL, Jr, Kern ER: J Natl Cancer Inst 60:659, 1978.
31. Hersh EM, Gutterman JU, Alexanian R, Lotzova E, Murphy SG: Proc Am Assoc Cancer Res 22:372, 1981.
32. Davies M-E, Field AK: J Interferon Res 3:89, 1983.
33. Talmadge JE, Adams J, Phillips H, Collins M, Lenz B, Schneider M, Chirigos M: Cancer Res 45:1066, 1985.
34. Djeu JY, Heinbaugh JA, Holden HT, Herberman RB: J Immunol 122:182, 1979.
35. Gidlund M, Orn A, Wigzell H, Senik A, Gresser I: Nature 273:759, 1978.
36. Djeu JY, Heinbaugh JA, Vieira WD, Holden HT, Herberman RB: Immunopharmacology 1:231, 1979.
37. Edwards BS, Borden EC, Smith-Zaremba K: Cancer Immunol Immunother 13:168, 1982.
38. Malatzky E, Ehrlich R, Finkler A, Koltin Y, Witz IP: In Serrou BJ, Rosenfeld C, Daniels JC, Saunders JP (eds): "Current Concepts in Human Immunology and Cancer Immunomodulation." New York: Elsevier, 1982, pp 371-378.
39. Talmadge JE, Adams J, Phillips H, Collins M, Lenz B, Schneider M, Schlick E, Ruffman R, Wiltrout RH, Chirigos MA: Cancer Res 45:1058, 1985.
40. Taramelli D, Varesio L: J Immunol 126:58, 1981.
41. Norlund J, Wolff S, Levy HB: Proc Soc Exp Biol Med 133:439, 1970.
42. Robinson RA, DeVita VT, Levy HB, Baron S, Hubbard SP, Levine AS: J Natl Cancer Inst 57:599, 1976.
43. Granados EN, Lewinski S, O'Malley J, Bello J: J Interferon Res 4:51, 1984.
44. Levy HB, Baer G, Baron S, Buckler CE, Gibbs CJ, Iadarola MJ, Gordon WT, Rice J: J Infect Dis 132:434, 1975.
45. Champney KJ, Levine DP, Levy HB, Lerner AM: Infect Immun 25:831, 1979.
46. Talmadge JE, Tribble HR, Pennington RW, Phillips H, Wiltrout RH: Cancer Res 47:2563, 1987.
47. Talmadge JE, Hartmann D: J Biol Response Mod 4:484, 1985.
48. Hartmann D, Adams JS, Meeker AK, Schneider MS, Lenz BF, Talmadge JE: Cancer Res 46:1331, 1985.
49. Quesada JR, Gutterman JU: J Natl Cancer Inst 70:1041, 1983.
50. Foon KA, Sherwin SA, Abrams PG, Longo DL, Fer MF, Stevenson HC, Ochs JJ, Bottino CS, Schoenberger CS, Zeffren J, Jaffe ES, Oldham RK: N Engl J Med 311:1148, 1984.
51. Bunn PA, Jr, Foon KA, Ihde DC, Longo DL, Eddy J, Winkler CF, Veach SR, Zeffren J, Sherwin S, Oldham R: Ann Intern Med 101:484, 1984.
52. Sherwin SA, Foon KA, Abrams PG, Heyman MR, Ochs JJ, Watson T, Maluish A, Oldham RK: J Biol Response Mod 3:599, 1984.
53. Kirkwood JM, Ernstoff MS: J Clin Oncol 2:336, 1984.
54. Krown SE, Burk MW, Kirkwood JM, Kerr D, Morton DL, Oettgen HF: Cancer Treat Rep 68:723, 1984.
55. Bonnem EM, Spiegel RJ: J Biol Response Mod 3:580, 1984.
56. Sherwin SA, Foon KA, Abrams PG, Heyman MR, Ochs JJ, Watson T, Maluish A, Oldham RK: J Biol Response Mod 3:599, 1984.
57. van der Burg M, Edelstein M, Gerlis L, Liang C-M, Hirschi M, Dawson A: J Biol Response Mod 4:264, 1985.
58. Schulof RS, Lloyd MJ, Stallings JJ, Magi D, Phillips TM, Jones GJ, Schechter GP: J Biol Response Mod 4:310, 1985.
59. Berek JS, Hacker NF, Lichtenstein A, Jung T, Spina C, Knox RM, Brady J, Greene T, Ettinger LM, Lagesse LD, Bonnem EM, Spiegel RJ, Zighelboim J: Cancer Res 45:4447, 1985.
60. Edwards BS, Merritt JA, Fuhlbrigge RC, Borden, EC: J Clin Invest 75:1908, 1985.
61. Vadhan-Raj S, Al-Katib A, Bhalla R, Pelus L, Nathan CF, Sherwin SA, Oettgen HF, Krown SE: J Clin Oncol 4:137, 1986.
62. Rinehart JJ, Malspeis L, Young D, Neidhart JA: J Biol Response Mod 5:300, 1986.
63. Levine AS, Sivulich M, Wiernik PH, Levy HB: Cancer Res 39:1645, 1979.
64. Krown SE, Kerr D, Stewart WE, Pollack MC, Cunningham-Rundles S, Hirshaut Y, Pinsky CM, Levy HB, Oettgen HF: In Hersh EM, Chirigos MA, Mastrangelo MJ (eds): "Augmenting Agents in Cancer Therapy." New York: Raven Press, 1981, p 165.
65. Lampson GP, Field AK, Tytell AA, Hilleman MR: J Interferon Res 1:539, 1981.

66. Chirigos MA, Schlick E, Piccoli M, Read E, Hartung K, Bartocci A: In Hadden J, Chedid L, Mullen T, Spreafico F (eds): "Advances in Immunopharmacology." Elmsford, N.Y.: Pergamon Press, 1982, pp 669–676.
67. Levine AS, Durie B, Lampkin B, Leventhal BF, Levy HB: In Terry WD, Rosenberg SA (eds): "Immunotherapy of Human Cancer" New York: Elsevier-North Holland, 1982, pp 411–418.
68. Stevenson HC, Abrams PG, Schoenberger CS, Smalley RB, Herberman RB, Foon KA: J Biol Response Mod 4:650, 1985.
69. Herberman RB, Pinsky CM: J Biol Response Mod 4:680, 1985.
70. Hart IR: Am J Pathol 97:587, 1979.
71. Talmadge JE, Fidler IJ: J Natl Cancer Inst 69:975, 1982.
72. Klein E, Klein G: J Natl Cancer Inst 32:547, 1964.
73. Dunn TB, Patter MJ: J Natl Cancer Inst 18:587, 1957.
74. Talmadge JE, Fidler IJ, Oldham RK: "Screening for Biological Response Modifiers: Methods and Rationale." Boston: Martinus Nijhoff, 1985.
75. Weinberg JB, Chapman HA, Jr, Hibbs JB: J Immunol 121:72, 1978.
76. Pace JL, Russell SW: J Immunol 126:1863, 1981.
77. Snedecor GW, Cochran WG: "Statistical Methods." Ames: Iowa State University Press, 1967.
78. Foon KA, Sherwin SA, Abrams PG, Stevenson HC, Holmes P, Maluish AE, Oldham RK, Herberman RB: Cancer Immunol Immunother 20:193, 1985.
79. Kurzrock R, Rosenblum MG, Sherwin SA, Rios A, Talpaz M, Quesada JR, Gutterman JU: Cancer Res 45:2866, 1985.
80. Huddlestone JR, Merigan TC, Jr, Oldstone MBA: Natura 282:417, 1979.
81. Einhorn S, Ahre A, Blomgren H, Johansson B, Mellstedt H, Strander H: Int J Cancer 30:167, 1982.
82. Golub SH, D'Amore P, Rainey M: J Natl Cancer Inst 68:711, 1982.
83. Hawrylowicz CM, Rees RC, Hancock BW, Potter CW: Eur J Cancer Clin Oncol 18:1081, 1982.
84. Maluish AE, Ortaldo JR, Conlon JC, Sherwin SA, Leavitt R, Strong DM, Wiernik P, Oldham RK, Herberman RB: J Immunol 131:503, 1983.
85. Maluish AE, Leavitt R, Sherwin SA, Oldham RK, Herberman RB: J Biol Response Mod 2:470, 1983.
86. Spina CA, Fahey JL, Durkos-Smith D, Dorey F, Sarna G: J Biol Response Mod 2:458, 1983.
87. Maluish AE, Ortaldo JR, Sherwin SA, Oldham RK, Herberman RB: J Biol Response Mod 2:418, 1983.
88. Ernstoff MS, Reigh S, Nishoda Y, Kirkwood JM: Immunology 26:280, 1985.

Gene Expression and Tumor Cell Escape From Host Effector Mechanisms in Murine Large Cell Lymphoma

Ronald A. LaBiche, Mitsuzi Yoshida, Gary E. Gallick, Tatsuro Irimura, Donald L. Robberson, Jim Klostergaard, and Garth L. Nicolson

Departments of Tumor Biology (R.A.L., M.Y., G.E.G., T.I., J.K., G.L.N.) and Genetics (D.L.R.), The University of Texas M.D. Anderson Hospital and Tumor Institute, Houston, Texas 77030

Using in vivo selection methods, we obtained metastatic sublines of the murine RAW117 large cell lymphoma that form multiple liver metastases. The highly metastatic subline RAW117-H10 has a low number of gp70 molecules expressed at the cell surface and low cytostatic sensitivity to activated syngeneic macrophages. This subline was infected with endogenous RNA tumor virus isolated from a high virus-expressing RAW117-P subline of low metastatic potential. After superinfection the H10 subline gradually increased its expression of cell surface gp70 and showed enhanced sensitivity to macrophage-mediated cytostasis, suggesting that gp70 might be involved in host macrophage-mediated surveillance. Culture of RAW117-P and H10 cells in media conditioned by activated macrophages indicated that parental cells are severely growth inhibited in a dose dependent fashion while H10 cells showed almost no effect. Examination of differentially expressed genes in the highly metastatic RAW117-H10 cells by analysis of RNA blots indicated that a mitochondrial gene was expressed at a level that was ~10 times higher in H10 cells than in parental cells. This gene was identified as ND5, which codes for a subunit of NADH dehydrogenase (complex I of the mitochondrial electron transport chain); this complex is the target for an activated macrophage-released cytostatic factor. Among other possibilities, the results are consistent with the suggestion that highly metastatic RAW117 cells may escape macrophage surveillance by decreasing the synthesis of specific cell-surface receptors for cytostatic molecules and increasing the synthesis of specific cellular targets for such molecules.

Key words: tumor metastasis, viral antigens, macrophage cytostasis, differential gene expression, mitochondrial genes

Presented at the ICN/UCLA Symposium "Tumor Progression and Metastasis," Keystone, April 6–12, 1987.

Received May 22, 1987; revised and accepted September 30, 1987.

© 1988 Alan R. Liss, Inc.

The interactions of a neoplasm with its host during tumor dissemination are complex and poorly understood [1–3]. Such interactions, for the most part, appear to be mediated at the level of the cell surface. Highly malignant cells express unique cell-surface properties that, in combination with host environment and responses, are important determinants in metastasis formation [1,2, 4–6]. Established tumor models have been used to study differences between nonmetastatic and metastatic neoplastic cells, as well as the role of host tumor surveillance mechanisms in metastasis [2, 3, 6]. Such research indicates that in many metastatic tumors the ability of highly malignant cells to escape host macrophage-mediated cytolysis and cytostasis is important in the metastatic process [3,7–13]. This is reinforced by studies showing that activated macrophages produce soluble respiratory-inhibiting factors (RIF) which inhibit the activity of complexes I and II of the tumor cell mitochondrial electron transport chain and thus cellular respiration [14,29,41,42].

One tumor model that has been useful in examining the role of host response in metastasis is the murine RAW117 large cell lymphoma [15,16]. This tumor system was established by Abelson murine leukemia virus (AbMuLV) transformation to yield parental RAW117-P cells of low malignant potential in syngeneic BALB/c mice. After ten sequential selections for liver colonization, a variant subline (RAW117-H10) was obtained that forms greater than 200 times as many gross liver tumors than does the parental cell line after intravenous or subcutaneous injection [15–17]. Highly metastatic RAW117-H10 cells possess differences in gene expression [18], exposures of cell surface proteins [19] and glycoproteins [17,20], lectin-binding sites [20,21], viral antigens [17,22], two-phase partitioning behavior [23], liver adhesion properties [24], and are less sensitive to macrophage-mediated cytolysis and cytostasis [8,13]. Here we report further studies of the role of macrophage-mediated cytostasis in the metastatic properties of RAW117 cells.

MATERIALS AND METHODS
Cell Lines and Metastasis Assays

RAW117 cells were cultured in petri dishes in Dulbecco-Modified Eagle's medium (DME) supplemented with high glucose (4.5 g/L), 10% fetal bovine serum (FBS), and 25 mM HEPES buffer except for the cells used for RNA isolation and growth curves with activated macrophage conditioned media which were cultured in a 50:50 mixture of DME and Ham's F12, 10% FBS. Cell cultures were used within ten passages (4–6 weeks) from frozen stocks to eliminate possible drift in metastatic properties [16]. All lines were negative for *Mycoplasmas* and other infections [18]. Metastatic potential was assessed by intravenous injection of 5×10^3 viable tumor cells (0.2 ml inoculum) in phosphate-buffered saline (PBS) into groups of 6–8-week-old BALB/c mice [15–18]. Twelve days after the injection mice were killed, and visible tumor nodules were counted and confirmed by histologic analysis [21].

Superinfection of RAW117 Cells

Some RAW117-P cells release infective AbMuLV and Moloney murine leukemia virus (MoMuLV) into culture medium [22]. Such released viruses can be isolated, purified, and used to reinfect susceptible cells such as NIH/3T3 by the procedure of Wong and Gallick [25]. With this method NIH/3T3 cells were completely transformed in vitro, indicating the presence of infectious AbMuLV, and MoMuLV structural proteins were found expressed in the transformed NIH/3T3 cells [22].

RAW117-H10 cells expressing low amounts of MoMuLV components [17] were superinfected with an equal volume of filtered culture supernatant from RAW117-P cells by suspending 10^6 cells in 2 ml of DME plus 56 μg/ml DEAE Dextran. After a 1-hr incubation at 37°C with mild shaking, the cells were resuspended in 30 ml of DME containing 10% FBS and allowed to grow for a few passages. Mock infections omitted the RAW117-P supernatants. Some of the cultures were further cloned [22].

Viral Glycoproteins

RAW117 cells were labeled metabolically with [^{3}H]-leucine, lysed in a buffered detergent solution, and immunoprecipitated with gp70 antiserum as described previously [22, 26]. Immune complexes were precipitated with formalin-treated *Staphylococcus aureus* and prepared for sodium dodecylsulfate-polyacrylamide gel electrophoresis (SDS-PAGE) using 8% polyacrylamide gels, followed by autoradiography [22]. For lectin staining of cellular glycoproteins separated by SDS-PAGE, the procedures of Irimura et al. [20] were used. Cells were lysed with 0.5% NP-40, 0.25 M sucrose, 50 μM $CaCl_2$, 0.4 mM phenylmethylsulfonyl fluoride, 10 mM Tris-HCl (pH 6.7), for 30 min. After centrifugation at 1,000g, the supernatant was collected, mixed with SDS sample buffer, heated at 100°C for 5 min, and subjected to SDS-PAGE using 7.5% polyacrylamide gels [20, 22]. After electrophoresis, the glycoproteins were transferred to nitrocellulose membranes [27], and detected by ^{125}I-concanavalin A (^{125}I-Con A) or peroxidase-Con A (Sigma Chemical, St. Louis, MO) staining [20].

Cytostasis in Macrophage Coculture

Syngeneic peritoneal exudate cells were obtained by intraperitoneal injection of 3 ml of thioglycollate (Difco Laboratories, Detroit, MI) into BALB/c mice [8]. Three days later the peritoneal cavities were flushed with PBS containing 100 μg/ml gentamicin, and the cell suspension was centrifuged at 400g for 5 min at 4°C. After resuspending the cells in DME, aliquots (0.1 ml) of the suspension were placed into wells of a 96-well plate (Costar, Cambridge, MA) at varying cell densities. After a 4-hr incubation at 37°C, the plates were washed twice to remove unattached cells, and 40 μg/ml of poly I:C (Sigma, St. Louis, MO) was added to each well. The DME was replaced after 24 hr with fresh medium containing poly I:C, and RAW117 cells were added. Cytostasis was determined in a 24-hr incubation period using the inhibition of [^{3}H]thymidine incorporation method of Germain et al. [28]. The results were expressed as follows: percent cytostasis = $1 - (E-T_1)/(C-T_2) \times 100$, where E and C are the [^{3}H]thymidine incorporation of target cells in the presence or absence of activated macrophages, respectively, and T_1 and T_2 are the background incorporation in the presence or absence of macrophages, respectively. Statistical significance was determined by one-way analysis of variance and the significance of differences between sublines by the Mann-Whitney U-test.

Cytostasis in Macrophage Conditioned Media

Activated macrophages release soluble factors that inhibit tumor cell growth by blocking mitochondrial electron transport and cellular respiration [14]. Media conditioned by activated macrophages was obtained as previously described [14]. Briefly, mice were immunized i.p. with 1×10^7 colony-forming units of BCG (*Bacillus calmette guerin*, strain *M. bovis*, Connaught Labs, Toronto, Ontario, Canada), 25 and 4 days before harvesting cells. The resulting plastic nonadherent cells were activated with 50 ng/ml endotoxin and the media conditioned by such cells was stored at $-20°C$ for further use. Macrophage-conditioned media (MCM) was concentrated tenfold by filtration over a YM10 ultrafiltration membrane (Amicon Corp., Lexington, MO) and added to cultures to produce the indicated effective concentration (e.g., 100% concentration was made by adding 0.1 vol of $10\times$ concentrate). These were then added to RAW117 cell cultures, and the effects on cell viability and growth determined [14].

Differentially Expressed RAW117 Genes

Total RNA was prepared from RAW117 cells [18] and the polyadenylated mRNA was separated by oligo(dT)-cellulose (type 30; Collaborative Research, Waltham, MA) chromatography [30]. RNA aliquots were heated at $60°C$ for 10 min, electrophoresed in a 2% agarose gel containing 6 M urea and 25 mM sodium citrate and visualized by staining with 1 μg/ml ethidium bromide for 30 min [31]. RNA was electrotransferred to freshly prepared DBM paper in 50 mM sodium acetate, pH 4.5 [32], and hybridized to plasmids containing specific gene sequences, labeled with ^{32}P-dCTP by the random primer method [33–35]. RNAs on DMB were probed using cloned mitochondrial DNA. RNA blots were prehybridized overnight in 50% formamide, 1% glycine, 0.2% SDS, $5\times$ SSPE (150 mM NaCl, 10 mM $NaH_2PO_4 \cdot H_2O$, 1 mM EDTA, pH 7.4), 100 μg/ml tRNA, and $2\times$ Denhardt's solution (0.02% Ficoll, 0.02% polyvinylpyrrolidone, and 0.02% bovine serum albumin). Hybridization was performed in the same solution as prehybridization except that $2–4 \times 10^7$ cpm of radioactive probe was added. After a 24-hr incubation, the blots were washed 5 times (250 ml each) in $2\times$ standard saline citrate (SSC: 150 mM NaCl, 15 mM sodium citrate, pH 7.0), 0.2% SDS; and five times in $0.1\times$ SSC, 0.1% SDS. The blots were then dried and exposed to Kodak XAR-5 film for 24-48 hr at $-80°C$.

Recombinant mitochondrial DNA clones were established from covalent closed circular DNA isolated from cultured mouse LA9 cells. The purified DNA was cleaved with either *Pst* I or *Hinc* II and recombinants were constructed using the vector pACYC177 [36] and transfected into *Escherichia coli* strain HB101. One of these clones was used in construction of a mitochondrial DNA vector [37]. The original clones were characterized only by their ethidium bromide-stained patterns in agarose gel electrophoresis. The clones have subsequently been confirmed by blot hybridization with nick-translated mouse mitochondrial DNA (D.L. Robberson and H. Eberspracher, unpublished results) and are designated according to an acronym of the restriction fragment they contain as follows: pMt1-Pst-1, pMt1-Pst-2, pMt1-Hnc-1 through pMt1-Hnc-5 in descending order of insert fragment size. We note that these designations are changed from those originally assigned [37]. These probes were synthesized using the random primer method from mouse mitochondrial genome fragments [33]. To make the ND5 gene probe, mitochondrial clone pMt1-Hnc-1 was restricted using *Hind* III and *Xho* I, and the resulting fragments were separated by electrophoresis on a 2.0% agarose gel in TBE (90 mM Tris base, 22 mM boric acid, 1 mM EDTA, pH 8.0) buffer. The band corresponding to gene ND5 was excised and electroeluted using Isco Model 1740 sample concentrators (ISCO, Lincoln, NB) in an

IBI model QSH gel electrophoresis apparatus (IBI Inc., New Haven, CT) as described [38] and the resulting DNA was labeled by the random primer method.

RESULTS
Superinfection of RAW117-H10 Cells

The biological properties of uninfected RAW117 sublines were similar to those previously described [15–18]. Intravenous injection of 5×10^3 RAW117-P cells produced few liver (median = 0) or lung (median = 0) tumor colonies, while RAW117-H10 cells produced large numbers (median > 200) of liver tumor colonies but few (median = 1) lung tumor nodules (Table I). Parallel studies showed that RAW117-H10 cells have a low level of expression of gp70 compared to RAW117-P cells [16,17,22].

To increase the expression of gp70 in low gp70-expressing RAW117-H10 cells we superinfected such cells with endogenous RNA tumor virus obtained from RAW117-P cells. Soon after superinfection, increases in gp70 were not found, but by 9–13 culture passages some superinfected RAW117-H10/P cultures showed increases in gp70 expression (Fig. 1) (the designation "/P" is used to indicate cultures superinfected by virus from the parental cells). In contrast, mock-infected H10 cells did not show increased expression of gp70 (Fig. 1). Superinfected H10/P cells heterogeneously expressed gp70, and cell clones derived from superinfected H10/P cells expressed from relatively low to high levels of gp70 (data not shown). Many cell clones showed substantially increased levels of gp70 with respect to mock-infected H10 cells (Fig. 2). Soon after infection the superinfected H10/P cells with a low expression of gp70 had metastatic properties similar to uninfected H10 cells (median liver tumor nodules > 200) (Table I), while several culture passages later some of the superinfected H10/P cells (e.g., cell line 4) had higher levels of gp70 expression (Fig. 2) and were less metastatic (median liver tumor nodules ~50), while mock-infected H10 cells were highly metastatic, similar to uninfected H10 cells (Table I).

Since H10 cells were found previously to be much less sensitive to activated macrophage-mediated cytolysis and cytotasis [8], we examined the abilities of poly I:C-activated macrophages to inhibit the growth of uninfected, mock-infected, and superinfected H10/P cells. At effector:target ratios > 10 there was little difference in activated macrophage-mediated cytostasis, but at lower effector:target ratios (3 to 7), the superinfected H10/P line 4 cells were significantly ($P < 0.001$) more sensitive to

TABLE I. Properties of Uninfected, Mock-Infected, and RNA Tumor Virus-Superinfected RAW117 Cells

RAW117 subline	Passage No.	Infection	Median liver tumors (range)[a]	Survival[a]
P	10	None	0 (0,5)	10/10
H10	10	None	>200 (>200)	0/10
H10/P(M)[b]	26	Mock infection	>200 (>200)	0/10
H10/P(4)[c]	12	Superinfection	>200 (80, >200)	3/10
H10/P(4)[c]	28	Superinfection	51 (18, >200)	8/10

[a]BALB/c mice (8 week old) were injected intravenously with 5×10^3 viable tumor cells and experimental metastases and survival determined 12 days later.
[b]Mock-infected RAW117-H10 cells from Figure 1.
[c]Line 4 superinfected RAW117-H10 cells from Figure 1.

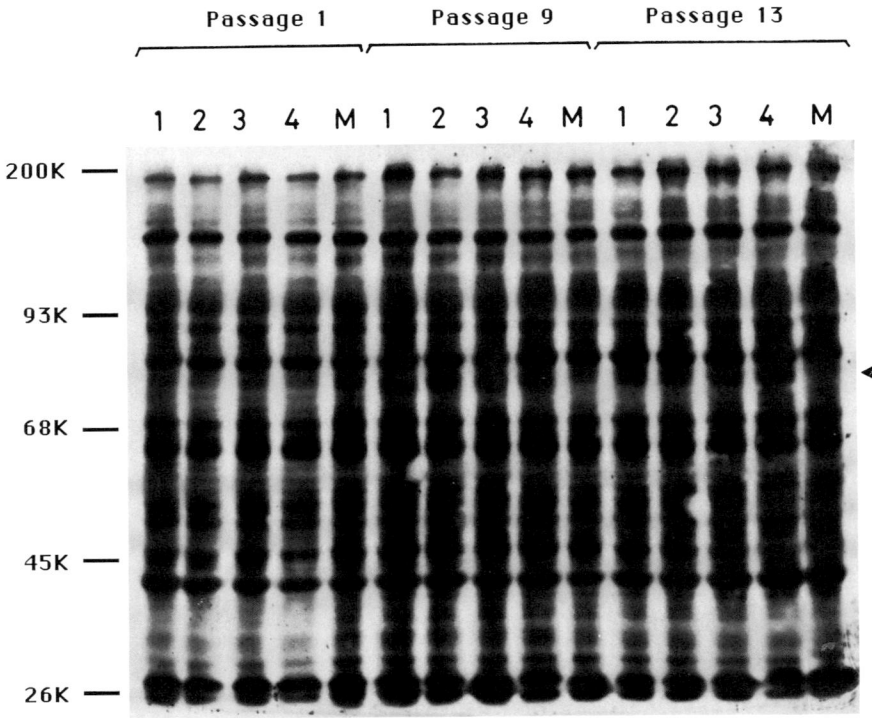

Fig. 1. Cellular levels of viral gp70 in RAW117-H10 cells at various passage numbers with or without endogenous virus superinfection. Superinfection was performed on five cultures of RAW117-H10 cells and electrophoresis, Western blotting, and ^{125}I-Con A staining were performed as described in Materials and Methods. **Lanes 1–4:** Superinfected RAW117-H10 cell lines 1 to 4. **Lane 5 (M):** Mock-infected RAW117-H10 cells. Arrow indicates position of gp70. Molecular weight markers are myosin (M_r ~200,000), phosphorylase b (M_r ~92,500), bovine serum albumin (M_r ~68,000), ovalbumin (M_r ~45,000), and alpha-chymotrypsinogen (M_r ~25,700).

macrophage-mediated growth inhibition (Fig. 3). Mock-infected H10/P cells behaved like uninfected H10 cells in such assays (Fig. 3).

Cytostasis in Macrophage-Conditioned Media

Activated macrophages synthesize and secrete factors that can inhibit tumor cell respiration [14]. By harvesting the culture supernatants of BCG/endotoxin-activated macrophage cultures and adding these to cultures of RAW117 cells, differences in susceptibility to such factors can be demonstrated. Growth rate experiments showed that RAW117-P cells were sensitive in a dose-dependent fashion to growth inhibition by macrophage culture supernatants, but RAW117-H10 cells were relatively resistant (Table II).

Differentially Expressed RAW117 Genes

Previous results indicated differences in gene expression between RAW117-P and -H10 cells [18]. Therefore, we examined some of the differentially expressed RAW117 cell genes to see if they encoded potential target molecules for macrophage cytostatic activities. Since mitochondrial respiration, specifically complexes I and II

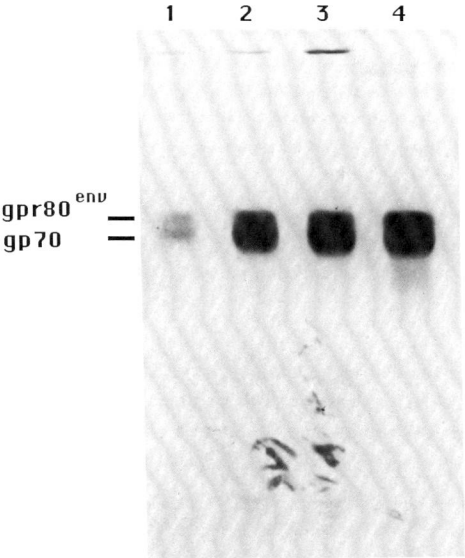

Fig. 2. SDS-PAGE- of RAW117-P, superinfected RAW117-H10, and mock-infected RAW117-H10 cell lysates and anti-gp70 immunoprecipitates. Cells were metabolically labeled with [^{3}H]-leucine and lysed as described in Materials and Methods, and precipitation was performed by adding anti-viral gp70 and protein-A. **Lane 1:** Mock-infected H10 (10 passages). **Lanes 2,3:** H10/P lines 2 and 4 (superinfected with MoMuLV) lines 2 and 4 (10 passages). **Lane 4:** RAW117-P.

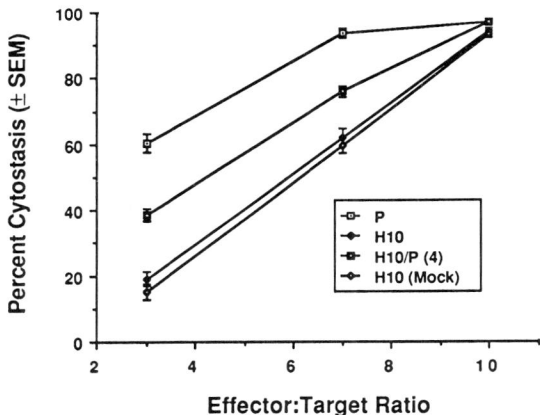

Fig. 3. Sensitivities of RAW117 cells to poly I:C-activated macrophage-mediated cytostasis. Macrophage-mediated cytostasis was performed at various effector:target cell ratios as described in Materials and Methods. At effector:target ratios of 3 and 7, superinfected RAW117-H10/P (line 4) is significantly different ($P < 0.001$) from RAW117-H10 by the Mann-Whitney U-test.

TABLE II. Growth Rates of RAW117-P and H10 Cells in Culture With Media Conditioned by Activated Macrophages

Cells	Effective MCM conc.[a] (%)	Doubling time (hr)
H10	0	9.41 (0.258)[b]
H10	33	11.15 (0.398)
H10	67	14.33 (0.651)
H10	100	15.05 (0.717)
P	0	9.12 (0.268)
P	33	18.81 (1.107)
P	67	30.10 (0.983)
P	100	44.66 (2.390)

[a]Effective concentration of macrophage-conditioned media (MCM) in culture.
[b](SEM).

of the mitochondrial electron transport chain, are the target for a class of macrophage mediators [14,42], we examined mitochondrial gene expression in RAW117-P and -H10 cells using probes derived from the entire mouse mitochondrial genome and portions of the mitochondrial genome. The resulting Northern analyses indicated that a mitochondrial gene, ND5, was expressed at higher levels in H10 than in parental RAW117 cells (Fig. 4). ND5 encodes a subunit of the NADH dehydrogenase of complex I [43,44]. Examination of Northern blots indicates that ND5 is expressed at ~10 times higher levels in H10 than parental cells, while the rest of the structural genes in the mitochondria are expressed at nearly equivalent amounts with the hybridization ratio of H10 to P approximately equal to 1.88 (range 1.2–2.8). Deviation of this ratio from unity is due to imprecision in the amount of RNA loaded on the gel.

DISCUSSION

When RAW117 cells are selected in vivo for enhanced metastatic properties, differences can be found in the cellular properties of the highly metastatic cells [8,13,16–24]. The most dramatic change is in the expression of Moloney leukemia virus-encoded gp70. In addition to in vivo selection for metastasis, highly malignant RAW117 cells have been selected in vitro for decreased binding to immobilized lectins [21], increased partitioning in dextran-polyethylene glycol two-phase systems [23], and increased binding to hepatic endothelial cells (R. Tressler and G.L. Nicolson, in preparation). Selected RAW117 cells and unselected cell clones show a good correlation (r = 0.93) between loss of gp70 and metastatic potential [16]. Highly metastatic RAW117 cells are also significantly less sensitive to activated macrophage-mediated cytolysis and cytostasis [8,13]. If macrophage-mediated effector systems are suppressed in vivo, the metastatic potentials of the low malignant RAW17 sublines are increased dramatically [13], suggesting a relationship between metastasis, gp70 expression, and macrophage-mediated surveillance mechanisms.

We therefore modified RAW117 cell surface gp70 by superinfection with endogenous RNA tumor virus. Superinfection had been used previously to alter the cell

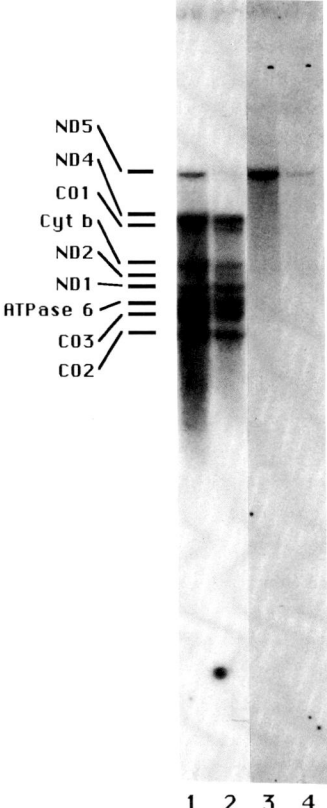

Fig. 4. Blot of RAW117-P and RAW117-H10 poly A+ RNA. **Lane 1:** RAW117-H10 probed with total mitochondrial DNA. **Lane 2:** RAW117-P probed with total mitochondrial DNA. **Lane 3:** RAW117-H10 probed with ND5 specific DNA. **Lane 4:** RAW117-P probed with ND5 specific DNA.

growth, antigenic [39], and malignant [40] properties of rodent cells. By superinfecting highly metastatic low gp70-expressing RAW117-H10 cells with endogeneous RNA tumor virus from some high-expressing low malignant parental cells, we were able to increase gp70 expression and sensitivity to macrophage-mediated cytostasis while lowering metastatic potential in vivo. This suggests that these properties are interrelated and that one of the steps in cytostasis is macrophage recognition of RAW117 cells through a viral-encoded or related structure at the cell surface.

To examine further the mechanism of macrophage-mediated growth inhibition of RAW117 cells, we tested for the ability of activated macrophages to release soluble factors that could differentially affect RAW117 cells [14,41,42]. We found that soluble factors from activated macrophages that are capable of inhibiting the respiration of tumor cells can inhibit significantly the growth of RAW117-P cells, but have little effect on highly metastatic RAW117-H10 cells. These factors are now being purified and characterized, and they have in common the ability to inhibit tumor cell respiration by blocking mitochondrial electron transport systems [14,42].

Previously we found that highly metastatic RAW117-H10 cells express differentially only a few genes compared to low metastatic RAW117-P cells [18]. We have identified one of these differentially expressed genes as a subunit of NADH dehydrogenase of complex I of the mitochondrial electron transport chain, the target for a macrophage-released cytostatic factor called respiration-inhibiting factor (RIF) [14,29,41,42]. The overexpression of mitochondrial gene ND5 could be related to the ability of H10 cells to escape macrophage-mediated cytostasis, but support for this notion must await further studies on the role of RIF-like molecules in inhibiting the respiration and growth of RAW117 cells.

The limitations in our studies are that the data are correlative and do not definitively prove that gp70 and electron transport components are directly involved in RAW117 cell escape from macrophage surveillance mechanisms. Additional experiments, such as blocking the ability of macrophage cytostatic molecules to bind to RAW117 cells and demonstrating that increased levels of mitochondrial NADH dehydrogenase or other complex I or II components can overcome the cytostatic action of molecules like RIF, will be necessary. Preliminary experiments indicate that there are differences in the steady-state levels of mitochondrial proteins in RAW117-P and -H10 cells, including those thought to be involved in electron transport. Further research should determine whether overproduction of specific respiration components can allow malignant cells to circumvent the action of molecules such as RIF.

Our studies suggest that highly metastatic RAW117 cells may be altered in several characteristics that allow these cells to disseminate and survive at secondary organ sites. In addition to the ability of highly metastatic RAW117 cells to escape host surveillance mechanisms, they also have the characteristics to adhere better to target organ sites [24] and respond differentially to paracrine growth factors released from different organs [45]. Collectively, these properties probably allow highly malignant RAW117-H10 cells to metastasize to liver with high efficiencies.

These studies were supported by National Cancer Institute Grant R01-CA29571 and R35-CA44352 (OIG) (to G.L.N.), R01-CA39319 (to T.I.), R23-CA39802 (to G.E.G.) and ACS IM-419 (to J.K.).

REFERENCES

1. Nicolson GL: Biochim Biophys Acta 695:113, 1982.
2. Nicolson GL, Poste G: Curr Probl Cancer 7(7):1, 1983.
3. North SM, Nicolson GL: In Herberman R, Wiltrout R, Gorelik E (eds): "Host Responses to Metastasis." Boca Raton, Florida: CRC Press, Inc., 1987, pp 1–22.
4. Nicolson GL: Exp Cell Res 150:3, 1984.
5. Turner GA: Invasion Metastasis 2:197, 1982.
6. Schirrmacher V: Adv Cancer Res 43:1, 1985.
7. Miner KM, Klostergaard J, Granger GA, Nicolson GL: J Natl Cancer Inst 70:717, 1983.
8. Miner KM, Nicolson GL: Cancer Res 43:2063, 1983.
9. North SM, Nicolson GL: Cancer Res 45:1453, 1985.
10. Pal K, Koppa L, Timor J, Rajnai J, Lopez K: Invasion Metastasis 5:159, 1985.
11. Yamashima K, Fulton A, Heppner G: J Natl Cancer Inst 75:765, 1985.
12. Schirrmacher V, Applehaus B: Clin Exp Metastasis 3:29, 1985.
13. Reading CL, Kramer PM, Miner KM, Nicolson GL: Clin Exp Metastasis 1:135, 1983.
14. Kilbourn RG, Klostergaard J, Lopez-Berestein G: Immunol 133:2577, 1984.
15. Brunson KW, Nicolson GL: J Natl Cancer Inst 61:1499, 1978.
16. Nicolson GL, Mascali JJ, McGuire EJ: Oncodev Biol Med 4:149, 1982.
17. Reading CL, Brunson KW, Torriani M, Nicolson GL: Proc Natl Acad Sci USA 77:5943, 1980.
18. Nicolson GL, LaBiche RA, Frazier ML, Blick M, Tressler RJ, Irimura T, Rotter V: J Cell Biochem 31:305, 1986.

19. Nicolson GL, Reading CL, Brunson KW: In Crispen RG (ed): "Tumor Progression." Amsterdam: Elsevier North-Holland, Inc., 1980, pp 31–48.
20. Irimura T, Tressler RJ, Nicolson GL: Exp Cell Res 165:403, 1986.
21. Reading CL, Belloni PN, Nicolson GL: J Natl Cancer Inst 64:1241, 1980.
22. Yoshida M, Gallick G, Irimura T, Nicolson GL: Cancer Res 47:2558, 1987.
23. Miner KM, Walter H, Nicolson GL: Biochemistry 20:6244, 1981.
24. McGuire EJ, Mascali JJ, Grady SR, Nicolson GL: Clin Exp Metastasis 2:213, 1984.
25. Wong PK, Gallick GE: Virology 25:187, 1978.
26. Naso RB, Arcement LJ, Arlinghaus RB: Cell 4:31, 1975.
27. Towbin H, Staehelin T, Gordon J: Proc Natl Acad Sci Usa 76:4350, 1979.
28. Geramin RN, Williams RM, Benacerrof B: J Natl Cancer Inst 54:709, 1975.
29. Hibbs JB, Jr, Lambert LH, Jr, Remington JS: Science 117:998, 1982.
30. Aviv H, Leder P: Proc Natl Acad Sci USA 69:1408, 1972.
31. Rosen JM, Woo SM, Holder JW, Means AR, O'Mally BW: Biochemistry 14:69, 1975.
32. Alwine J, Kamp D, Stark G: Proc Natl Acad Sci USA 74:5350, 1977.
33. Feinberg AP, Vogelstein B: Anal Biochem 132:6, 1983.
34. Rotter V, Wolf D, Nicolson GL: Clin Exp Metastasis 2:199, 1984.
35. Rigby PW, Dieckmann M, Rhodes C, Berg P: J Mol Biol 113:237, 1977.
36. Chang ACY, Cohen SN: J Bacteriol 134:1141, 1978.
37. Manire MK, Legerski RJ, Robberson DL: Second Annual Congress on Recombinant DNA Research, Los Angeles, CA, 1982.
38. Zassenhaus HP, Butow RA, Hannon YD: Anal Biochem 125:125, 1982.
39. Todaro GJ, Habel K, Green H: Virology 27:179, 1965.
40. Vesely P, Wyke J, Kren V: Folia Biol (Prague) 28:185, 1982.
41. Granger GA, Taintor RR, Cook JL, Hibbs JB, Jr: J Clin Invest 65:357, 1980.
42. Granger GA, Lehninger AL: J Cell Biol 95:527, 1982.
43. Chomyn A, Marriottini P, Cleeter MWJ, Ragan CI, Matsuno-Yagi A, Hatefi Y, Doolittle RF, Attardi G: Nature 314:592, 1985.
44. Mariottini P, Chomyn A, Riley M, Cottrell B, Doolittle RF, Attardi G: Proc Natl Acad Sci USA 83:1563, 1986.
45. Nicolson GL: Exp Cell Res 168:572–577, 1987.

Increased Content of Chondroitin Sulfate Proteoglycan in Human Colorectal Carcinoma Metastases Compared With the Primary Tumor as Determined by an Anti-Chondroitin-Sulfate Monoclonal Antibody

Takao Yamori, David M. Ota, Karen R. Cleary, and Tatsuro Irimura

Departments of Tumor Biology (T.Y., T.I.), Surgery (D.M.O.), and Pathology (K.R.C.), The University of Texas M.D. Anderson Hospital and Tumor Institute at Houston, Houston, Texas 77030

To determine if the amount of chondroitin sulfate proteoglycan (CSPG) in human colorectal tumor tissue correlates with the tumor's aggressiveness we immunochemically determined the CSPG levels in colorectal carcinomas at different stages. A total of 50 specimens—4 polyps, 15 stage B tumors, 9 stage C tumors, 12 stage D tumors, 7 liver metastases, and 3 lymph node metastases—were examined. Tumor tissues were extracted with 4 M guanidine hydrochloride containing protease inhibitors. The extracts were serially diluted and blotted onto nitrocellulose membranes. Reactivity of a chondroitin sulfate-specific mouse monoclonal antibody (CS-56) was determined by biotinylated goat antimouse Ig and avidin-biotin-peroxidase complex. After comparing tissues from tumors at different stages (classified by the presence or absence of metastasis), we could not find a positive or negative correlation between the amount of CSPG in primary colorectal carcinoma tissues and the tumor's metastatic potential. However, the metastatic foci in the liver or lymph node contained higher amounts of CSPG than the primary tumors did. Immunohistochemical staining of colon carcinoma tissue with CS-56 revealed that CSPG is predominantly localized in fibrotic portions in the tumor tissues. Two-year follow-up studies indicated that a high level of CSPG in primary tumors was not predictive of recurrence.

Key words: human colorectal cancer, metastasis, chondroitin sulfate proteoglycan, dot-blot analysis

The prognosis for cancer is often directly related to the presence or absence of metastases. This is particularly true of colorectal cancer, in which the five-year survival rate is greater than 60% for patients with localized disease (Dukes' stage B)

Received May 18, 1987; revised and accepted September 11, 1987.

© 1988 Alan R. Liss, Inc.

and smaller than 5% for those with disseminated metastases (Dukes' stage D) [1,2]. Dukes' classification system is a good indicator of survival [3,4]; however, stage of disease is not sufficient for prediction of recurrence or development of metastasis in individual patients, especially in those without apparent metastases at the time of surgical removal of primary colorectal tumors. The search for a specific marker for those tumor cells most likely to metastasize may lead to the development of a new prognostic indicator.

Recent work with experimental animals has shown that highly metastatic tumor cells have a variety of specific biochemical properties different from those of normal cells, e.g., cell surface glycoproteins [4–6], cell adhesiveness [7,8], specific enzymes for the degradation of basement membranes, and extracellular constituents [8–10]. However, little is known about biochemical properties associated specifically with human colorectal carcinoma cells having higher metastatic potentials. We were interested in examining if biochemical changes known to occur on cell surface and extracellular molecules during malignant transformation also influence the metastatic potential of colorectal cancer. We have already shown that the expression of high molecular weight fucosylated glycoproteins in the distal colon and rectum [11] and sulfated glycoproteins [12] tends to decrease upon progression of carcinomas. On the other hand, we have found that collagenolytic activity of human colorectal carcinoma is not related to the stage of disease [13].

Proteoglycans are major constituents of the connective tissue stroma of most organs and are involved in tissue organization and other biological processes, such as cell proliferation and migration [14–16]. Altered levels of proteoglycan production and release and changes in the structure of glycosaminoglycan chains have been reported in a variety of transformed cells and tumor tissues [17,18]. Increased production of chondroitin sulfate proteoglycan (CSPG) has been reported in transformed fibroblasts [19] and hepatocytes [20] as well as in more tumorigenic melanoma and mammary carcinoma [21,22]. Iozzo et al. recently demonstrated an increased amount of CSPG in human colon carcinoma tissues compared with normal colonic epithelium [23]. Iozzo has also shown that colon carcinoma cells produce factors that stimulate the production of CSPG by colonic fibroblast cells in culture [24]. Such a tumor cell–host interaction comparable with desmoplastic response may influence the metastatic propensity of tumors [25]. However, correlation of proteoglycan alterations in colorectal carcinoma tissues with the tumor's metastatic potential has not been shown.

We have demonstrated by metabolic ^{35}S labeling and biochemical analysis of sulfated glycoconjugates that the production of sulfomucin by colorectal carcinoma decreases during the tumor's progression and metastasis [12]. The amount of sulfated proteoglycans slightly increases at the same time. Since this proteoglycan consists mainly of CSPG, we focused on CSPG as a potential marker of human colorectal carcinoma metastasis. We measured the amount of CSPG in the extracts of colorectal tumors at different stages by using an anti-chondroitin-sulfate monoclonal antibody (CS-56) [26]. After examining the amount of CSPG in colorectal primary carcinomas that did or did not metastasize and comparing the amount of CSPG in primary carcinoma with that in metastasis, we could not find a correlation between the content of CSPG in the bulk of primary colorectal carcinoma and its aggressiveness or metastatic potential.

MATERIALS AND METHODS

Selection of Patients and Staging

Patients with histologically proven polyps and adenocarcinoma of the colon and rectum were selected for this study. Those who had undergone previous radiotherapy or chemotherapy or who had had colon carcinoma previously were excluded. Staging was based on the Dukes' classification system [3].

Specimen Processing

Tumor specimens of approximately 0.5–1.0 g were obtained from the intraluminal edge of colorectal tumors. Specimens of liver and lymph node metastases from colorectal carcinoma were obtained when available. The surface portion of the metastasis was removed to eliminate the possible influence of fibrotic tissues on the analytical data. Necrotic portions of the tumors also were excluded. Tumor tissues were immediately frozen in liquid nitrogen and stored at $-70°C$ until use. Thirty milligrams of the tissue was minced and mixed with 300 μl of proteoglycan extracting buffer (PG buffer) containing 4 M guanidine-HCl, 4% Zwittergent 3–12 (Calbiochem Behring, La Jolla, CA), 0.1 M sodium acetate buffer (pH 6.0), and protease inhibitors [10 mM ethylenediaminetetraacetate, 10 mM benzamidine (Sigma Chemical Co., St. Louis, MO), 25 mM ϵ-aminocaproic acid (Sigma), 5 mM phenylmethylsulfonylfluoride (Sigma), 10 μg/ml N-tosyl-L-phenylalanine chloromethyl ketone, 10 μg/ml Nα-P-tosyl-L-lysine chloromethyl ketone (Sigma), 20 mU/ml aprotinin (Sigma), and 2 mM N-ethylmaleimide (Sigma)]. After ultrasonication on ice for 10 sec (Ultrasonic Cell Disrupter, Heat System Ultrasonics, Inc., Farmingdale, NY), the mixture was incubated on ice for 18 hr with occasional gentle mixing. Supernatant was collected by centrifugation at 13,000g for 10 min. Protein concentration was determined by the method of Lowry et al. [27].

Preparation of ^{35}S-sulfated Proteoglycans

A ^{35}S-sulfated proteoglycan fraction was prepared from colon carcinoma tissue as described below and used to assess whether dot-blot analysis could be employed for the measurement of proteoglycans. One hundred milligrams of fresh tumor obtained from a 73-yr-old man with stage C sigmoid colon adenocarcinoma was rinsed with Dulbecco's phosphate-buffered saline (DPBS) containing 50 units/ml of penicillin, 50 μg streptomycin, and 1.25 μg/ml of amphotericin B; minced with scalpel blade into small pieces; and incubated in 1 ml of a one-to-one mixture of Dulbecco's modified Eagle's medium and Ham's F12 medium containing 10% fetal bovine serum, 50 units/ml of penicillin, 50 μg/ml streptomycin, 1.25 μg/ml of amphotericin B, and 50 μCi/ml of [^{35}S]Na$_2$SO$_4$ under humidified conditions in 5% CO$_2$ at 37°C for 48 hr. The tissue was removed by centrifugation, and ^{35}S-sulfated materials were extracted with 1 ml of PG buffer as described above. The extract was applied to a Sephadex PD-10 column (Pharmacia Fine Chemicals, Piscataway, NJ) equilibrated with 50 mM sodium acetate buffer (pH 6.0) containing 50 mM NaCl, 8 M urea, 1 mM phenylmethylsulfonylfluoride, and 0.02 U/ml of aprotinin and eluted with the same buffer. Each 0.1-ml fraction was collected, and radioactivity was measured after small aliquots of each fraction were mixed with Liquiscint (National Diagnostics, Somerville, NJ). Radioactive materials eluted at the void volume fractions were pooled and diluted with nine parts per volume of 8 M urea containing buffer A [50 mM sodium acetate buffer (pH 6.0), 50 mM NaCl, and 0.2% CHAPS] and then applied to a DEAE-Sephacel column (1.2 × 3 cm) equilibrated with the same buffer. The column was washed with about 20 ml of buffer A, and the ^{35}S-sulfated molecules were eluted first with 10 ml buffer B of [0.1 M acetate buffer (pH 6.0), 0.2 M NaCl in 8 M urea, and 0.2% CHAPS] and second with buffer C [15 ml of 0.23 M acetate buffer (pH 6.0), 0.5 M NaCl in 8 M urea, and 0.2% CHAPS]. Radioactivity in each 1-ml effluent fraction was measured. The fractions eluted with buffers B (peak I) and C (peak II) were respectively pooled, dialyzed against distilled water, and lyophilized. Peak I was mostly sulfated mucin, and peak II was proteoglycans including chondroitin sulfate and heparan sulfate as major components [12].

Recovery of Proteoglycans After Transfer Onto Nitrocellulose Membrane Under Various Conditions

Proteoglycans labeled with ^{35}S from 100-mg tumor tissue samples were dissolved in 0.5 ml of distilled water and used for testing recovery of these molecules after blotting onto nitrocellulose membranes. Five-microliter aliquots of ^{35}S-labeled proteoglycans were mixed with 95 µl of 6 M urea, 1% CHAPS, and 4 M guanidine-HCl containing 0.1 M sodium acetate (pH 6.0), 2% sodium dodecyl sulfate (SDS), or 90% ethanol and blotted onto a nitrocellulose membrane on Hybri Dot (Bethesda Research Laboratories, Inc., Gaithersburg, MD) under moderate negative pressure generated by water aspirator. After being rinsed in DPBS each dot was separated and incubated in 0.5 ml of NCS (Amersham Corp., Arlington Heights, IL) at 37°C for 18 hr. The samples were then mixed with 10 ml of Liquiscint (National Diagnostics) and their radioactivity was measured by a 1214 RACKBETA liquid scintillation counter (LKB Instruments, Gaithersburg, MD).

In order to test the effect of the protein concentration of the samples on the recovery of proteoglycans on nitrocellulose membranes, an extract prepared from tumor tissue derived from a 60-yr-old woman with Duke's stage D sigmoid colon adenocarcinoma was diluted with 4 M guanidine-HCl containing 0.1 M sodium acetate (pH 6.0) into different concentrations (7.4–0.12 mg protein/ml). A fixed amount of radiolabeled proteoglycans (2,000 cpm) was added to each diluted extract (100 µl), which was then transferred onto a nitrocellulose membrane and processed as described above.

Chondroitinase ABC Treatment of Tumor Tissue

To confirm the specificity of the antibody in our experimental system, an extract from a chrondroitinase avidin-biotin-peroxidase complex (ABC)-treated tissue was prepared. Thirty milligrams of fresh liver metastasis tissue obtained from a 58-yr-old woman with colon carcinoma was rinsed with DPBS, minced, and incubated at 37°C for 18 hr with 2 U/ml of chondroitinase ABC (ICN Radiochemicals, Irvine, CA) in 1 ml of 50 mM Tris-HCl (pH 8.0) containing 60 mM sodium acetate, 50 mM NaCl, 0.01% bovine serum albumin (BSA), 0.02% sodium azide, and 2 mM phenylmethyl-sulfonylfluoride. Control samples were incubated without chondroitinase ABC. After incubation, tumor tissues were removed by centrifugation at 13,000g for 10 min and extracted with 300 µl of PG buffer as described above. The extracts were diluted, transferred to a nitrocellulose membrane, and allowed to react with anti-chondroitin-sulfate monoclonal antibody as described below.

Semiquantitative Determination of CSPG in Tissue Extracts by Monoclonal Antibody CS-56

The anti-chondroitin-sulfate IgM monoclonal antibody CS-56 was kindly supplied by Dr. Benjamin Geiger (Department of Chemical Immunology, The Weizmann Institute of Science, Rehovot, Israel). The nature of this antibody has been described by Avnur and Geiger in detail elsewhere [26]. The tumor extracts were serially diluted twice with 4 M guanidine-HCl containing 0.1 M sodium acetate (pH 6.0) and blotted onto nitrocellulose membranes. The membranes were rinsed in phosphate-buffered saline (PBS), incubated in PBS containing 2% normal goat serum at 25°C for 18 hr, and allowed to react with 200 µg/ml of CS-56 at 25°C for 1 hr. The membranes were washed in PBS for 1 hr, allowed to react with biotinylated antimouse IgM (Vector Laboratories, Burlingame, CA), diluted in PBS containing 1% BSA, washed in PBS for 1 hr, and allowed to react first with ABC-peroxidase reagent (Vector Labs) and then with 4-chloro-1-naphthol as peroxidase substrates. The maximum dilution of the antibody to give visible reactivity (i.e., Fig. 1, row a, dot 6) was recorded as titration score.

Immunohistochemical Localization of CSPG

Immunohistochemical localization of CSPG was studied with a primary adenocarcinoma of left colon and liver metastasis from a 52-yr-old man. Four-micron sections were made from a formalin-fixed and paraffin-embedded permanent pathological specimen. The sections were treated with 0.2% hydrogen peroxide to destroy endogeneous peroxidase, rehydrated, presoaked with 5% BSA (RIA grade) in PBS overnight at 4°C, and reacted with CS-56 (200 µg/ml diluted in 1% BSA) for 1 hr. The sections were then processed under the same conditions as dot-blot assay described above, except that 3,3'-diaminobenzidine were used for a peroxidase substrate.

RESULTS
Optimal Conditions for Dot-Blot Analysis of Proteoglycans

We have recently shown that colon tumor tissue synthesizes two different classes of sulfated macromolecules (slightly acidic peak I and highly acidic peak II) in vitro, which were separated by DEAE-Sephacel ion-exchange chromatography [12]. The less acidic peak I was sulfated mucin, and highly acidic peak II was proteoglycans

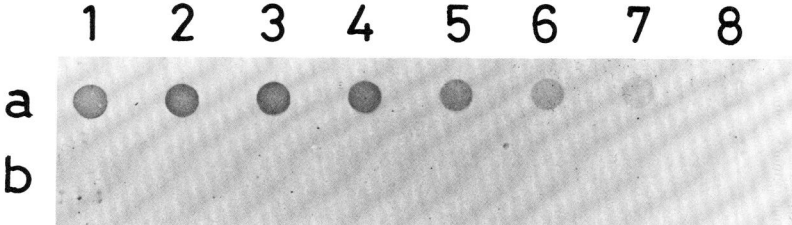

Fig. 1. Effect of the absence (**a**) or presence (**b**) of chondroitinase ABC treatment on the reactivity of CS-56 to tissue extract. Thirty milligrams of fresh tumor tissue obtained from colon carcinoma metastasis was incubated with or without chondroitinase ABC and extracted with 10 volumes of PG buffer, blotted onto a nitrocellulose membrane, and allowed to react with CS-56 as described in Materials and Methods. The starting concentration of the extracts in the twofold dilution was 0.25 mg protein/ml.

containing chondroitin sulfate and heparan sulfate [12]; [^{35}S]-sulfate-labeled proteoglycans (2,000 cpm/ml) were used to compare their binding to nitrocellulose membrane under the different conditions described below. Radiolabeled proteoglycans were dissolved or uniformly suspended in 6 M urea, 1% CHAPS, 4 M guanidine-HCl, and 2% SDS or 90% ethanol, and 100 µl of each sample was blotted onto nitrocellulose membranes. The 4 M guanidine-HCl containing 0.1 M sodium acetate (pH 6.0) allowed maximum binding of proteoglycans to nitrocellulose membranes (60% of input radioactivity). Other allowed less than 20% binding efficiency, so 4 M guanidine-HCl was used thereafter for the dot-blot analysis of proteoglycans. To examine the effect of protein concentration on the efficiency of dot-blot analysis of proteoglycans, we diluted the extract to different concentrations (7.4–0.12 mg protein/ml) with 4 M guanidine-HCl. Radiolabeled proteoglycans were added to the various dilutions of the tumor extracts and blotted. The bound radioactivities were 5, 26, 44, and 47% of total at concentrations of 7.4, 0.93, 0.46, and 0.12 mg protein/ml, respectively. The maximum binding of radiolabeled proteoglycans was observed at a protein concentration of 0.12 mg/ml. The binding efficiency was extremely low at protein concentrations more than 1 mg/ml. As protein concentration decreased, the binding efficiency of proteoglycans appeared to increase, reaching a plateau at protein concentrations ranging between 0.12 and 0.42 mg/ml. Therefore, the dot-blot analyses of proteoglycans described below were done with protein concentrations of less than 0.25 mg/ml.

Specificity of CS-56

The monoclonal antibody CS-56 used in the present study was directed to chondroitin sulfate [26]. Its specificity was confirmed by the results shown in Figure 1. The CS-56 reacted to colon tumor extract blotted onto a nitrocellulose membrane (Fig. 1, row a), but the reactivity was completely eliminated when the tumor tissue had been treated with chondroitinase ABC, which degrades chondroitin 4- and 6-sulfates, prior to extraction (Fig. 1, row b).

Semiquantitative Determination of CSPG in Colorectal Carcinoma Tissues at Different Stages

Extracts were prepared from four polyps, 36 primary colorectal carcinoma tissues, and ten metastases at a ratio of 100 mg wet tissue/10 ml buffer. The protein concentration of these extracts ranged between 12.0 and 20.4 mg/ml and thus we diluted them with the same buffer to 0.25 mg/ml. The extracts were serially diluted twofold and blotted onto nitrocellulose membranes. The samples were allowed to react with CS-56 and were immunochemically stained and the titration score was recorded (Fig. 2). The reactivity of primary cancer tissue extracts to this antibody varied from one specimen to another and seemed slightly higher in stage C and D tumors than in stage B disease. However, there was no statistically significant correlation between antibody reactivity and the stage of colorectal carcinomas. The reactivity of metastases to this antibody was compared with that of the corresponding primary carcinoma tissues (Fig. 3); the metastases appeared to contain slightly greater amounts of CSPG than the primary carcinomas from which they were derived ($P < .027$).

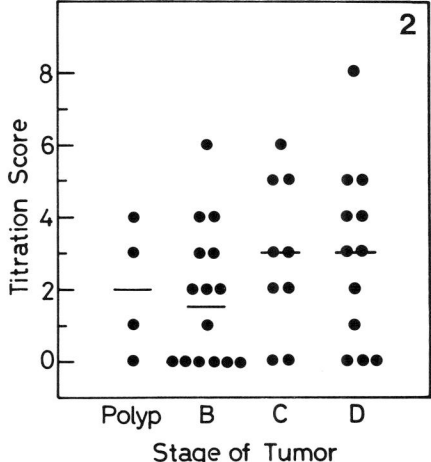

Fig. 2. Amount of CSPG in the extracts of tumors at different stages as determined by CS-56. Tumor extracts were prepared, blotted onto nitrocellulose membranes, allowed to react with CS-56, and scored as described in Materials and Methods. The starting concentration of the extracts in the twofold dilution was 0.25 mg protein/ml. Staging was based on the Dukes' classification system [3]. In case the first well showed no reactivity, the titration score of the extract was defined as 0. Bars show the mean volumes of the scores.

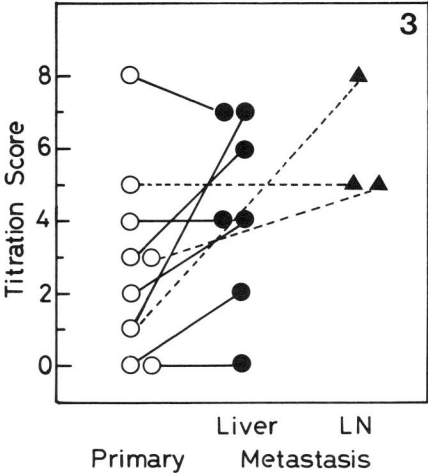

Fig. 3. Differences between CSPG content in primary tumor and in metastasis. The CSPG content in extracts from metastases was compared to those from the corresponding primary tumors. Experimental conditions were the same as those described in the legend for Figure 2. ○, primary tumor; ●, liver metastasis; and ▲, lymph node (LN) metastasis. The corresponding primary tumor and metastasis were tied with a solid line (liver metastasis) or a dotted line (lymph node metastasis) (P < .027 by Wilcoxon signed-rank test).

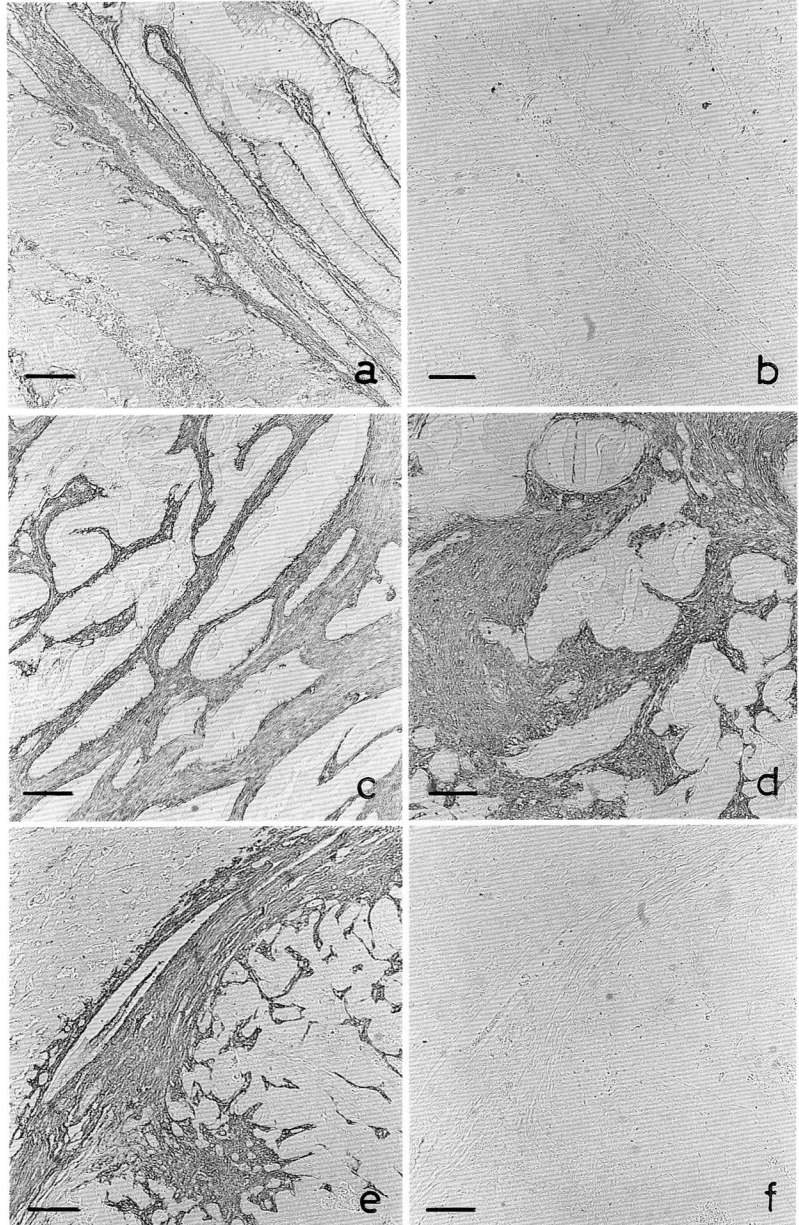

Fig. 4. Immunohistochemical localization of CSPG. Adenocarcinoma of left colon and liver metastasis from a 52-yr-old man was used. **a**: Superficial portion of primary carcinoma stained with CS-56 followed by biotinylated goat antimouse IgG and avidin-biotinyl peroxidase complex; 3,3′-diaminobenzidine was used as a substrate. Positive staining is seen associated with fibrotic tissues in carcinoma and adjacent colonic mucosa. **b**: Another serial section stained under the same condition as a except that CS-56 was omitted. **c**: Deep portion of the same tumor stained with CS-56. This antibody binds predominantly to desmoplastic portions in carcinoma tissue. CSPG is apparently produced by host-derived cells in the fibrotic tissues. **d**: Hepatic metastasis from the same patient. CS-56 bound to fibrotic tissues, which appeared more extensively than in the primary tumor. **e**: Border of liver metastatic tumor and adjacent liver tissue (top left). **f**: The same field in another serial section processed without CS-56. Bars indicate 100 µm.

Immunohistochemical Localization of CSPG in Colorectal Carcinoma Tissues Using CS-56

Immunohistochemical localization of CS-56 was studied with tissue sections of primary adenocarcinoma of left colon and hepatic metastasis. CSPG localized in lamina propria in colonic mucosa adjacent to carcinoma tissues (top right, Fig. 4a). In carcinoma tissues adjacent to normal mucosa desmoplastic response was not extensive, and weak CS-56 reactivity was seen (bottom left, Fig. 4a). On the other hand, at the deep portion of the same tumor, extensive desmoplasia was observed, and CS-56 bound to these fibrotic tissues (Fig. 4c). Extensive desmoplasia was also seen associated with hepatic metastasis from the same patient (Fig. 4d,e). These results clearly indicated that CSPG is predominantly localized in fibrotic tissues in colorectal carcinomas and that there was a intratumoral heterogeneity in CSPG contents.

Patient Follow-Up

Recurrence of colorectal cancer within 2 yr after the initial surgery was followed up for those patients classified as stage B or C. The status was available for 19 patients. Figure 5 shows the amount of CSPG in primary tumors using CS-56. Three patients died of recurrence with liver metastasis. The CSPG contents of the primary tumors of these patients having recurrence were not significantly different from those who were disease-free for 2 yr.

DISCUSSION

Proteoglycans are considered to be dynamic components that influence fundamental biological processes including cellular proliferation, recognition, and differentiation. Changes in proteoglycan production by tumor cells have been suggested to be related to tumorigenicity, disease progression, and metastasis [18,28,29]. In-

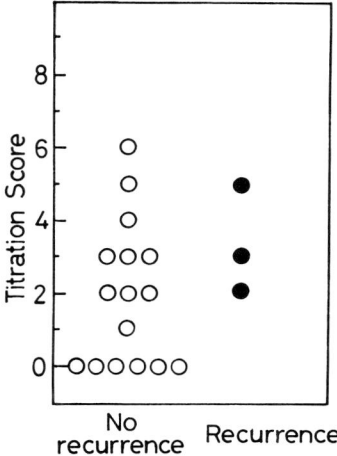

Fig. 5. Two-year follow up of those patients diagnosed as stage B or C at the time of surgery of the primary tumors. The titration scores with CS-56 were plotted according to the clinical status of the patients.

creased amounts of CSPG have been reported in carcinomas of the lung [30,31], liver [32,33], prostate [34], and colon [23,35,36]. Chondroitin sulfate is also known to stimulate the growth of mammary carcinoma cells in vitro [37], of Ehrlich ascites tumor cells in vivo [38], and of chondroitinase to inhibit the growth of Ehrlich ascites tumor cells [39]. This evidence indicates significant involvement of CSPG in malignant transformation and progression. However, little is known regarding the importance of CSPG production in determining the metastatic potential of human tumors in vivo or its potential use as a prognostic marker.

We have been interested in elucidating the determinants of colorectal cancer metastases. We have previously shown that there is no correlation between size of the primary colorectal carcinoma and the stage of disease as classified by the presence of metastasis [40]. Therefore, primary colorectal carcinomas at different stages should contain tumor cells that express cellular or extracellular phenotypes related to different metastatic potentials. Production of CSPG might be one of these phenotypes.

We recently analyzed metabolically labeled $[^{35}S]$-sulfated macromolecules of human colorectal carcinoma and showed that metastases produce slightly higher amounts of $[^{35}\text{-}S]$-labeled proteoglycans than the primary tumors do when CSPG accounted for approximately 50% of the radioactivity in the primary carcinomas [12]. In this study the amount of CSPG detected by CS-56 in tumor tissue extracts did not differ with the stages of the tumor. Although the amount of CSPG tended to be slightly higher in stage C and D tumors than in stage B tumors, the differences were not statistically significant. On the other hand, we observed higher amounts of chondroitin sulfate detected by CS-56 in metastases than in primary carcinoma tissues. It is not known whether these differences were due to the selective colonization of colorectal carcinoma cells having higher capacity to stimulate CSPG production by the host tissue or to the stimulation of CSPG production by the different host tissue microenvironment. Also, it remains possible that the portion of primary tumors responsible for producing metastases was a small fraction, and the analysis of randomly taken tumor tissues from the superficial edges did not reflect the phenotypes related to the formation of metastases. In such an event, even if there had been a higher content of CSPG in the portion of tumors responsible for the metastasis formation, that content would have been diluted by the noncontributing population. Therefore, we have studied histochemical localization of CS-56 using peroxidase methods (Fig. 4). In carcinoma tissues, CS-56–positive sites were seen associated with extracellular fibrotic portions which was more extensively developed in the invasive edge of the primary tumors and metastasis (Fig. 4). As an additional method, we also used high iron diamine (HID) staining [41] in combination with chondroitinase ABC treatment to localize CSPG in histological sections of formalin-fixed tumor tissues, which gave a similar result. The results clearly show that there was an intratumoral heterogeneity in CSPG contents. Whether they reflect heterogeneous tumor cell populations, and whether one of these subpopulations is responsible for the formation of metastasis, remain to be answered.

Our study is based on semiquantitative dot-blot assay of CSPG in guanidine-HCl extracts. Preliminary attempts to use other methods in immunochemical measurement of CSPG using CS-56 were not successful. For example, binding assay with enzyme-linked second antibody or radiolabeled second antibody could not be applied because we could not quantitatively immobilize CSPG extracted from tumor tissues on plastic plates. Guanidine-HCl extraction which was suitable for quantitative solubilization of CSPG from tissues followed by dot-blot analysis in the same solution gave highly reproducible and quantitative recovery of ^{35}S-labeled materials from colorectal carcinoma tissues.

In conclusion, we compared the amount of CSPG measured using CS-56 extracts from primary colorectal carcinoma tissue at different Dukes' stages. The amount of CSPG in the primary carcinoma did not correlate with presence or absence of metastasis. On the other hand, the amount in metastases was significantly higher than the amount in primary tumor tissues. Although CSPG appeared to be an extracellular component of host origin as shown in Figure 4 and as previously described [18,24], this molecule may play a functionally important role in determining metastasis. As an example, histological observation indicated that vascular invasion as well as liver colonization of colon carcinoma were accomplished not by a single cell but as aggregates possibly including host-derived stromal constituents [42].

ACKNOWLEDGMENTS

This work has been supported by United States Public Health Service grant RO1-CA39319. We thank Dr. Garth L. Nicolson for suggestions and encouragement on this work; Dr. Benjamin Geiger for his generous gift of the monoclonal antibody CS-56; Eleanor Felonia, Susan Lyman, and Debora A. Carlson for their help in preparation of this manuscript; and Tania Busch for her help in the preparation of illustrations.

REFERENCES

1. Olson RM, Perencevich NP, Malcolm AW, Chaffey JT, Wilson RE: Cancer 45:2969, 1980.
2. Eisenberg B, DeCosse JI, Hartford F, Michalek J: Cancer 49:1131, 1982.
3. Dukes CE: J Pathol Bacteriol 35:323, 1932.
4. Nicolson GL: Biochim Biphys Acta 695:113, 1982.
5. Irimura T, Nicolson GL: Cancer Res 94:791, 1984.
6. Nicolson GL: Exp Cell Res 150:3, 1986.
7. Irimura T, Gonzalez R, Nicolson GL: Cancer Res 41:3411, 1981.
8. Irimura T, Nakajima M, Nicolson GL: Gann Monogr 29:35, 1983.
9. Liotta LA, Thorgeirsson UP, Garbisa S: Cancer Metastasis Rev 1:277, 1982.
10. Nakajima M, Irimura T, Di Ferrante N, Nicolson GL: J Biol Chem 259:2283, 1984.
11. Irimura T, Ota DM, Cleary KR: Cancer Res 47:881, 1987.
12. Yamori T, Kimura H, Stewart K, Ota DM, Cleary KR, Irimura T: Cancer Res 47:2741, 1987.
13. Irimura T, Yamori T, Bennett SC, Ota DM, Cleary KR: Int J Cancer 40:24, 1987.
14. Hay ED: In Brinkley B, Porter K (eds): "International Cell Biology." New York: Rockefeller University Press, 1977, pp 50–57.
15. Toole BP, Jackson G, Gross J: Proc Natl Acad Sci USA 69:1384, 1978.
16. Comper WD, Laurent TC: Physiol Rev 58:255, 1978.
17. Turley E: Cancer Metastasis Rev 3:325, 1984.
18. Iozzo RV: Lab Invest 53:373, 1985.
19. Chiarugi VP, Dietrich CP: J Cell Physiol 99:201, 1979.
20. Ninomiya Y, Hata R, Nagai Y: Biochim Biophys Acta 629:349, 1980.
21. Heany-Kieras J, Kieras FJ: JNCI 65:1345, 1980.
22. Angello JC, Danielson KG, Anderson H: Cancer Res 42:2207, 1982.
23. Iozzo RV, Bolender RP, Wight TN: Lab Invest 47:124, 1982.
24. Iozzo RV: J Biol Chem 260:7464, 1985.
25. Barsky SH, Gopalakrishna R: Cancer Res 47:1663, 1987.
26. Avnur Z, Geiger B: Cell 38:811, 1984.

27. Lowry OHL, Rowebrough NJ, Farr AL, Randall RJ: J Biol Chem 193:265, 1959.
28. Pauli BU, Schwartz DE, Thomas EJ-M, Kuettner KE: Cancer Metastasis Rev 2:129, 1983.
29. Takeuchi J, Sobue M, Sato E, Shamoto M, Miura K, Nakagaki S: Cancer Res 36:2133, 1976.
30. Hatae Y, Atsuta T, Makita A: Gann 68:59, 1977.
31. Horai T, Nakamura N, Tateishi R, Hattori S: Cancer 48:2016, 1981.
32. Kojima J, Nakamura N, Kanatani M, Ohmori K: Cancer Res 35:542, 1975.
33. Kojima J, Nakamura N, Kanatani M, Ohmori K: Cancer Res 42:2857, 1982.
34. De Klerk DP, Lee DV: J Urol 131:1008, 1984.
35. Iozzo RV, Wight TN: J Biol Chem 257:1135, 1982.
36. Isemura M, Munakata H, Ototani N, Goto K, Yoshizawa Z: Gann 73:721, 1982.
37. Ozzello L, Lasfargues EY, Murray MR: Cancer Res 20:600, 1960.
38. Takeuchi J: Nature 207:537, 1965.
39. Takeuchi J: Br J Cancer 26:115, 1972.
40. Miller W, Ota DM, Giacco G, Guinee V, Irimura T, Nicolson GL, Cleary K: Clin Exp Metastasis 3:189, 1985.
41. Spicer SS: J Histochem Cytochem 13:211, 1965.
42. Irimura T, Ota DM, Cleary KR, Nicolson GL: In Mastromarino A (ed): "Biology and Treatment of Colorectal Cancer Metastasis." Boston: Martinus Nijhoff Publishing, 1986, pp 57–72.

In Vivo Metastatic Progression of an H-*ras* Transformed Mouse 10T1/2 Cell Line

M.-C. Gingras, L. Jarolim, J.A. Wright, and A.H. Greenberg

Manitoba Institute of Cell Biology, University of Manitoba, Winnipeg, Manitoba R3E 0V9, Canada

Experiments from this laboratory have demonstrated that the metastatic efficiency of a series of H-*ras* transfected fibroblasts correlates with the expression of the oncogene. We now tested the hypothesis that the ability of a *ras*-transformed line to survive in the lung may be related to *ras* expression. If this were the case, then preferential selection of high H-*ras*-expressing, increasingly metastatic variants may be observed during early lung growth. A T-24 H-*ras* transformed mouse 10T1/2 fibroblast clone was injected i.v. into C3H/HeN mice and tumor cells were recovered from the lungs at different times (30 min, 1, 9, and 21 days) from the lungs by selective growth in G418 sulfate. Their metastatic efficiency was tested in vivo and *ras* expression evaluated by Northern blotting. We report that lung-derived tumor cells show a gradual increase in their metastatic ability over the first 9 days of implantation, and that this is an unstable characteristic which is lost with prolonged growth in vivo or in vitro. No increase in the transcriptional activity of the *ras* gene was detected in variants with a 27-fold increase in metastatic ability. We conclude that while the metastatic efficiency of in vitro transformed lines is dependent on the expression of the *ras* gene, metastatic progression in vivo can be independent of *ras* transcription. It was previously reported by this laboratory that natural killer (NK) cells can control the number of metastatic cells surviving in the lung. The same experimental protocol was repeated in natural-killer-cell-deficient bg/bg mice. A similar pattern of metastatic potential of tumor cells recovered from bg/bg mice and normal bg/+ mice was observed, which permits us to exclude the possibility that the selection process was the result of increased survival of NK cell-resistant variants.

Key words: lung-derived tumor cells, metastatic efficiency, H-*ras* transcription

Two theories have been proposed to explain the origin of metastatic cells. The first was advanced by Fidler, in which metastasis formation was considered a nonrandom selective process where metastatic variants possessing a defined phenotype emerge from inherently unstable parental primary tumor with characteristics that will permit them to migrate and proliferate in distant organs [1,2]. The theories of Weiss [3] and Harris et al. [4] described metastasis formation also as a selection event, but in their model, the

Received May 4, 1987.

© 1988 Alan R. Liss, Inc.

metastatic phenotype is only expressed transiently and can be rapidly lost under non-selecting conditions.

Little information is available concerning the mechanism(s) involved in selection and survival of metastatic tumor cells. Using gene transfection, it has been established that the members of the *ras* family of oncogenes can confer metastatic ability to non-senescing and diploid fibroblasts, and that tumorigenicity [5,6] and efficiency of lung colonization [7] correlates with the expression of the gene. In the present study, we have tested the hypothesis that the ability of H-*ras* transfected fibroblasts to survive in the lung can also be related to *ras* expression. If the *ras* gene can confer any growth advantage, it is possible that cells giving rise to metastases are either preexisting variants with enhanced H-*ras* expression that have emerged from the in vivo selection pressures, or cells which have increased their *ras* expression in vivo and preferentially survive after lung implantation. We report here that while the metastatic efficiency of in vitro *ras* transformed lines was dependent on the expression of the *ras* gene, the metastatic progression we observed in vivo was independent of *ras* expression, at least at the transcriptional level.

MATERIALS AND METHODS
Animals

C3H/HeN mice were purchased from Charles River Laboratories (Quebec). C3H/HeJ bg/+ and bg/bg mice were bred at the University of Manitoba vivarium from breeders that were purchased from Jackson Laboratories (Bar Harbour, ME).

Cell Line

Mouse 10T1/2 fibroblast transfection was previously described [7]. The pSV2neo plasmid containing a 6.6 kb BamH1 T-24 H-*ras* insert (plasmid pAL8A), permitted the selection of transformed foci which were subsequently shown to be G418-resistant and contained multiple copies of the H-*ras* gene [7]. One of these clones, named CIRAS-1, which was poorly metastatic and expressed an intermediate *ras* RNA level [7], was chosen for the present study. Its characteristics would allow us to identify the in vivo selection of variants with enhanced *ras* expression and lung colonizing ability.

Lung-derived Tumor Cells

The CIRAS-1 lung-derived tumor cells (C1-LDT) were obtained by the following procedures. A CIRAS-1 inoculum of 10^6 cells in a 0.2 ml volume of Hanks balanced salt solution (Gibco Laboratories, Grand Island, NY) was injected into the tail vein of C3H/HeN mice. At different times after injection (30 min, 1, 9, and 21 days), tumor cells in the lungs were recovered by enzymatic treatment (660 µg/ml of collagenase type 1 (Sigma), 8.3 U/ml of hyaluronidase type 1-S (Sigma), 0.05% trypsin-EDTA (Gibco)) of mechanically disaggregated fragments of lung [8]. Using selective growth conditions for plasmid-carrying cells, that is, 400 µg/ml of G418 sulfate (Gibco) in the F12 medium (Gibco) supplemented with 10% FCS (Gibco), permitted the recovery of pure CIRAS-1 cells. Recovered lung-derived tumor cells were then analyzed for experimental lung metastasis formation, and *ras* expression by Northern blot analysis. Control cells were the CIRAS-1 parental tumor submitted to the same culture conditions as those applied to the C1-LDT cells after their recovery from lung. Initially, they were cultured at a low plating concentration in the presence of G418 and maintained over a period of 9 days, which represents the maximum time that the C1-LTD cells were grown in the presence of the drug.

Experimental Metastasis Assays

Metastatic efficiency of the C1-LDT cells recovered at different times after lung implantation, was tested by i.v. injection of an inoculum of 3×10^5 cells per mouse in C3H/HeN mice. Metastasis formation was evaluated by counting lung foci under a dissecting microscope which had previously been stained with Bouin's solution [7].

Evaluation of In Vivo NK Selection

CIRAS-1 cells were injected i.v. (10^6 cells/mouse, into natural-killer-cell-deficient C3H/HeJ bg/bg mice and their normal bg/+ littermates. The C1-LDT cells were recovered at 1 and 9 days as described above, and their metastatic efficiency was tested at 21 days in the normal bg/+ mice following i.v. injection of 3×10^5 cells/mouse.

Northern Blot Analysis

Total RNA was prepared by the guanidinium-cesium chloride method [9], and 20μg was electrophoresed on 1% formaldehyde gels [10] using ethidium bromide staining to confirm equal loading. The RNA was then electrophoretically transferred to nylon membrane, as described in the protocol of the Biorad Company, and hybridized for 24 h to a 32p-labelled (Klenow extension [11]; 3×10^8 cpm/μug) v-H-*ras* probe (Oncor Inc., Gaithersburg, MD) at 42°C in 50% formamide. The filter was washed in $2\times$ SSC, 0.5% SDS (5 min at room temperature), followed by $2\times$ SSC, 0.1% SDS (15 min at room temperature), and finally $0.1\times$ SSC, 0.1% SDS (2×30 min at 65°C). Autoradiography was performed at $-70°C$ with Kodak X-Omat AR film and Cronex lighting plus intensifying screen.

RESULTS

The evaluation of the metastatic potential of the C1-LDT cells (Fig. 1) clearly demonstrated that the metastatic efficiency of these cells varied according to the time they were in the lung. Tumor cells recovered after 30 min possessed a slightly higher but significant metastatic potential than in vitro controls (2.7-fold, P=0.053), while those taken after 1 and 9 days' implantation were increasingly metastatic (7.7-fold and 26-fold, respectively, P=0.002). However, the enhanced metastatic rate was significantly reduced by 21 days, almost reaching the 1-day level (9.8-fold, P=0.025), suggesting that the selection process was unstable. A similar instability of the metastatic potential was observed in vitro when the 9-day-C1-LDT cells were maintained in culture over a 27-day period (data not shown). Metastatic potential decreased to 3.7-fold (P=0.021) from the 7th to the 27th day in culture.

Since it was previously shown in this laboratory that NK cells can control the metastatic efficiency of the *ras* transformed 10T1/2 fibroblasts [7,8], the possibility that the selection process could be the result of increased survival to the attack of these immune effector cells also had to be tested. For this purpose, CIRAS-1 cells were injected into normal C3H/HeJ bg/+ mice and natural-killer-cell-deficient C3H/HeJ bg/bg mice. As illustrated in Table I, the cells recovered from both bg/bg and bg/+ lungs possessed increased metastatic potential compared to the in vitro control. This increase in the absence of functional NK cells in the bg/bg mice indicates that the selection cannot

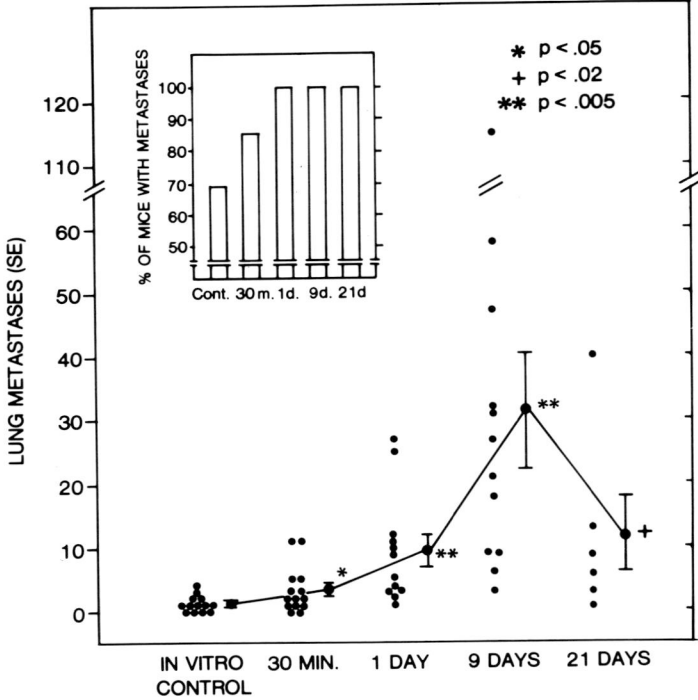

Fig. 1. Metastatic efficiency of CIRAS-1 lung-derived tumor cells (CI-LDT) recovered at different times after implantation in the lung. Metastatic potential of the C1-LDT from two experiments was tested by reinjecting cells (3×10^5) recovered from lungs and selected in G418 sulfate to eliminate all normal lung tissue. The graph illustrates both individual points which represent metastasis formation in one mouse, in addition to the mean of each group. The insert (upper left) is the percentage of mice with metastasis at each time point.

be the result of the preferential survival of NK-resistant variants. Evaluation of the NK lytic sensitivity of these lung-derived tumor cells in vitro confirmed this result. Cells recovered from the bg/+ and bg/bg mice showed no difference in NK sensitivity in vitro (data not shown). Therefore, the enhanced metastatic potential of the lung-derived tumor cells recovered from normal mice is not dependent on an NK selection event.

A direct relationship had been observed between *ras* expression and metastasis formation in a series of *ras* transformed 10T1/2 fibroblast lines described in an earlier publication [7]. In evaluating the C1-LDT cells recovered between 30 min and 21 days after lung implantation, Northern blot analysis did not reveal any increase in the expression of the *ras* gene for all the tested times (Fig. 2) The enhanced metastatic efficiency of the C1-LTD cells is therefore not correlated with *ras* expression.

DISCUSSION

In this study, we observed that a poorly metastatic H-*ras* transfected 10T1/2 line (CIRAS-1) recovered from lungs after i.v. injection gradually increased in metastatic

TABLE I. Enhanced Metastatic Potential of CIRAS-1 Lung-Derived Tumor (CI-LDT) Is Not Dependent on an NK Selection Event

Cells	Tumor recovered from C3H/HeJ bg/+		Tumor recovered from C3H/HeJ bg/bg	
	Lung metastases		Lung metastases	
	Mean ± SE	Frequency	Mean ± SE	Frequency
In vitro control	7.0 ± 2.2	6/7	7.0 ± 2.2	6/7
CI-LDT 1 day	80.0 ± 26.2*	6/6	29.2 ± 8.1*	6/6
CI-LDT 9 days	62.8 ± 28.5**	5/6	48.5 ± 21.9**	5/6

*$P < 0.01$
**$P < 0.08 > .05$

CIRAS-1 cells were injected i.v. into C3H/HeJ bg/+ or C3H/HeJ bg/bg mice, then recovered 1 and 9 days later. These cells and in vitro controls were then injected into bg/+ mice and experimental metastases counted 21 days later.

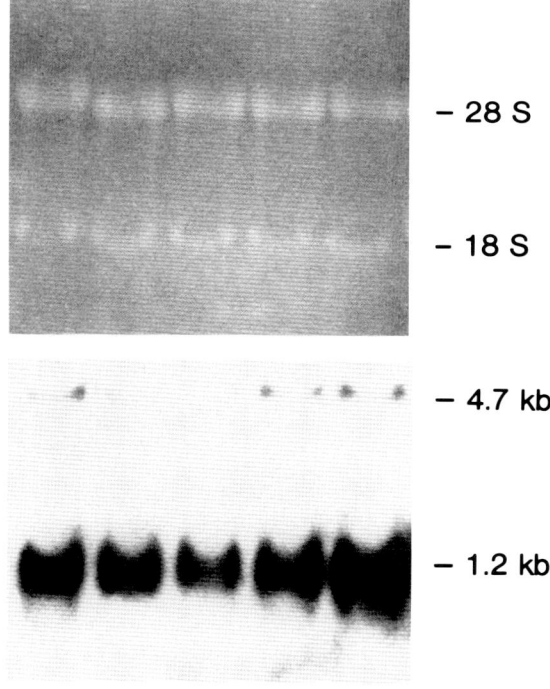

Fig. 2. Northern blot analysis of CIRAS-1 lung-derived tumor cells recovered at different times after implantation in the lung (bottom panel). The top panel shows ribosomal RNA stained with ethidium bromide after electrophoresis of 20 μg of total RNA extracted from C1-LDT cells, and indicates equal loading of RNA on gels.

efficiency over the level of the in vitro-passaged parental line between 30 min and 9 days of lung implantation. A similar observation was made by Young and Hill [12] for two different cell lines, KHT fibrosarcoma and B16 melanoma cells. They noted an increase of 50-100-fold in metastatic efficiency of cells recovered after 5 days' lung implantation. In their study, as in ours, instability of the metastatic efficiency of the lung-derived tumor cells was observed as the metastatic growth progressed, resulting in an eventual decrease to the level characterizing the parental lines. As mentioned earlier, two theories have been advanced that could explain the enhanced metastatic efficiency; selection of preexisting variants or preferential outgrowth of a transiently expressed phenotype under selection pressure. Recovery of highly metastatic variants in the lung would be consistent with in vivo selection occurring over the first day(s) after injection of a small subpopulation and the appearance of tumor expressing a favorable phenotype for implantation and proliferation in the lung. However, our experiments selected for an unstable characteristic(s), suggesting that the phenotype was necessary for initial tumor development but was lost as metastasis formation progressed. The transient nature of the increase in metastatic ability we observed would certainly argue against the selection of a specific low frequency variant of high metastatic ability in the initial inoculum, and in favor of the model of Harris et al., [4] and Weiss [3].

Experiments with radioactively labelled cells have shown that most tumor cells are arrested in the lung after i.v. injection and gradually cleared during the first days (unpublished data, [13–15]). A cell population recovered a few days after implantation would be derived from the surviving implanted cells and would, therefore, have to be a selected population. The subsequent loss of metastatic efficiency in these cells, that is, their instability, suggests only that the characteristic which is selected is likely not a stable genetic event. This is in contrast to our earlier studies which identified rare lung-derived metastases from another poorly metastatic *ras*-transfected 10T1/2 cell line, called NR3, that were stable, highly metastatic variants. These lines had amplified and rearranged H-*ras* sequences and greatly enhanced H-*ras* expression [7], indicating that in vivo selection of H-*ras* amplified metastases had occurred. However, in the present study, CIRAS-1 cells, which successfully implanted in the lung and gave rise to metastases, neither arose from preexisting variants with an increased expression of the *ras* gene, nor did they subsequently develop enhanced *ras* expression. Therefore, even though *ras* was required for the metastatic conversion of the 10T1/2 to the CIRAS-1 tumor, a further increase in the expression of *ras* was not required for the in vivo selection and survival of this line.

In a previous study from this laboratory [7] we observed that metastatic efficiency of a series of H-*ras* transfected 10T1/2 and NIH/3T3 lines correlated with the expression of the oncogene and we suggested that *ras* directly regulated metastatic behavior in these fibroblasts. The unaltered *ras* RNA levels in the 9-day-C1-LTD cells suggests that we could be dealing with selection for another locus of control. One possibility is that the *ras* pathway may still be involved but at the posttranscriptional level. For example, in vivo surviving cells may be regulatory variants for p21 production. Recent observations indicate that the *ras* oncogene, which is a G protein [16], can also alter phosphatidylinositol turnover [17,18] and protein phosphorylation [18], and these could constitute other potential sites of regulation. One could postulate, therefore, that the unstable or "epigenetic" regulation of metastasis of in vivo-derived *ras*-transfected lines may be a result of selection of variants with altered and unstable metabolic regulation downstream from the transcription of the *ras* gene. It is also possible, however, that in vivo selection favors the appearance of variants which are regulated outside of this pathway. This remains to be answered in future experiments.

ACKNOWLEDGMENTS

This work was supported by the National Cancer Institute of Canada, the Manitoba Health Research Council, and the Winnipeg Childrens' Hospital Research Foundation. M.C.G. is supported by a Winnipeg Childrens' Hospital Research Foundation fellowship. A.H.G. and J.A.W. are Terry Fox Cancer Research Scientists.

REFERENCES

1. Fidler IJ, Kripke ML: Science 197:893–895, 1977.
2. Poste G, Fidler IJ: Nature 283:139–146, 1980.
3. Weiss L: Invasion Metastasis 3:193–207, 1983.
4. Harris JF, Chambers AF, Hill RP, Ling V: Proc Natl Acad Sci USA 79:5547–5551, 1982.
5. Monoharan TH, Burgess JA, Ho D, Newell CL, Fahl WE: Carcinogenesis 6: 1295–1301, 1985.
6. Pulciani S, Santos E, Long LK, Sorrentino V, Barbacid M: Mol Cell Biol 5: 2836–2841, 1985.
7. Egan SE, McClarty GA, Jarolim L, Wright JA, Spiro I, Hager G, Greenberg AH: Mol Cell Biol 7: 830–837, 1987.
8. Greenberg AH, Egan SE, Jarolim L, Gingras M-C, Wright JA: Cancer Res 47:4801–4805, 1987.
9. Chirgwin JM, Przbyla AE, McDonald RJ, Rutter WJ: Biochemistry 18: 5294–5299, 1979.
10. Lehrach H, Diamond D, Wozney JW, Baldtker H: Biochemistry 16: 4743–4751, 1977.
11. Feinberg AP, Vogelstein B: Anal Biochem 132:613, 1983.
12. Young SD, Hill RP: Clin Expl Metastasis 4:153–176, 1986.
13. Brown JM, Parker ET: Br J Cancer 40:677–688, 1979.
14. Conley F: J Natl Cancer Inst 69:465–472, 1982.
15. Fidler IJ: J Natl Cancer Inst 45:773–782, 1970.
16. Gibbs JB, Sigal IS, Scolnick EM: Trends Biochem Sci 10:350–353, 1985.
17. Fleischman LF, Chahwala SB, Cantley L: Science 231:407–410, 1986.
18. Wolfman A, Macara IG: Nature 325:359–361, 1987.

Application of Gene Transfer to the Study of Tumor Progression and Metastasis

Carol Waghorne, Martin L. Breitman, and Robert S. Kerbel

Division of Cancer and Cell Biology, Mount Sinai Hospital Research Institute (C.W., M.L.B., R.S.K.) and Department of Medical Genetics, University of Toronto (M.L.B., R.S.K.), Toronto, Ontario, Canada

Some of the applications of utilizing gene transfer into neoplastic cells as a means of studying tumor progression and metastasis are reviewed. Foremost among these is the finding that random insertion of foreign DNA sequences can be exploited as clonotypic markers to study complex tumor cell interactions and lineage relationships in vivo. Using this approach it can be shown that metastases are actively selected from genotypically distinct tumor cell subpopulation(s) and that primary tumors can become overgrown with these same subpopulations.

Key words: metastasis, gene transfer, *ras*, clonal selection

Unravelling the biological complexities of the metastatic process and the metastatic phenotype remains one of the most challenging and important goals of cancer research. Its importance lies in the fact that the lethality of most types of cancer is related to their ability to disseminate from one site to another throughout the body, and thereby establish multiple lesions in crucial organs or tissues. Whereas the localized primary tumor may be amenable to control—usually by surgical removal—distant metastases usually are not. Hence, successful treatment of "cancer" usually means successful control of metastatic disease.

In 1973, Fidler reported evidence which suggested that the metastatic process was nonrandom and that metastases probably derive from rare specialized variants which arose during the growth of primary tumors [1]. This provocative paper proved to be a landmark in the development of basic metastasis research for two reasons. First, it demonstrated an approach to more accurate and rigorous study of the inherently complex process of metastasis (prior to 1973 good animal models of metastasis were uncommon). Second, the results clearly implied that there must be specific genes and gene products which control, or influence, the metastatic phenotype. This stimulated a major worldwide effort to try to identify these relevant genes and the phenotypes they specify.

It is ironic that, despite the stimulus this work provided to the metastasis field, Fidler's results and hypothesis remain highly controversial. A number of investigators have been unable to confirm his results using other tumor models [2–4] and argue that

Received September 2, 1987.

the metastatic phenotype is highly unstable [5], or that the process is nonselective [2–4]. Resolving this controversy is by no means an intellectual triviality. As this is largely a genetic problem, it would seem logical to use molecular genetic methods and approaches to achieve a resolution to the controversy. We have attempted to do so, and summarize here some of our recent findings.

Molecular Genetic Approach to Study Metastasis: Transfer of Oncogenes Into Nonmetastatic Neoplastic Cells

Transfection of DNA into primary embryonic diploid fibroblasts or "immortalized" cell lines such as NIH-3T3 or C3H 10T 1/2 has been used extensively to identify oncogenes [6,7]. In the case of the H-*ras* oncogene, expression of the transfected gene can also lead to the induction of a fully malignant-metastatic phenotype [8–11]. However, such an approach does not allow one to study the metastogenic potential of a gene independent of its oncogenic potential. It seemed reasonable therefore to assess the effect of certain transfected genes on the metastatic behavior of tumor cells which are normally benign. This also provides one with the opportunity to discern phenotypic changes that accompany malignant conversion from those which are simply characteristic of neoplastic transformation.

This line of reasoning has been adopted by us (Waghorne et al.) [12] as well as other investigators, e.g., Vousden et al. [13], and Collard et al. [14]. In all of these studies the basic approach was to transfect an activated (or normal) gene into a tumor cell line which was known to be deficient in metastatic ability, and then assess the transfectants to determine if they had acquired high-grade metastatic potential. As Table I shows, all of these studies had an underlying consistent finding: transfection of an activated H-*ras* gene was successful in either inducing—or amplifying—the metastatic potential of the various tumor cell lines studied. Using the BW5147 T cell lymphoma Collard et al. [14] noted a direct correlation between the level of activated *ras* gene expression and the extent of metastatic aggressiveness, whereas no such correlation was

TABLE I. Effect of Transfer of Activated *ras* Gene Into Established Mouse Tumor Cell Lines on Their Metastatic Potential

Recipient tumor cell line (and reference)	Effect of transfer of activated c-H-*ras*	Remarks
MT1 C1.5 mouse mammary adenocarcinoma	Significant increase in spontaneous metastatic potential	Control pSV$_2$neo or normal c-H-*ras* transfections had little or no effect on metastasis
SP1 mammary adenocarcinoma	Induction of spontaneous metastatic potential	Similar effect observed, at much lower frequency, after pSV$_2$neo control transfection
BW5147 T cell lymphoma	Induction of spontaneous metastatic potential	Control pSV$_2$neo transfection had no effect

observed by Vousden et al. [13] or Waghorne et al. [12] when studying the MT1C1. 5/7 and SP1 mouse mammary carcinomas, respectively. In the latter two cases [12,13], it also appeared that expression of the normal ras gene was not sufficient to trigger metastatic potential. It must be noted, however, that not all cell lines are equally susceptible to the metastatic effects of activated ras oncogenes. The mouse epithelial line C127, for example, when transformed by the viral H-ras gene was tumorigenic but not metastatic [9]. At present this differential response of different cell types is not understood.

It also remains to be determined what changes induced by transfection of the H-ras oncogene result in acquisition of the metastatic phenotype. One possibility is increased cell invasiveness due to secretion of basement membrane collagenase, as suggested by Liotta and colleagues [15]. Another possibility is alterations in cell surface glycoproteins, which are thought to be involved in cell adhesion, invasion, and metastasis [16] and which have been shown to be affected by expression of activated ras oncogenes [17,18]. The generation of stably metastatic tumor cell populations by DNA transfection has allowed us to compare specific biochemical properties of these cells with the nonmetastatic parental SP1 population. We have, in a recent study, found a direct correlation between the apparent metastatic potential of SP1 transfected clones and the extent of β-1–6 linked branching of complex type oligosaccharides on a particular cell surface glycoprotein, gp130 [19].

Induction/Modulation of the Metastatic Phenotype by Transfection Procedures

The activated ras oncogene results summarized in Table I can be, as we discovered, occasionally complicated by the fact that the experimental controls can manifest metastatic behavior. For example, in the case of the SPI mammary carcinoma, transfection with the pSV_2neo plasmid itself was associated with induction of spontaneous metastatic behavior in almost 20% of the $G418^r$ transfectant clones [20]. Moreover, subsequent experiments, as shown in Table II, demonstrated that $CaPO_4$ treatment without any precipitated DNA present could achieve the same result [20]. Similar results were reported independently by Verrelle et al. using the RMS/8 rat rhabdomyosarcoma [21], and by Nicolson and Fidler using the rat K13576 mammary tumor and K1735 mouse melanoma respectively (personal communication). Thus the phenomenon is clearly not restricted to one type of tumor cell.

TABLE II. Summary of Metastatic and Tumorigenic Properties of Various Sources of Cloned SP1 Cells

Source of clones tested	# tum$^-$ clones / # clones tested	# met$^+$ clones / # clones tested
SP1 clones (nontransfected control)	0/20	0/20
SP1 clones obtained after $CaPO_4$ treatment	0/20	5/20
SP1 pSV_2neo transfected clones	3/16	3/16
SP1 pSV_2gpt transfected clones	1/18	3/18
SP1 clone 31 pSV_2neo transfected clones[a]	0/6	1/6
SP1 clone 32 pSV_2neo transfected clones[a]	0/6	2/6
SP1 clone 33 pSV_2neo transfected clones[a]	0/6	1/6

[a]Three individual clones of SP1 were transfected with pSV_2neo and six $G418^r$ colonies from each were grown to mass culture and assessed for their tumorigenic and metastatic growth in vivo.

These results highlight one potential pitfall of employing certain gene transfection protocols to study metastasis, especially when aneuploid neoplastic cells are used as the recipients. As it turns out, however, DNA insertions can be exploited as unique molecular tags to study tumor progression and metastasis in vivo. This is discussed in the following section.

Analysis of Growth, Selection, and Metastasis of Tumor Cell Populations In Vivo Using Random Insertions of Foreign DNA as Genetic Tags

Southern blot analysis of pSV$_2$neo transfectants of the SP1 mammary adenocarcinoma revealed that the majority of transfectants contained a limited number of copies of the inserted plasmid DNA. Because the insertions are random, the size of the fragments generated by a restriction enzyme such as BamH1 (for which there is only one recognition site within the pSV$_2$neo plasmid) will almost always vary from one transfectant clone to another. Thus each transfectant will manifest a unique restriction pattern by Southern analysis using pSV$_2$neo as a probe. In other words, each transfectant has a unique, readily identifiable genetic marker.

Pooling a large number (e.g., 50–100) of such transfectants, each having a unique DNA marker, and injecting the mixture into animals facilitates complicated lineage analyses in vivo during tumor growth and metastasis. Initially the DNA from the mixture will manifest a faint "smear" in a Southern gel, as the "signal" for any one transfectant will be too weak to be seen. But if a strong selection pressure has occurred during tumor growth so that only a small number of clones grow or predominate, this would be evident by the appearance of distinct hybridizing bands in a Southern gel. A similar picture would be seen if a metastasis was ultimately derived from a single or small number of tumor cells.

The results shown in Figure 1 demonstrate the potential of exploiting this approach. Female CBA/J mice were injected subcutaneously with a pooled population of 10^5 cells obtained after pSV$_2$neo transfection of SP1 mammary adenocarcinoma cells. Between 50 and 100 independent G418-resistant colonies were pooled [20]. As expected, DNA from this pooled population (the "inoculum") presented as a faint broad smear on a Southern gel when probed with pSV$_2$neo (Fig. 1, lane 1). However, when the "primary" tumors were removed 4–6 weeks later and the DNA extracted and analyzed, evidence was obtained for the presence of a single clone of SP1 cells[20] (Fig. 1, lanes 2, 4, 6). Moreover, DNA isolated from spontaneous lung metastases obtained from several different mice manifested the *same* restriction pattern (Fig. 1, lanes 3, 5, 7). The results showed that the metastases were derived from a genotypically distinct subpopulation (clone) of tumor cells. More important, this clone also seemed to have overgrown the primary tumor.

It could be argued that these results and/or conclusions are erroneous because of possible artifacts. It may be that only one or a small number of the transfected clones could grow in vivo. Thus there was not any authentic selection for a dominant clone. This is not so, however, because we have found that 10 independently isolated (in vitro) pSV$_2$neo transfectants were all equally tumorigenic [20]. Second, a time-course analysis of primary tumors removed 2–5 weeks after injection revealed evidence for the presence and growth of multiple clones during the first 2–3 weeks of tumor growth. This heterogeneity was eventually displaced by the homogeneous pattern seen in Figure 1. Again it was the *same* clone (called "SP1neo5") which overtook the primary tumors (Waghorne et al., in preparation).

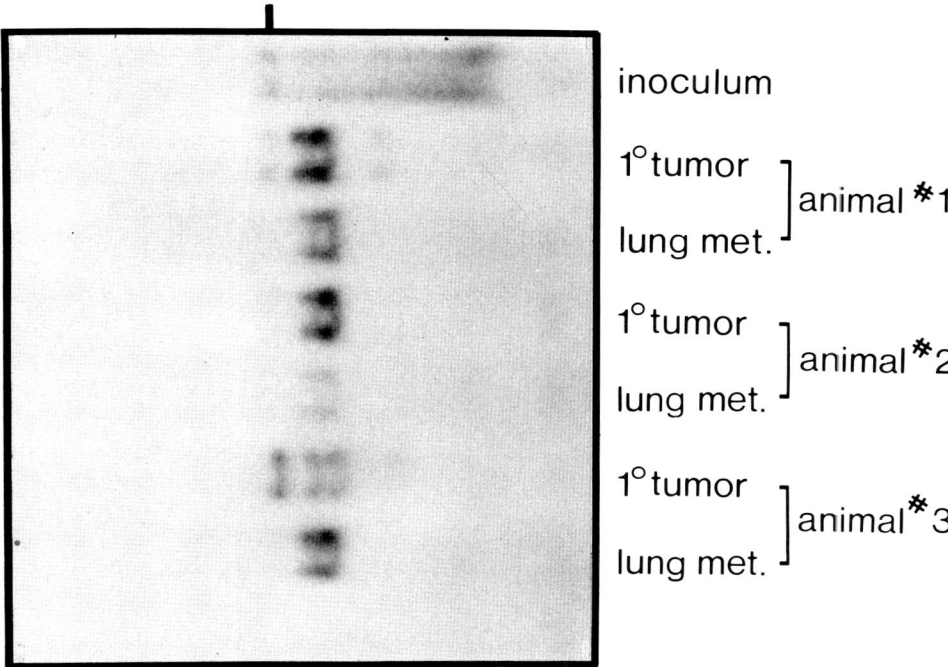

Fig. 1. Southern blot analysis of primary tumors and lung metastases obtained from 3 CBA/J mice injected with a pool of 50–100 independent G418^r pSV$_2$neo transfected SP1 mammary carcinoma cells. 5 μg of genomic DNA digested with BamH1 was electrophoretically fractionated, transferred to nitrocellulose, and hybridized to a ^{32}P-labeled linear pSV$_2$neo probe. Adapted from Kerbel et al. [20].

A second possible explanation of these results derives from the use of subcutaneous inoculations in these experiments. There is evidence that the tumorigenic/metastatic potential of tumor cell populations can be profoundly influenced by the type of tissue into which the cells are injected [22–24]. Thus breast carcinomas may grow considerably better when implanted into breast tissue (mammary fat pads), i.e., an "orthotopic" site as opposed to an inappropriate or ectopic site such as the subcutis [25]. Hence, overgrowth of a single clone from a breast tumor cell line such as SP1 at a subcutaneous injection site may simply reflect the fact that *only* that clone manifests a growth advantage in the subcutis; in contrast it may be that many more clones might grow progressively when injected into mammary fat pads of the same mice. Indeed the SP1 tumor *does* grow much better when injected into mammary fat pads than subcutaneously (e.g., 2,000 cells will give 100% tumor takes when injected into breast tissue, whereas 20,000–50,000 cells are required for a 100% tumor take at a subcutaneous site). Nevertheless we still found that the same clone (i.e., "SP1neo5") overgrew these primary tumors after injection of the pooled SP1 population of 50–100 pSV$_2$neo transfectants (Waghorne et al., in preparation).

Implications of the Results With Respect to Metastasis

At a general level, it is apparent that random insertions of limited numbers of foreign DNA sequences into the genome of tumor cells can be exploited to investigate a range of important (and often complex) biological problems associated with tumor progression and metastasis. These include: 1) the genetic relationship of metastases to primary tumors; 2) the rate and extent of selection of tumor subpopulations in vivo; 3) the clonal origin of tumors; 4) the nature and effects of tumor cell clonal interactions during tumor growth. Talmadge and Zbar, for example, have also recently exploited this type of genetic approach to show the monoclonal origin of spontaneous B16 mouse melanoma metastases [26].

This approach has already helped to clarify many of the discrepancies and controversies surrounding Fidler's 1973 "metastasis-selection" model and hypothesis. It is clear from our results that spontaneous SP1 metastases were derived from a genotypically distinct progenitor subpopulation of tumor cells. Thus, the process was *not* random. However, because this subpopulation (or clone) also eventually overgrew the primary tumor, comparison of late or advanced stage primary tumors with distant metastases for relative metastatic potential may not reveal any difference, because, in this case, the late stage tumor is the equivalent of a metastatic nodule. In contrast, metastases *will* be more metastatic than early stage primary tumors which have not been overgrown by the dominant malignant clone. In short, it is not possible to select a metastatic population of cells from a population that is *already* metastatic. This fact could resolve many of the discrepancies in the literature where investigators have been unsuccessful in isolating variants having increased metastatic potential: the starting or "wild-type" cell population may already have been "malignant" even though it was recovered as a "primary" tumor.

Thus it is clear that careful attention will have to be paid to the *stage* at which primary tumors—be they autochthonous or transplanted, spontaneous or induced—are removed from their hosts and analyzed. In general it may turn out that late stage, advanced primary tumors (e.g., Duke's level D colon carcinomas or Clarke's level IV melanoma) will behave identically or very similarly to distant metastases derived from these tumors, whereas early stage tumors will not.

ACKNOWLEDGMENTS

We thank Micki Thomas for her excellent technical assistance and Astrid Eberhart for her excellent secretarial assistance. This work was supported by grants from the NCIC to MLB and RSK and NIH grant RO1-CA41233 to RSK. RSK and MLB are respectively a Research Associate of the NCIC and a Research Scholar of the MRC.

REFERENCES

1. Fidler IJ: Nature (New Biol) 242: 148–149, 1973.
2. Milas L, Peters LJ, Ito H: Clin Exp Metastasis 1: 309–318, 1983.
3. Weiss L, Holmes JC, Ward PM: Br J Cancer 47: 81–91, 1983.
4. Weiss L: Pathobiol Annu 10: 51–81, 1980.
5. Ling V, Chambers AF, Harris JF, Hill RP: Cancer Metast Rev 4: 173–194, 1985.
6. Shih C, Padhy LC, Murry M, Weinberg RA: Nature 290: 261–264, 1981.
7. Perucho M, Goldfarb M, Shimizu K, Lama C, Fogh J, Wigler M: Cell 27: 467–476, 1981.
8. Thorgeirsson UP, Turpeenniemi-Hujanen T, Williams JE, Westin EH, Heilman CA, Talmadge JE, Liotta LA: Mol Cell Biol 5: 259–262, 1985.
9. Muschel RJ, Williams JE, Lowy DR, Liotta LA: Am J Pathol 121: 1–8, 1985.
10. Egan SE, McClarty GA, Jarolim L, Wright JA, Spiro I, Hager G, Greenberg AH: Mol Cell Biol 7: 830–837, 1987.
11. Pozzatti R, Muschel R, Williams J, et al.: Science 232: 223–227, 1986.

12. Waghorne CG, Kerbel RS, Breitman ML: Oncogene 1: 149–155.
13. Vousden KH, Eccles SA, Purvies H, Marshall CJ: Int J Cancer 37: 425–433, 1986.
14. Collard JG, Schijven JF, Roos E: Cancer Res 47: 754–759, 1987.
15. Spiridione G, Pozzatti R, Muschel RJ, et al.: Cancer Res 47: 1522–1528, 1987.
16. Schirrmacher V, Altevogt P, Fogel M, et al.: Invas Metast 2: 313–360, 1982.
17. Santer UV, Gilbert F, Glick MC: Cancer Res 44: 3730–3735, 1984.
18. Collard JG, Van Beek WP, Janssen JWG, Schijven JF: Int J Cancer 35: 207–214, 1985.
19. Dennis JW, Laferte S, Waghorne CG, Breitman ML, Kerbel RS: Science 236: 582–585, 1987.
20. Kerbel RS, Waghorne CG, Man MS, Elliott B, Breitman ML: Proc Natl Acad Sci USA 84: 1263–1267, 1987.
21. Varelle P, Lascaut V, Poupon MF, Hillova J: Anticancer Res 7: 181–186, 1987.
22. Giavazzi R, Jessup JM, Campbell DE, Walker SM, Fidler IJ: J Natl Cancer Inst 77: 1303–1307, 1986.
23. Ibranhiem EHI, Nigan VN, Brailovsky CA, Elhilali PM, Elhilali M: Cancer Res 43: 617–622, 1983.
24. Tan MH, Holyoke ED, Goldrosen MH: J Natl Cancer Inst 59: 1537–1544, 1977.
25. Miller FR: Invasion Metastasis 1: 220–226, 1981.
26. Talmadge JE, Zbar B: J Natl Cancer Inst 78: 315–320, 1987.

Malignant Progression of Human Breast Cancer

Helene S. Smith, Charles M. Dollbaum, Britt-Marie Ljung, Brian Mayall, and Adeline J. Hackett

Peralta Cancer Research Institute, Oakland, California 94609 (H.S.S., C.M.D., A.J.H.), Department of Pathology (B.-M.L.), and Department of Laboratory Medicine (B.M.), University of California, San Francisco, San Francisco, California 94143

Cell culture offers a systematic approach to investigate human breast cancer at the cellular level. We utilized a short-term culture system that supports extensive proliferation of both normal and malignant human mammary epithelial cells. Cells cultured from primary breast cancers were compared to nonmalignant mammary epithelium to study early stages of malignancy. The tumor cells differed from nonmalignant cells by a number of criteria including invasiveness and sensitivity to tumor necrosis factor. To study later stages in malignant progression, primary breast cancers were compared to metastatic lesions. Cells cultured from primary lesions were mostly diploid, while those cultured from late stages in malignant progression were uniformly aneuploid. These results are best explained by the hypothesis (Nowell PC: Science 194:23–28, 1986) that diploid neoplastic cells generate nonviable cells with grossly abnormal chromosomal contents. Only occasionally does this process generate viable aneuploid cells with growth advantage allowing them to selectively populate the original tumor or subsequent metastases. We hypothesize that this evolving malignant process is quite slow in breast cancer so that diploid neoplastic cells, nonviable aneuploid cells, and viable aneuploid cells all coexist in the primary lesion. This model makes the following predictions, all of which were found to be true: 1) many aneuploid cells will be nonviable; 2) aneuploidy will be associated with malignant progression; 3) metastases will be highly variable because they arise from multiple random genetic changes; and 4) diploid neoplastic cells will be found in the primary tumors. The relative proportion of viable aneuploid and diploid tumor cells in vivo was unclear, since the predominantly diploid population observed after culture may be the result of selective proliferation. The diploid tumor cells may provide important insights into fundamental differences between normal and malignant mammary epithelium because they lack secondary but irrelevant karyotypic change which would confound the analysis.

Key words: malignant progression, human breast cancer, ploidy, antigenicity

Human specimens taken directly from the operating room have limited value for biochemical and molecular comparisons between tumor and normal tissues. Besides the

Received May 15, 1987.

cell type of interest, these tissues contain varying amounts of other cells and tissue components, including lymphocytes, blood vessels, and stromal fibroblasts, which interfere with comparisons. When attempts are made to dissociate the tissue and isolate the particular cell type of interest, usually too few cells are obtained for study. In vitro culturing to amplify the number of available cells is one approach to this dilemma. Unfortunately, only occasional tumor specimens develop into cell lines with infinite growth potential, while most primary carcinomas and all normal tissues do not. This is particularly true for breast cancer where the vast majority of cell lines have been derived from effusion metastases. Only very rarely have breast cancer cell lines been derived from primary carcinomas. Furthermore, the few lines that have been established from primary tumors were derived from specimens with unusual histopathologies rather than infiltrating duct carcinomas which represent the majority of human breast cancers (for review see reference 1).

The human mammary gland is a good system for studying malignant progression, since specimens representing at least some stages of progression are readily available as discard material from surgical specimens. Reduction mammaplasties are an excellent source of normal epithelial cells as there is little, if any, pathology of the epithelial cells in such cases. Tissues peripheral to carcinomas in mastectomy specimens are another source of nonmalignant cells. Malignant lesions usually provide sufficient discard tissue for the culture of carcinoma cells; malignant effusions are a readily available source of metastatic cells, since they are often removed for the comfort of the patient.

Our laboratory has been involved in developing techniques for short-term culture of malignant and normal human mammary epithelium [2–8]. Our goal has been to isolate, to culture with high efficiency, and to identify the cultured epithelial cells from every specimen regardless of stage in malignant progression. Here we describe our progress to date and illustrate how these cultures provide unique insights into the nature of malignant progression.

PROPERTIES OF CELLS CULTURED FROM PRIMARY CARCINOMAS

One of the problems with culturing breast carcinoma cells is that mammary tumors are desmoplastic. It is difficult to isolate the tumor cells free from the reactive stroma. Some breast cancer cells are only loosely attached to the stromal matrix so that they can be dissociated mechanically. These cells represent a minority population within the tumors, characterized by low viability [9]. The majority of breast carcinoma cells can only be released after enzymatic digestion of the stromal matrix with collagenase. With such treatment, part of the tumor is dissociated to single cells but most remains as tightly associated clumps. These conditions result in dissociation of the stromal fibroblasts and blood vessels to single cells. The tumor clumps can then easily be isolated free from fibroblasts by sedimentation at unit gravity [10] or by filtration through nylon mesh filters [2]. The tumor cells proliferate to some degree in a variety of culture conditions [11–15]. Serum-free media which also allow significant growth have been recently described [16,17].

We use a medium formulation which supports considerable proliferation in mass cultures [2,3] and which permits both normal and tumor cell growth in a highly efficient clonogenic assay when cells are plated sparsely on a fibroblast feeder layer [4]. A number of criteria have been used to demonstrate the epithelial nature of cells grown under these conditions. The cultured cells possess a typical cuboidal morphology with the formation of secretory domes and ductlike, three-dimensional ridges at confluence. Ultrastructurally, the cells show junctional complexes and evidence of secretory activity [2]. The cells are positive for cytokeratins [18], have a diminished punctate pattern of cell-associated fibronectin [19] typical of epithelium, and express epithelial membrane antigens as defined by antibodies raised to milk-fat globule membrane [4].

There is some controversy as to whether the carcinoma-derived cultures are bona fide tumor cells or nonmalignant cells originating from tissue peripheral to the malignancy [20,21]. It is unlikely that cellular clumps dissociated from tumors originate from nonmalignant peripheral tissue, since they tend to be much smaller and less structured than clumps digested from nonmalignant tissue [22]. Furthermore, there are a number of consistent differences between cultures derived from malignant and nonmalignant tissues. Asaga et al. [23] reported a significant increase in multinucleated cells after incubation of human mammary carcinoma cultures with cytochalasin when compared with cultures derived from various benign tissues. Similar results were reported for cultured rodent mammary tissues [24]. Carcinoma-derived cultures also showed increased variability in surface antigen expression when compared to nonmalignant tissue from the same donor [25]. We have compared malignant and nonmalignant cultures using a polyvalent antiserum prepared by Edgington and colleagues [26,27] to a 19.5 kilodalton glycoprotein reported to be tumor-specific; all tumor-derived cultures were positive, and all nonmalignant cultures tested were negative [18]. Additionally, in an in vitro assay for invasion utilizing denuded human amnions [28], we found that the tumor cells retained their malignant phenotype in culture by being capable of invasive growth while nonmalignant cells did not [29].

Recently we compared tumor and normal cells for sensitivity to tumor necrosis factor (TNF) [30]. Although the response of the tumors varied from specimen to specimen, the vast majority were very sensitive to TNF. In 13 of 18 cases, the TNF concentration which kills 90% of the cells (LD90) was <500 units/ml. In contrast, all of the specimens derived from normal breast epithelium had LD_{90} values >5,000 units/ml (Table I). In three cases, this differential sensitivity to TNF was seen in nonmalignant and malignant mammary epithelium from the same patient.

MODEL FOR MALIGNANT PROGRESSION

It has been hypothesized by Nowell [31] that increased capacity for genetic instability is a fundamental aspect of malignancy. He suggested that the gross chromosomal abnormalities observed in most cancers are the result of this genetic instability occurring in conjunction with selective pressures over a long period of time. In this model, the initial malignant changes usually occur without detectable cytogenetic abnormalities. Diploid neoplastic cells generate nonviable cells with grossly abnormal chromosomal

TABLE I. Response to TNF of Cultured Human Normal and Malignant Mammary Epithelium

Cultures	LD_{90} Values[a]		
	<500 units/ml	500–5000 units/ml	>5000 units/ml
Breast carcinoma	13/18(72%)	3/18(17%)	2/18(11%)
Nonmalignant breast epithelium	0/8(0%)	0/8(0%)	8/8(100%)

[a]Data are presented as follows: $\frac{\text{number of specimens with the indicated LD90 values}}{\text{total number of specimens examined}}$.

contents. Only occasionally does this process generate a viable aneuploid cell whose growth advantage allows it to populate the original tumor and or subsequent metastases.

There may be marked differences in the time course of these events in tumors of different tissues and organs. In some instances, the sequence occurs in a compressed time frame so that only a population with a grossly abnormal karyotype is present by the time of initial diagnosis. In other cases this evolutionary process may be slower so that the original diploid cells, the nonviable aneuploid cells, and the viable aneuploid subpopulations with growth advantages (i.e., at metastatic sites) all coexist in the primary lesion. We suggest that the latter situation occurs for breast cancers. This model makes predictions which have been verified by work reported from a number of laboratories as well as our own studies on breast cancer in culture. These predictions are summarized and discussed below.

Prediction 1: Diploid cells will be found in primary breast cancers and aneuploidy will be associated with malignant progression.

The majority of studies on the cellular DNA content of breast cancers have utilized either flow cytometry or microspectrophotometry on in situ material [for reviews, see references 1,8,32]. In these studies, the majority of breast cancers contain a cell population with diploid DNA content. In approximately 30% of the cases, all of the tumor cells are indistinguishable from true diploidy [33–38]. Auer et al. [35], using microspectrophotometry, described three additional types of primary breast cancer specimens. Besides diploid malignancies, a second type of cancer shows either a distinct modal value in the tetraploid region or has two well-defined peaks around the 2C and 4C regions. Whether those cells in the 4C regions are truly tetraploid cells or diploid cells in the G_2 phase of the cell cycle cannot be distinguished. The third type contains both 2C and 4C peaks but also includes cells with intermediate values for DNA content. The cells with intermediate DNA content may be either aneuploid or in the S phase of the cell cycle. The fourth group of cancers, which comprise only 30% of specimens, shows a pronounced and irregular aneuploidy with DNA content per cell ranging from levels near 2C up to values beyond 6C.

The tumors with more aneuploid and aberrant DNA ploidy levels tend to be more dedifferentiated and negative for estrogen receptors indicating a poor prognosis for the patient [35]. Auer et al. [39] undertook a retrospective study of fine-needle aspiration biopsy material from 112 patients with primary mammary carcinoma. They divided the specimens into those from patients who were alive after 10 years and those who were dead after 2 years. The vast majority of patients with long survival times had cancers with DNA values within the limits of normal mammary epithelial cells, while the majority of patients with apparently highly malignant breast carcinomas and poor survival exhibited DNA profiles with significant deviation from normal.

Cytometric analysis is limited by inability to detect small deletions, rearrangements, or other subtle deviations from diploidy. Direct karyotypic analysis of breast cancers has been difficult because of their slow growth rate. Most of the earlier studies on breast cancer karyotypes describe a single breast cancer; hence, it is difficult to evaluate how representative these are of most breast cancers. In two recent studies [40,41], approximately 40% of primary breast cancers were karyotyped. Both of these studies detected aneuploid cells in the tumors. However, it is most notable that, in the vast majority of cases, from 2 to 75% (median 9%) of the observed spreads were diploid. While the authors interpret these diploid cells as being of normal lymphocytic origin, they present no evidence that excludes the possibility that they are bona fide tumor cells. If lymphocytes were indeed proliferating, we would expect to see them in S or G-2 phase by microspectrophotometry. In our studies, only 4 lymphocytes were seen with S phase DNA contents among over 800 lymphocytes examined from 10 consecutive breast cancer cases; and none had G-2/M DNA contents (unpublished observations). Furthermore, there is no evidence in the literature that lymphocytes continue proliferation within tumors.

We have found that the vast majority of cells in short-term cultures from 15 different primary breast carcinomas were diploid [42]. In contrast, all of the cells cultured from effusion metastases were aneuploid [29,42]. Only an occasional cell within these cultures showed minimal and nonclonal karyotypic deviations from normal. As discussed above, similar (in some cases identical) short-term diploid cultures of primary breast carcinomas differed from cultured nonmalignant breast cells by a number of criteria including invasion, sensitivity to TNF, glycoprotein expression, expression of antigenic heterogeneity, and cytochalasin-induced heterokaryon formation. These observations provide strong evidence that the cells cultured from primary carcinomas indeed represent malignant cells and indicate that at least some malignant populations need not have gross karyotypic rearrangements. These diploid tumor cells may represent an early stage of malignancy which will provide important insights into fundamental differences between normal and malignant cells. By the time cancer cells reach the very deviant stage characteristic of effusion metastases such initial changes may be masked by numerous secondary changes.

Prediction 2: Many aneuploid cells in primary breast cancers are nonviable.

Some breast cancer cells are only loosely attached to the stromal matrix so that they can be easily dissociated by mechanical manipulation. These cells represent a population, within the tumor, characterized by low viability using dye exclusion tests. Mechanically separated populations are enriched in aneuploid cells, while cells released after enzymatic digestion of minced tumor tissue are predominantly viable and diploid [9]. These observations are predicted if the proposed model is correct, since one would expect populations enriched in aneuploid cells to be largely nonviable. However, it is important to be certain that the nonviable cells were present in vivo and not the result of artifacts arising during tissue processing. In the published studies, the mechanically dissociated cells were subjected to sheer stress in order to create a single cell population. More recently, we have mechanically dissociated tumors in a very gentle manner, making no attempt to dissociate tumor cell clumps. Even under these conditions, many preparations contained a large percentage of nonviable cells. We also ruled out the possibility that the mechanically dissociated cells are viable in vivo, but die during the period from initiation of surgery to dissociation in the laboratory. To approach this question, we examined cells immediately after needle aspiration of the lesion prior to commencement of surgery. We found a similar proportion of nonviable cells as with gentle mechanical dissociation of the tumor biopsy [43]. It is noteworthy that the mechanical dispersion techniques are the ones that are frequently used for analyzing DNA contents [39] and karyology [40] of tumor specimens; hence many reports of aneuploidy within breast cancers may overestimate the percentage of aneuploid cells within the tumor.

Prediction 3: Metastases will be highly variable because they arise after accumulation of many random genetic alterations.

To gain insight into the properties of cells representing later stages of malignant progression, we have begun to study malignant effusions. In culture, the effusion metastases are much less predictable than primary carcinomas even when they are handled in an identical manner [5]. For example, one effusion metastasis will attach well to the plastic substrate, proliferate until confluence, and then form domes and ridges characteristic of normal mammary epithelium. In contrast, a second effusion will not attach to the plastic, but will proliferate slowly in suspension [illustrated in ref. 5]. Cellular morphology and growth properties differ dramatically among pleural effusion specimens. In the samples we studied, the short-term cultures of malignant effusions often grew more slowly than primary cancer cultures and very few were able to clone on irradiated fibroblasts. Many malignant effusions grew better with medium M199 plus 10% fetal calf serum than with the medium formulation derived for normal mammary epithelium, although sometimes the reverse was true. Thus, each effusion seems to have a combination of properties in culture that deviate in a unique way from the uniform and predictable behavior of most primary carcinomas. These observations suggest that effusions have diverged from primary carcinomas via differing pathways, as would be predicted by our hypothesis.

Another example of the variability of metastatic specimens is seen in the derivation of established cell lines. Almost all breast cancer cell lines in existence have been derived from effusion metastases [for reviews, see 44-46]. Although the majority of metastatic specimens from pleural effusions can be cultured for a few population doublings, only approximately 5% of these cultures even under the best conditions, develop into cell lines. In one case, we examined the properties in culture of three breast cancer effusions from the same patient. Despite repeated attempts with cryopreserved cells, only the last specimen reproducibly exhibited immortality in culture. The first two specimens grew initially, but failed to develop into cell lines. Each specimen was also unique in morphology and growth properties, although karyotypic markers indicated a common origin [47]. These observations also suggest that the ability to develop cell lines from a human breast cancer is not random, either in relation to culture technique or to tumor progression. Furthermore, the capacity for infinite life in vitro is not a characteristic of all malignant breast cancer cells, rather it is an example of another phenotype which is sometimes acquired by some breast cancer cells at a late stage of malignant progression.

CONCLUSION

In these studies, we have demonstrated the utility of short-term cultures to investigate the biology of breast cancer at the cellular level. Most cultures from primary breast cancers are apparently diploid while those of metastatic effusions are uniformly aneuploid. We have also demonstrated that a significant but variable proportion of cells in primary breast cancers are biologically unimportant because they are no longer viable as measured by dye exclusion. These findings are consistent with the model stated by Nowell [31] in which malignancy arises in diploid cells which coexist in the early tumor with unstable and often irrelevant aneuploid cells.

ACKNOWLEDGMENTS

This study was supported by grants from ACS (PDT-282), NCI (RO1-CA38739, PO1-CA44768), and Cetus Corporation.

REFERENCES

1. Smith HS, Wolman SR, Hackett AJ: Biochim Biophys Acta 738:103–123, 1984.
2. Stampfer MR, Hallowes RC, Hackett AJ: In Vitro 16:415–425, 1980.
3. Stampfer MR: In Vitro 18:531–537, 1982.
4. Smith HS, Lan S, Ceriani R, Hackett AJ, Stampfer MR: Cancer Res 41:4637–4643, 1981.
5. Hackett AJ, Smith HS: In Webber and Sekeley (ed): "In Vitro Models for Cancer Research." Vol. III. Boca Raton, FL: CRC Press, 1986, pp 31–49.
6. Smith HS, Hackett AJ: Lab Clin Med 109:236–243, 1987.
7. Smith HS, Hackett AJ: NY Acad Sci 464:288–300, 1986.
8. Smith HS, Wolman SR, Auer G, Hackett AJ: In Rich MA, Hager JC, Taylor-Papadimitriou J (eds): "Breast Cancer: Origins, Detection and Treatment." Boston: Martinus Nijhoff, 1986, pp 75–89.
9. Chassevent A, Daver A, Bertrand G, Coic H, Geslin J, Bridabe MCl, George P, Larra F: Cytometry 5:263–267, 1984.
10. Easty GC, Easty DM, Monaghan P, Ormerod MG, Neville AM: Int J Cancer 26:577–584, 1980.
11. Stoker MGP, Pigott D, Taylor-Papadimitriou J: Nature 264:764–767, 1976.
12. Taylor-Papadimitriou J, Purkiss P, Fentimen IS: J Cell Physiol 102:317–321, 1979.
13. Soule HD, McGrath CM: In Vitro 22:6–12, 1986.
14. Kirkland WL, Yang H, Jorgensen T, Langley C, Furmanski P: J Natl Cancer Inst 63:29–42, 1979.
15. Yang J, Richards J, Guzman R, Omagawa W, Nandi S: PNAS 77:2088–2092, 1980
16. Biran S, Horowitz AT, Fuks Z, Vlodavsky I: Int J Cancer 31:557–566, 1983.
17. Hammond SL, Ham RG, Stampfer MR: PNAS 81:5435–5439, 1984.
18. Stampfer MR, Hackett AJ, Hancock M, Leung JP, Edgington TS, Smith HS: Cold Spring Harbor Symposium on Cell Proliferation 9:819–829, 1982.
19. Stampfer MR, Vlodavsky I, Smith HS, Ford R, Becker FF, Riggs, J: JNCI 67:253–261, 1981.
20. Hallowes RC, Millis R, Pigott D, Shearer M, Stoker MGP, Taylor-Papadimitriou J: Clin Oncol: 3:81–90, 1977.
21. Taylor-Papadimitriou J, Fentimen IS, Burchell J: In McGrath C, Brennan MJ, Rich MA (eds): "Problems and Directions in Cell Biology of Breast Cancer." New York: Academic Press, 1980, pp 347–362.
22. Smith HS, Dairkee SH, Ljung BM, Mayall B, Sylvester SS, Hackett AJ: In Medina D, Kidwell W, Heppner G, Anderson E (eds): "Biology of Experimental Mammary Cancer." New York: Plenum Press, in press.
23. Asaga T, Suzuki K, Takemiya S, Okamoto T, Tamura N, Umeda MB: Gann: 74:95–99, 1983.
24. Medina D, Osborn CJ, Ash BB: Cancer Res 40:329–333, 1980.
25. Ceriani RL, Peterson JA, Blank EW: Cancer Res 44:3303–3039, 1984.
26. Leung JP, Plow EF, Nakamura RM, Edgington TS: J Immunol 121:1287–1296, 1978.
27. Leung JP, Borden GM, Nakamura RM, DeHeer DH, Edgington TS: Cancer Res 39:2057–2061, 1979.
28. Russo RG, Thorglirsson UP, Liotta LA: In Liotta LA, Hart IR (eds): "In Vitro Quantitative Assay of Invasion Using Human Amnion." The Hague: Martinus Nijhoff, 1982, pp 173–187.
29. Smith HS, Liotta LA, Hancock MC, Wolman SR, Hackett AJ: PNAS 82:1805–1809, 1985.
30. Dollbaum C, Smith HS, Hiller AJ, Creasey A, Lin L, Rudolph A: Proc Am Assoc Cancer Res: 28:401, 1987.
31. Nowell PC: Science 194:23–28, 1976.
32. Meyer JS, McDivitt RW, Stone KR, Prey MU, Baur WC: Breast Cancer Res Treat 4:79–88, 1984.
33. Fossa SD, Marton PF, Knudson OS, Kaalhus O, Bormer O, Vaage S: Human Pathol 13:626–630, 1982.
34. Fossa SD, Thorud E, Vaage S, Shoaib MC: Acta Pathol Microbiol Immunol Scand Section A 91:235–243, 1983.
35. Auer GU, Caspersson TO, Wallgren AS: Anal Quant Cytol 2:161–165, 1980.

36. Krug H: Cell Mol Biol 22:309–312, 1977.
37. Kute TE, Muss HB, Anderson D, Crumb K, Miller B, Burnes D, Dube LA: Cancer Res 41: 3524–3529, 1981.
38. Olszewski W, Darzynkiewicz Z, Rosen PP, Schwartz MK, Melamed MR: Cancer 48:980–984, 1981.
39. Auer G, Eriksson E, Azavido E, Caspersson T., Wallgren A: Cancer Res 44:394–396, 1984.
40. Rodgers CS, Hill SM, Hulten MA: Cancer Genetics Cytogenetics: 13:95–119, 1984.
41. Gebhart E, Bruderlein S, Tulusan AH, Maillot KV, Birkmann J: Int J Cancer: 34:369–373, 1984.
42. Wolman SR, Smith HS, Stampfer HS, Hackett AJ: Cancer Genetics Cytogenetics 16:49–64, 1985.
43. Ljung BM, Mayall BH, Lottich C, Boyer C, Leight GS, Siegler HF, Sylvester SS, Smith HS: Proc Am Assoc Cancer Res 28:34, 1987.
44. Engel LW, Young MA: Cancer Res 38:4327–4339, 1978.
45. Cailleau R, Olive M, Cruciger QVJ: In Vitro 14:911–915, 1978.
46. Smith HS, Dollbaum C: In Barserga R (ed): "Handbook of Experimental Pharmacology: Tissue Growth Factors." 57:451–478, 1982.
47. Smith HS, Wolman SR, Dairkee SH, Hancock MC, Lippman M, Leff A, Hackett AJ: JNCI: 78:611–615, 1987.

Role of Inflammatory Cells in Tumor Progression and Diversification

Gloria H. Heppner

Michigan Cancer Foundation, Detroit, Michigan 48201

Tumor progression is believed to result from the generation of variant tumor cell populations ("tumor heterogeneity") that gradually proliferate and change the population distribution of cells with varying phenotypic traits within the growing neoplasm. The basis of tumor heterogeneity is thought to be an underlying "genetic instability" in tumor cells. It has been suggested that genetic instability itself increases with progression so that the most malignant (metastatic) tumor cells are the most unstable. Using a series of tumor lines derived from a single mouse mammary tumor, we were unable to show that metastatic ability and spontaneous mutation rate were correlated. However, we did find metastatic ability to be associated with sensitivity to the action of an exogenous mutagen, ethyl methanesulfonate. We have also found that metastatic mammary tumors, in contrast to nonmetastatic counterparts, are preferentially infiltrated with relatively mature, activated macrophages, known to be the source of potentially mutagenic oxygen metabolites. We postulate that there is some sort of a cause-effect relationship among sensitivity to mutagen, ability to metastasize, and free-radical-producing, infiltrating macrophages. To this end, we have shown that tumor-associated macrophages are mutagenic in the Ames assay and are able to induce stable, drug-resistant variants in mammary tumor populations. The mutagenic activity of macrophages is dependent on their stage of activation and is prevented by inhibitors of H_2O_2, $OH\cdot$, and superoxide. The variants induced by macrophages are biochemically similar to those induced by a standard chemical mutagen.

Key words: tumor progression, tumor heterogeneity, mutagenic macrophages

The idea that tumor heterogeneity and progression are reflections, at least in part, of multiple, sequential genetic changes in emerging neoplastic populations has its strongest origins in the works of Foulds [1] and of Nowell [2], both of whom emphasized the importance of change and variability in cancer behavior. My own interest in this area has two starting points. As a graduate student I was exposed to the work of Ken DeOme and "Ranu" Nandi on the development of mouse mammary cancers. A favorite saying of DeOme was "There is no such thing as *a* cancer cell," and he stressed the necessity of studying cancer on the tissue level. My own graduate advisors were David Weiss and Phyllis Blair, immunologists who did pioneering studies on the host responses to

Received April 9, 1987.

© 1988 Alan R. Liss, Inc.

neoplasia. These themes—the multicellular biology of cancer and the interrelationships between cancer and host—continue to shape my approach to cancer research.

TUMOR HETEROGENEITY AND PROGRESSION

The idea that cancers are composed of multiple subpopulations of neoplastic cells—variants derived from some, perhaps lost, "initiated" cell—has become commonly accepted. Similarly, the notion that tumor progression is due to the development and ascendance of additional variants, each bringing new biological and therapeutic characteristics into the "mix," is recognized as reasonable. Attention has now shifted from the mere description of tumor heterogeneity to a search for the mechanisms which bring it about. One hypothesis is that cancer cells per se are "genetically unstable," that is, prone to experience genetic errors that translate into new phenotypic potentials. A corollary of this hypothesis is that genetic instability is itself a progression characteristic such that the "most progressed" or malignant variants are the most unstable. Direct evidence for this has been presented in several types of tumors [3]. Kenji Yamashina and I decided to test this corollary in our system, which is a series of phenotypically diverse tumor lines, all of which were derived from the same, autochthonous strain BALB/cf C_3H mouse mammary tumor [4].

GENETIC STABILITY OF MAMMARY TUMOR LINES

Following the precedent of Cifone and Fidler [3], we tested lines of our series that differed in ability to metastasize for the rate at which they developed resistance to two drugs, 6-thioguanine (6-TG) and ouabain. Although there was a 9–10-fold difference among our lines in rates of spontaneous mutation to drug resistance, mutation was not notably frequent (rates were in the range of 0.5–30×10^{-7}/cell/generation) and, most importantly, there was no correlation between mutation rate and ability to metastasize (nor with other potentially confounding characteristics such as cell size, shape, ploidy, or ability to participate in metabolic cooperation) [5].

Of course one can argue that mutations that involve alterations at the level of single base pairs are just one, perhaps irrelevant, type of genetic error and that our failure to reproduce, in our system, the results of Cifone and Fidler is not very meaningful. Although we certainly accept that argument, Yamashina and I decided to look at genetic instability from another perspective—not as a spontaneous event, but as susceptibility to an exogenous mutagen.

For our experiments we chose the mutagen, ethyl methanesulfonate (EMS), and we worked out the experimental protocol to optimize the factors for inducing mutation, again to 6-TG and to ouabain, in our mammary tumor line system. In this case our results were different from those of the spontaneous assays. The frequency of EMS-induced mutation to 6-TG resistance was highest in those lines that were able to metastasize spontaneously from a subcutaneous or mammary fat pad site to lung and was undetectable (frequency $<10^{-5}$) in lines that were nonmetastatic. The frequency of EMS-induced mutation to ouabain resistance also was highest in those lines that could metastasize spontaneously, as well as in one line that could colonize the lung after intravenous injection. Induced mutation was below detectability in nonmetastatic lines [5].

As a consequence of these results, we turned our attention away from "spontaneous instability'' and toward ''induced'' mutations as a mechanism for genetic variation in our system. This shift required that we identify sources in situ, in the tumor environment, that might be such inducers. Other work in our laboratory pointed to a possible source.

TUMOR ASSOCIATED MACROPHAGES (TAMS) IN MOUSE MAMMARY TUMORS

As stated at the outset, one of my concerns is the role of host cells in the development and behavior of tumors, in particular, mammary tumors. Work done in collaboration with Scott Loveless, Keith Mahoney, and Amy Fulton had characterized the macrophage infiltrates of tumors produced by the same mammary tumor lines that Yamashina and I had used above. To our surprise we found that TAMs from metastatic tumors are *qualitatively* different from those of nonmetastatic tumors, even though the numbers of infiltrating TAMs are similar. TAM populations from primary implants of metastatic tumors are skewed in the direction of large dense cells, with ectoenzyme and prostaglandin profiles of mature macrophages, and with the ability to kill tumor cells in in vitro assays. By contrast, TAMs from nonmetastatic tumors are smaller, less dense, have immature profiles, and are poorly tumoricidal, if at all [6–8].

These observations on TAM characteristics of metastatic versus nonmetastatic tumors were important to our work on genetic instability for two reasons: 1) more mature, ''activated'' macrophages are known to release a variety of active oxygen metabolites, such as superoxide anion, OH·, and H_2O_2 [9]; 2) these same oxygen metabolites are hypothesized to be involved in, among other things, inducing the genetic changes of tumor initiation and promotion [10].

In a perhaps unjustifiably large leap of faith, we hypothesized that TAMs might be the source of oxidative mutagens which could fuel tumor progression by inducing the production of new variant populations. The association of free-radical-producing TAMs with metastatic tumors could have a cause-effect basis—in either direction: 1) those tumor cells that already had some part of the necessary metastatic associated phenotype might attract or retain that subpopulation of TAM which could induce new mutations, some of which would complete the repertoire necessary for full metastatic capability, or 2) mutagenic TAMs could enhance the rate at which tumor cells gain metastatic capability per se, and, in that way, actually contribute to the definition of a ''metastatic tumor.'' This possibility may be most easily related to the ''dynamic heterogeneity'' model in which high vs low metastasis is seen, not in terms of the acquisition of stable, absolute characteristics, but rather as a relative difference in the frequency with which basically unstable metastatic ability is gained and lost [11]. In either event, our hypothesis requires that one visualize metastasis as a tissue phenomenon involving multiple cell types of both cancer and host origin.

MUTAGENIC MACROPHAGES AND MOUSE MAMMARY TUMORS

Over the past couple of years various associates and I have tried to address our hypothesis. Suffice it to say that we are not proposing that mutagenic macrophages are ''the,'' or even ''a'' *major* determinant in metastasis in all systems; we know that mutagenic activity *alone* is not enough for metastasis to occur; we suspect that mutagenic macrophages are not a factor at all in some tumor systems. Nevertheless, we feel that we have gotten hold of a big-enough piece of the total picture to warrant further study. What we have found so far is that 1) TAMs can increase the mutation rate in the Ames assay, using bacterial tester strains TA 98 and TA 100 [12], and that 2) macrophages, including TAMs, can induce 6-TG resistant variants in mouse mammary tumor cells in vitro [13]. This latter activity is seen after coincubation of tumor cells and macrophages in vitro for 7–9 days, followed by cloning in selective, 6-TG-containing medium. Activity requires macrophage activation. In our assay system the ratio of macrophages to tumor cells must be at least 50:1 for consistent results. The activity is reproducible and 2 to 15 times above background levels. The 6-TG variants that are cloned after macrophage exposure behave like EMS-induced variants, both in regard to the biochemical alteration (decreased hypoxanthine-guanine phosphoribosyltransferase activity) and in the low frequency of reversion to parental type ($\sim 2 \times 10^{-7}$). We find no evidence that the basis of our results is macrophage-mediated selection of 6-TG resistant variants. Thus, we think that macrophages are acting as true mutagens in our system.

We are not alone in drawing attention to the possible role of inflammatory cells as sources of genetic alterations in neoplasia. Troll and Wiesner [14] have recently reviewed the role of oxygen radicals in promotion and have discussed the links between oxygen-radicals and inflammatory phagocytes and between inflammatory cells and promotion. Weitzman, Stossel, and associates have reported extensively on the mutagenic activity of human peripheral monocytes [15–18] and have also shown that such leucocytes can induce both morphological transformation of 10T 1/2 cells and the ability of these cells to grow as tumors in nude mice [19].

As indicated above, the mechanism whereby inflammatory cells cause genetic change is thought to involve production of active oxygen species. In our studies we found that inhibitors of superoxide, OH·, and H_2O_2, all could inhibit macrophage induction of 6-TG resistant mammary tumor variants [13]. Macrophages can produce oxygen metabolites by two routes—the respiratory burst and arachidonate metabolism. The metabolites must then somehow interact with the target cell. The most likely mechanism is lipidperoxidation of cell membranes, an event which is known to generate intracellular free radicals and other DNA-altering substances collectively known as clastogenic factors [10,20]. How all this results in genetic error is a complicated subject beyond the scope of this presentation.

FUTURE PLANS

It is becoming clear that the relationship of macrophages to heterogeneity and progression is exceedingly complex. From our perspective we are in immediate need of two things (other than more money). One is a fast, relatively inexpensive, relatively easy way of measuring macrophage mutagenicity in vitro. To this end, Leslie Dorcey and Amy Fulton have begun to adapt Birnboim's DNA strand break assay [21] to our system. So far they have shown that enzyme-generated oxygen metabolites can cause strand breaks in mammary tumor cells, as can TPA-treated macrophages. We have high hopes that this assay will prove to be a useful tool to test inflammatory cell activity under a variety of conditions.

A second need is a reproducible in vivo system to study the mutagenic role of inflammatory cells in neoplasia. Weitzman's lab has described a colon cancer model in which ulcerative colitis is induced by repeated enemas of leucocyte-attracting peptides in mice given the carcinogen 1,2 dimethylhydrazine [22]. Preliminary results show that inflammation of the colon increases cancer incidence and that vitamin E might reverse this effect.

For our part, we are continuing to investigate the role of mutagenic macrophages in metastasis but we are also turning our attention to another in vivo model of tumor progression, the spontaneous development of mammary adenocarcinomas from mammary fat pad implants of preneoplastic hyperplastic alveolar nodule (HAN) lines. Wei-Zen Wei has found that active NK cells, which also produce oxygen radicals, are in high numbers in HANs, in contrast to the cancers that develop from them [23]. It is possible that the NK cells are involved directly, or indirectly through effects on infiltrating macrophages, in the generation of tumorigenic variants in the preneoplastic line and thus on the benign to cancerous progression. If so, it will once again illustrate "there is no such thing as *a* cancer cell."

ACKNOWLEDGMENTS

These studies are supported by NIH grants CA 27437 and CA 27419, by a grant from Concern Foundation, by the United Foundation of Detroit, and by the E. Walter Albachten bequest to the Michigan Cancer Foundation.

REFERENCES

1. Foulds L: Neoplastic Development, Vols 1 and 2. New York: Academic Press, 1969, 1975.
2. Nowell PC: Science 194:23–28, 1976.
3. Cifone MA, Fidler IJ: Proc Nat Acad Sci USA 78:6949–6952, 1981.
4. Dexter DL, Kowalski HM, Blazer BA, Fligiel Z, Vogel R, Heppner GH: Cancer Res 38:3174–3181, 1978.
5. Yamashina K, Heppner GH: Cancer Res 45:4015–4019, 1985.
6. Loveless SE, Heppner GH: J Immunol 131:2074–2078, 1983.
7. Mahoney KH, Fulton AM, Heppner GH: J Immunol 131:2079–2085, 1983.
8. Mahoney KH, Miller BE, Heppner GH: J Leuk Biol 38:573–585, 1985.
9. Nathan CF, Brukner LH, Silverstein SC, Cohn ZA: J Exp Med 149:84–99, 1979.
10. Cerutti PA: Science 227:375–381, 1985.
11. Harris JF, Chambers AF, Hill RP, Ling V: Proc Natl Acad Sci USA 79:5547–5551, 1982.
12. Fulton AM, Loveless SE, Heppner GH: Cancer Res 44:4308–4311, 1984.
13. Yamashina K, Miller BE, Heppner GH: Cancer Res 46:2396–2401, 1986.
14. Troll W, Weisner R: Annu Rev Pharmacol Toxicol 25:509–529, 1985.
15. Weitzman SA, Stossel TP: Science 212:546–547, 1981.
16. Weitzman SA, Stossel TP: J Immunol 128:2770–2772, 1982.
17. Weitzman SA, Stossel TP: Cancer Lett 22:337–341, 1984.
18. Weitberg AB, Weitzman SA, Destrempes SA, Latt SA, Stossel TP: N Engl J Med 308:26–30, 1983.
19. Weitzman SA, Weitberg AB, Clark EP, Stossel TP: Science 227:1231–1233, 1985.
20. Lewis JG, Hamilton T, Adams DO: Carcinogenesis 7:813–818, 1986.
21. Birnboim HC: Science 215:1247–1249, 1982.
22. Chester JF, Gaissert HA, Ross JS, Malt RA, Weitzman SA: J Natl Cancer Inst 76:939–942, 1986.
23. Wei W-Z, Heppner G: Br J Cancer 55:589–594, 1987.

Interactions Between Genetic Constitution of Metastatic Tumour Cells and Host Factors

D. Tarin

Nuffield Department of Pathology, John Radcliffe Hospital, Oxford University, Oxford OX3 9DU, England

The work of this laboratory is based on the conception that the driving force of the metastatic process is created by regulatory genomic disturbances in a small population of cells within the primary tumour and that the success or failure of such cells to form a deposit in distant organs is not random, but is dictated by interactions between the tumour cells, showering out from the primary neoplasm, and metabolic conditions encountered in the microenvironment of other organs in the body, where they lodge. Superimposed on such local interactions are systemic effects exerted by the immune and endocrine systems, the magnitude of which depends on the type and quantity of exposed antigens and receptors on the disseminating tumour cells, as well as on the constitutional vigour of the host.

Our work began several years ago, with studies on spontaneous murine mammary tumours, which we found to have differing capabilities to colonise the lungs, after intravenous inoculation into syngeneic recipients. The degree of colonisation was characteristic of the individual tumour and was broadly the same whether its cells were inoculated into the original donor (which had previous acquaintance with the tumour) or a naive recipient (which had not). (See review in [1]). Some tumours heavily colonised the lungs of every inoculated animal, while others could not form deposits in any recipient. Such findings indicated that pulmonary colonisation (experimental metastasis) after intravenous inoculation, is dependent on intrinsic properties of the tumour cells.

In further work we found that cells from a given primary tumour could reproducibly form secondary deposits in certain organs and not in others and that the combination of permissive sites for secondary tumour growth varied with each tumour [2]. Further work on this, with labelled tumour cells, showed that regardless of whether the tumour cells were inoculated intravenously or intraarterially, they were distributed to all organs within 1 hr, even though they only formed secondary tumour colonies in certain sites. This suggested that microenvironmental factors in the organs where the tumour cells arrested influenced whether they could form secondary deposits, even though cells from the same

Received May 15, 1987.

© 1988 Alan R. Liss, Inc.

tumour were known to be capable of forming tumour deposits in other organs. Thus, it was concluded that the growth of tumour cells can be regulated by the host organ microenvironment and that they are not invincible [3,4].

In recent years the introduction of a new form of therapy for patients with malignant ascites has provided direct confirmation of these observations and conclusions. These patients have been treated with the technique of peritoneovenous shunting, in which the malignant ascites (containing tumour cells) is returned to the circulation, to palliate the pain and discomfort caused by the accumulating fluid in the abdomen. In a series of 22 patients subsequently autopsied, approximately half were found to have no evidence of haematogenous metastases, despite surviving for periods of up to 3 years, while the remainder had seedling metastases in many sites, sometimes within 1 month. Again, it would appear that the capability to colonise distant sites is an intrinsic property of the tumour cells and that not all malignant neoplasms can necessarily do so. In some of these patients, who had clinically evident deposits before introduction of the shunt, we saw no evidence of metastases in any other site, corroborating the interpretation that the widely disseminated cells can grow only in certain organs [5].

Murine mammary tumour cells preferentially form secondary deposits in the lungs, and Horak et al. [6] found that their survival in vitro is improved when cocultured with lung fragments, but that they die or are dramatically reduced in number when cocultured with other organs. Further studies showed that this effect of the organ on cocultured cells can also be mediated by organ-conditioned medium, transferred to tumour cells cultured in separate dishes. The pattern of encouragement or inhibition of tumour cell growth and survival reflected the site specificity of growth of mammary tumour cells in vivo and provided further support for the interpretation that the host microenvironment can modulate secondary tumour formation. As the effect can be exerted by organs or by cell-free conditioned media from immunologically naive animals, it seems unlikely that these effects are related to immune suppression of tumour growth.

In our investigations of intrinsic properties which may endow tumour cells with the capability to migrate from the primary tumour and form secondary deposits elsewhere, we have examined protease output, cell surface properties, and clonogenicity. We found that there is a strong association between the output of collagenase and the capability of tumour cells to colonise the lungs [7]. On the other hand, we did not find any cell surface properties which correlated with the metastatic phenotype [8,9]. Now, however, we feel that these cellular characteristics are merely indicators of the prevailing pattern of gene activation at the time of study and are not prime movers in the metastatic process. We have therefore turned our attention to examination of the genetic constitution of the tumour cells, within the population in the primary tumour, which might become capable of migrating to distant sites and setting up metastases.

We have adopted a number of different approaches in an attempt to identify the gene or genes involved. The first approach has been to introduce a defined gene with known oncogenic potential into previously nonmetastatic cells and to observe for phenotypic change. This involved transfection of the c-Harvey-*ras* oncogene into nontumourigenic, nonmetastatic cells. A second approach we are using involves transfection of total genomic DNA from metastatic into nonmetastatic cells. Finally, we have examined whether treatment of weakly metastatic cells, with agents known to influence tumour progression and gene expression (e.g., tetra-phorbol acetate or 5-azacytidine) can affect metastatic capability. The results to date show that while successful incorporation and expression of the activated c-Ha-*ras* oncogene did not induce nonmetastatic

3T3 cells to become spontaneously metastatic [10], transfection of weakly metastatic tumour cells with DNA from highly metastatic human and animal cell lines did markedly augment their spontaneous metastatic capability and their lung colony-forming potential and induce them to form deposits in many extra pulmonary sites [11]. We have also found that treatment of some tumour cell lines with azacytidine and TPA increases their metastatic behaviour after subcutaneous inoculation. As several cell divisions must have occurred in producing the subcutaneous tumour before the cells disseminated, we consider the change of phenotype to be heritable and probably caused by alterations in gene expression.

These results suggest that components of the metastatic phenotype are heritable, highly conserved in evolution, and can be conferred on previously nonmetastatic tumour cells by transfer of genomic DNA. They also indicate that investigation of the genetic basis of metastatic behaviour is now technically feasible. However, the process is so complex that there is need for caution in interpretation, and the process of analysis will be long and difficult.

ACKNOWLEDGMENTS

This study was supported by the Cancer Research Campaign of Great Britain.

REFERENCES

1. Price JE, Carr D, Jones LD, Messer P, Tarin D: Invasion Metastasis 2:77–112, 1982.
2. Tarin D, Price JE: Cancer Res 41:3604–3609, 1981.
3. Juacaba SF, Jones LD, Tarin D: Invasion Metastasis 3:208–220, 1983.
4. Potter KM, Juacaba SF, Price JE, Tarin D: Invasion Metastasis 3:221–233, 1983.
5. Tarin D, Price JE, Kettlewell MGW, Souter RG, Vass ACR, Crossley B: Cancer Res 44:3584–3592, 1984.
6. Horak E, Darling DL, Tarin D: J Nat Cancer Inst 76:913–922, 1986.
7. Tarin D, Hoyt BJ, Evans DJ: Br J Cancer 46:266–278, 1982.
8. Sargent NSE, Price JE, Tarin D: Br J Cancer 48:569–577, 1983.
9. Sargent NSE, Price JE, Darling DL, Flynn MP, Tarin D: Br J Cancer 55:21–28, 1987.
10. Wallace JS, Syms AJ, Hayle AJ, Fleming KA, Tarin D: Proc Am Assoc Canc Res 27:59, 1986.
11. Hayle AJ, Darling DL, Whittaker PA, Fleming KA, Tarin D: Proc Am Assoc Canc Res 28:70, 1987.

Differences Among Endothelial Cells: Their Relation to Tumor Growth and Metastasis

Marek Kaminski and Robert Auerbach

Laboratory of Developmental Biology, Department of Zoology, University of Wisconsin, Madison, Wisconsin 53706

The observation that vascular endothelial cells of different organ origins differ in their cell surface antigens and lectin binding sites leads us to the hypothesis that heterogeneity among vascular endothelial cells may influence site-specific metastasis. Recent experiments from our laboratory indicate that tumors differ in their relative adhesion to murine endothelial cell monolayers depending on the organ from which they were derived. Selective affinity of specific tumors appears in general to conform to their behavior in vivo, albeit with some exceptions. Adhesion to cell monolayers protects tumor cells from the cytocidal action of natural killer cells, with adhesion to endothelial cell monolayers reducing NK-mediated lysis by as much as 75%. These experiments suggest that endothelial heterogeneity may play an important role in influencing differential tumor cell adhesion and survival, requisite to organ-specific metastasis.

Key words: endothelium, metastasis, adhesion, natural cytotoxicity, tumors

We have proposed that vascular endothelial cells may represent a heterogeneous population of cells manifesting organ specificity [1,2]. We based our initial hypothesis on the finding that mouse brain-derived microvascular endothelial cells expressed brain-specific antigens including Thy-1 but lacked class II antigens, whereas, in contrast, microvascular cells derived from the epididymal fat pad or ovary lacked Thy-1 but showed constitutive expression of Ia antigens [1,2]. Subsequently we were able to demonstrate through the use of monoclonal antibodies that lung endothelial cells shared antigens with lung fibroblasts, and that common cell surface antigens were expressed on ovary fibroblasts and ovary microvascular endothelium [3].

These initial experiments have prompted us to investigate in more detail the heterogeneity of endothelial cells, with special emphasis on the possible role of that heterogeneity in influencing tumor cell metastasis. Our research in this area, reviewed in this report, leads us to the conclusion that endothelial cell specificity can materially influence tumor cell adhesion. Moreover, adhesion of tumor cells to endothelium correlates well with in vivo metastatic behavior, suggesting that selective metastasis may

Received June 19, 1987.

© 1988 Alan R. Liss, Inc.

in part be due to selective adhesion to vascular endothelium [4,5]. Additional experiments will also be reviewed which demonstrate that endothelial cells afford protection to tumor cells from the cytocidal action of natural killer (NK) cells and that this protection is directly correlated with the extent of tumor cell adhesion to these endothelial cells [6]. Together our observations suggest that the vascular endothelial cells play a significant role in regulating the selective survival and metastatic spread of tumors.

MATERIALS AND METHODS

Vascular endothelial cells were isolated from different adult mouse organs by the basic collagenase protocol described in detail previously [2,3]. In brief, a 0.5% solution of collagenase (type II or mixed) in Dulbecco's phosphate-buffered saline (PBS) and 1% chicken or fetal bovine serum (FBS) was added to minced tissue fragments. The preparation was incubated for 30–60 min followed by mechanical dispersion. Microvascular fragments were concentrated on a 30 micron mesh Nitex filter and cultured directly to permit outgrowth of endothelial cells. Alternatively, the fragments were isolated and subjected to further collagenase digestion to obtain single cells.

Purification of endothelial cells was accomplished by cell sorting techniques [3,7]. Cells obtained initially or from subcultures were labelled either with a fluoresceinated monoclonal antibody to angiotensin-converting enzyme [7] or a fluorogenic derivative of acetylated low density lipoprotein (diIacLDL) [8], and sorted using a FACS-IV cell sorter operating with an argon ion laser with output at 488 nm (for fluorescein) or 514 nm (for diIacLDL).

Cell adhesion assays were carried out by adding ^{3}H-thymidine-labelled tumor cell suspensions to endothelial cell monolayers and assessing the extent of adhesion over 10, 20, 30, and 45 min following addition of tumor cells [4,5]. In brief, tumor cells in rapid growth phase were labelled with ^{3}H-thymidine for 18–24 hr to achieve maximal labelling, endothelial cells or control fibroblasts were plated in 24-well plates and permitted to grow to confluence, adhesion was permitted to occur under continuous agitation of the culture wells. Radioactivity retained on the monolayers was determined by first gently rinsing the plates to remove nonadhering tumor cells and then determining residual radioactivity by lysis of cells using ammonium hydroxide.

Natural cytotoxicity was determined by a standard NK assay using ^{51}chromium-labelled YAC-1 cells as NK targets, P815 tumor cells as a negative control target, syngeneic adult splenocytes as a source of NK cells, and syngeneic endothelial cells as a substrate monolayer. Endothelial cells were permitted to come to confluence in 96-well plates. Tumor cells and splenocytes were added simultaneously, and the amount of chromium released into the medium was determined after 4 hr. Maximum release data were obtained by 1N NH$_4$OH lysis of aliquots of labelled tumor cells, and background release data were determined by assessment of chromium release from cultures in which splenocytes were not included [6].

RESULTS

Selective Adhesion of Tumor Cells to Endothelium

We initially compared the adhesion of GL-26 glioma cells and OTT 6050 ovary-seeking teratoma cells to endothelial cells derived from perinatal brain and adult ovary microvessels (Fig. 1A). Adhesion of glioma cells was significantly greater to brain-derived

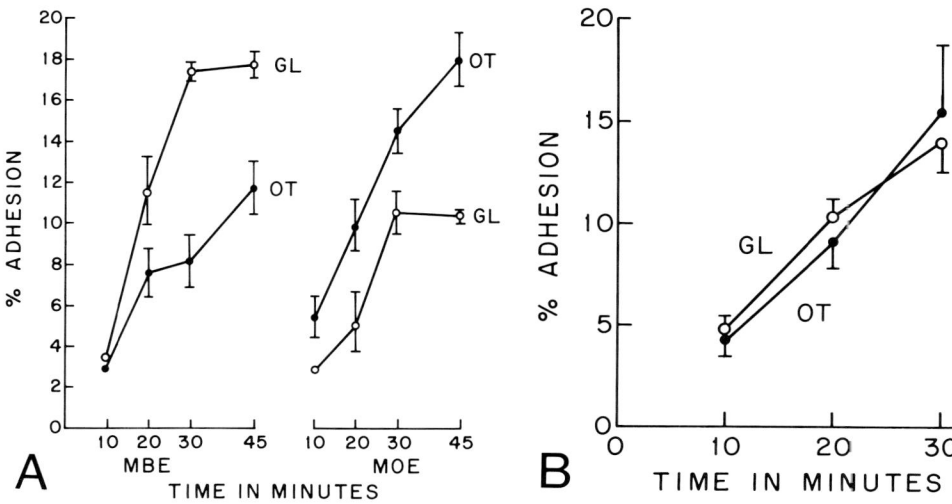

Fig. 1. Comparison of glioma (GL) and ovarian teratocarcinoma (OT) cell adhesion to **A:** mouse brain endothelial (MBE) and mouse ovary endothelial (MOE) cells; **B:** L929 fibroblasts (from ref. 4).

endothelial cells than to ovary-derived ones. Conversely, teratoma cells adhered more readily to ovary-derived endothelial cells than to those from brain. In parallel experiments, the adhesion of glioma cells and teratoma cells to fibroblasts was assessed. No differences were found in the ability of the GL-26 and OTT 6050 tumor cells to adhere to L929 fibroblasts (Fig. 1B).

To extend these findings we expanded both the panel of tumor cells and the number of different endothelial cell monolayers to be tested. In general, adhesion of tumor cells to different endothelial cell monolayers conformed to the prediction that selectivity would correlate with in vivo preferential metastatic or growth behavior. For example, when compared to the H7777 rat Morris hepatoma cell line, glioma cells once again showed preferential adhesion to brain endothelial cells. Conversely, the H7777 hepatoma cells adhered selectively to liver-derived endothelium (Fig. 2). A similar preferential adhesion to hepatic endothelial cells was shown by a second hepatoma cell line [5]. Mammary carcinoma cells manifested preferential adhesion to lymphatic endothelium, a result consistent with the fact that mammary tumor cells are disseminated via the lymphatic route. On the other hand, there were other tumors, such as the S180 sarcoma, that appeared to show little if any selectivity. Some other adhesive preferences remain totally unexplained: both the H7777 hepatoma and endothelioma cell lines showed maximal affinity for 3T3 cells, while other tumors such as the GL-26 glioma resisted adhesion to 3T3 monolayers [4,5,9].

Effect of Endothelial Cells on Lymphocyte-Mediated Immune Surveillance

Since natural cytotoxic reactions play an important role in the host defense against spontaneous tumors [10,11], we tested the influence of endothelial cell substrata on the ability of unstimulated splenocytes to lyse NK-cell sensitive tumor target cells. The experiments, summarized by the data included in Figure 3, show that compared to lysis of tumor cell targets in the standard plastic well assay, cell monolayer substrata can

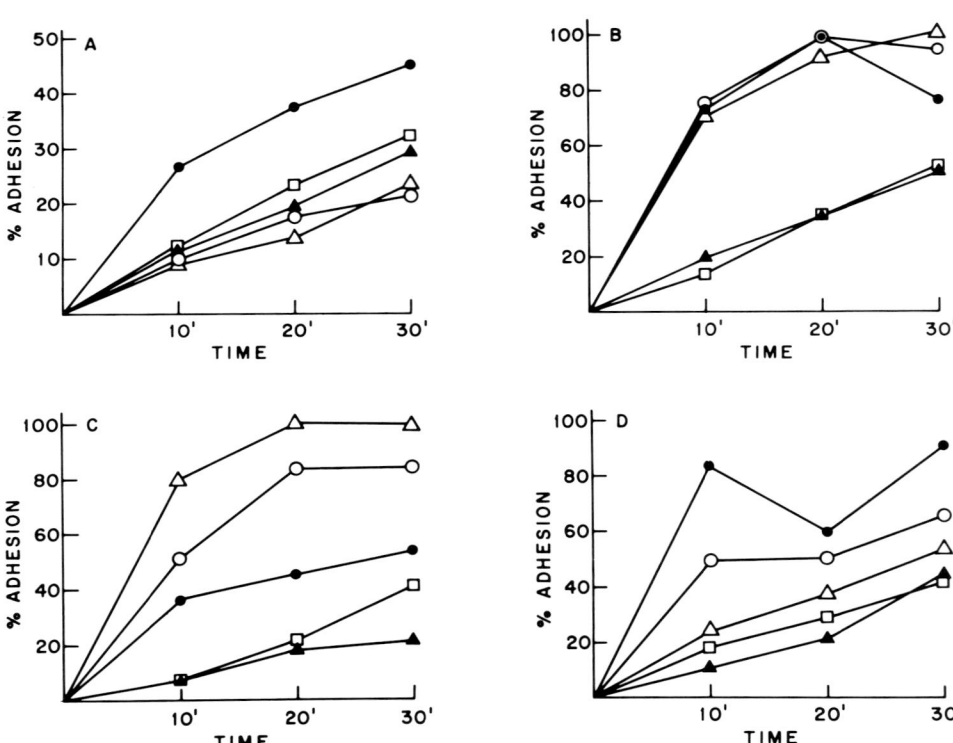

Fig. 2. Adhesion of different mouse tumors (**A**: endothelioma; **B**: sarcoma 180; **C**: teratoma OTT 6050; **D**: MBT-2 bladder tumor) to different murine confluent culture monolayers; (●) liver endothelial cells; (□) thoracic duct lymphatic endothelial cells; (△) lung endothelial cells; (○) 3T3 fibroblasts; (▲) brain endothelial cells (from ref. 5).

exert a strong protective effect on NK-mediated tumor cell killing. Moreover, fibroblasts and bovine aortic endothelial cells were found to be less effective than mouse lymphatic or lung microvascular endothelial cells (Fig. 3).

Further studies were carried out in which we assessed the extent of tumor cell adhesion to the monolayers during the course of the assay. These studies [6] showed a direct correlation between the extent of adhesion of the target cells to the monolayer substratum and the degree of protection from cytocidal action of the splenocytes. Moreover, when different tumor cells were used as targets for cytolysis this correlation was maintained. Thus, glioma cells were most protected by brain-derived microvascular endothelial cells [12,13], a result consistent with our earlier studies on the selective adhesion of different tumor cells to specific endothelial cell monolayers.

DISCUSSION

Site-specific selective adhesion of tumor cells has been demonstrated by several laboratories [e.g., 14–20]. While the earlier studies did not identify a particular cell type as having primary responsibility for this adhesion, subsequent studies both from our own laboratory and others [4,5,21–23] focused attention on the endothelium and

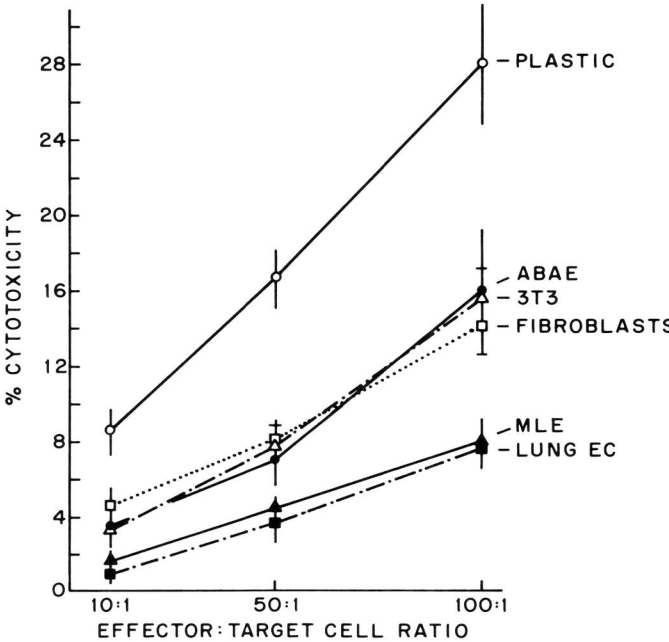

Fig. 3. Cytotoxicity of mouse splenocytes against YAC-1 tumor cells on different monolayers (data from six separate experiments, n = 3 for each data point for each experiment; results expressed as mean +/− S.E. [from ref. 6]). Adult bovine aortic endothelial cells (ABAE) and mouse lymphatic endothelial cells (MLE).

the subendothelial matrix. Since tumor dissemination is primarily through the vascular route, the relevance of endothelial cell selectivity is readily apparent: the probability of metastasis to a given site is directly related to the likelihood of tumor cell arrest by the endothelial cells of that site.

The fact that endothelial cell monolayers provide protection against natural immune surveillance by lymphocytes provides a further means of promoting selectivity of the metastatic process. It has always seemed remarkable that the efficacy of NK cell activity, as measured in vitro, should not be adequate to protect the organism in vivo from the development of metastases. Our results, however, provide an explanation of why tumor cells may survive in specific sites, since adhesion to endothelial cells appears to render the tumor cells less susceptible to NK-mediated lysis. Moreover, preliminary observations in our laboratory suggest that adhesion to endothelial cells is protective also against immune-mediated, antibody-dependent cytotoxicity (unpublished observations).

We do not yet have any clear understanding of the molecular basis for either the selective adhesion of tumor cells to endothelial cells or for the means by which endothelial cell/tumor interactions alter the susceptibility of the tumor cells to cytotoxic destruction [see ref. 5 and 7 for discussion]. A major goal of our research program is to identify the factors mediating these events.

Tumor metastasis represents a complex process involving a broad spectrum of events, including genetic and phenotypic alterations of the primary tumor cells, vascular dissemination, adhesion to endothelium, extravasation, induction of angiogenesis, and subsequent growth and differentiation at the metastatic site. We believe that heterogeneity of endothelial cells may play an important role in tumor cell metastasis, both directly and indirectly. Our in vitro experiments indicate that the tumor cell phenotype includes the capacity to differentiate among endothelial cell targets, so that the heterogeneity of the endothelium becomes a basis for selective retention of tumor cells released into the circulation. In turn, this retention permits these tumor cells to escape from immune surveillance and affords the cells time to penetrate the endothelial cell barrier. To what extent endothelial cell heterogeneity further influences the process of metastasis, as for example, by a differential response to angiogenic factors or by the production and release of specific growth factors, prostaglandins, or extracellular materials, remains to be determined.

ACKNOWLEDGMENTS

The authors acknowledge with gratitude the many contributions to these studies made by colleagues in the laboratory: Francine Gumkowski, Jane Bielich, Vivienne Woods, Wei Cheng Lu, Jorge Obeso, Louis Kubai, Joanne Weber, Larry Morrissey, Grazyna Kaminska, and Jack Rozental. The research studies have been supported by grants CA 28656 and EY 3243 from the National Institutes of Health and grant DCB 86-2751 from the National Science Foundation.

REFERENCES

1. Auerbach R, Joseph J: In Jaffe EA (ed): "The Biology of Endothelial Cells," The Hague: Martinus Nijhoff, 1983, pp 393–400.
2. Joseph J, Tu M, Alby L, Grieves J, Houser B, Kubai L, Morrissey L, Sidky Y, Watt SL, Auerbach R: In Thilo-Korner, DGS, Freshney RI (eds): "The Endothelial Cell, a Pluripotent Control Cell of the Vessel Wall," Basel: Karger, 1983, pp 55–66.
3. Gumkowski F, Kaminska G, Kaminski M, Morrissey LW, Auerbach R: Blood Vessels 24:11, 1987.
4. Alby L, Auerbach R: Proc Natl Acad Sci USA 81:5739, 1984.
5. Auerbach R, Lu WC, Pardon E, Gumkowski F, Kaminska G, Kaminski M: Cancer Res 47:1492, 1987.
6. Kaminski M, Auerbach R: Int J Cancer (in press).
7. Auerbach R, Alby L, Grieves J, Joseph H, Lindgren C, Morrissey LW, Sidky Y, Tu M, Watt SL: Proc Natl Acad Sci USA 79:7891, 1982.
8. Voyta JC, Via DP, Butterfield CE, Zetter BR: J Cell Biol 99:2034, 1984.
9. Auerbach R: In Rifkin DB, Klagsbrun M (eds): "Angiogenesis: Mechanisms and Pathobiology." Cold Spring Harbor Laboratory, 1987, pp 131–133.
10. Ortaldo JR, Herberman RB: Ann Rev Immunol 2:359, 1984.
11. Kay NE: CRC Crit Rev Clin Lab Sci 22:343, 1986.
12. Rozental JM, Kaminska GM, Kaminski MJ: Soc Neurosciences (Abstr) 1987.
13. Kaminska GM, Rozental JM, Kaminski MJ: 7th Conf Brain Tumor Res Therapy (Abstr) 1987.
14. Nicolson GL, Winkelhake JL: Nature 255:230, 1975.
15. Poste G, Fidler IJ: Nature 283:139, 1980.
16. Hart IR, Fidler IJ: Biochim Biophys Acta 651:37, 1981.
17. Fidler IJ, Hart IR: Science 217:998, 1982.
18. Schirrmacher V: Adv Cancer Res 83:1, 1985.
19. Sugarbaker ED: Cancer 5: 606, 1952.
20. Kahan B: Somatic Cell Genet 5:763, 1979.
21. Nicolson GL: J Histochem Cytochem 30:214, 1982.
22. Schirrmacher V, Cheingson-Popov R, Arnheiter H: J Exp Med 151:984, 1980.
23. Kramer RH, Vogel GL, Nicolson GL: In Jamieson GA (ed): "Interactions of Platelets and Tumor Cells," New York: Alan Liss, 1982, pp 333–351.

Immunologic Factors Influencing the Metastasis of Skin Cancers

Margaret L. Kripke and Cynthia A. Romerdahl

Department of Immunology, University of Texas M. D. Anderson Hospital and Tumor Institute, Houston, Texas 77030

Recent studies have demonstrated that several different populations of immune cells reside in the skin. In addition, a variety of immunologic mediators are produced by keratinocytes. Exposure of the skin to UV radiation can bring about changes in immune responsiveness by altering the quantity and activity of these immune cells and mediators. Studies with experimental animals have demonstrated that exposure to UV radiation also causes systemic alterations in immune function, some of which are important in the development of skin cancer. These findings raise the possibility that immunologic factors may play an important role in the pathogenesis of skin cancer and cutaneous metastases.

Key words: cutaneous immunity, skin cancers, UV radiation, photoimmunology

This report focuses on the local immunological factors that might influence the progression and metastasis of cutaneous tumors. The reasons for concentrating on these particular factors is that the field of cutaneous immunobiology has undergone a major revolution in the past few years. What has been learned recently about the immunology of the skin is undoubtedly of considerable significance for the metastasis of skin cancers and for the development of cutaneous metastases from primary tumors arising in other organs. However, at present, these advances in the immunology of the skin are only beginning to be applied to the problems of carcinogenesis and tumor progression. Therefore, the full implications of these findings for metastasis have not yet been determined.

FINDINGS FROM STUDIES OF UV-INDUCED SKIN CANCERS

A line of research that focused attention on cutaneous immunology was the study of skin cancers induced in mice by repeated exposure to UVB (280–320 nm) radiation. Most of these skin cancers are highly antigenic, in that they are rejected when transplanted into syngeneic animals and can only be transplanted successfully in immunosuppressed recipients [1]. The failure of the UV-induced tumors to grow in normal, syngeneic mice raised the question of how such highly antigenic skin cancers ever survived immunologic destruction in their original hosts.

Received June 11, 1987.

© 1988 Alan R. Liss, Inc.

Studies to address this question have shown that repeated exposure to UV radiation converts normal mice into tumor susceptible hosts [2]. This UV-induced alteration is systemic, because treatment of the dorsal skin with UV radiation renders the mice susceptible to tumors implanted on unexposed, ventral sites and to tumor cells injected intravenously. Additional experiments indicated that the failure of UV-irradiated animals to reject transplanted skin cancers was due to the presence of suppressor T lymphocytes that prevented the normal immunologic response to these tumors [3–6]. Suppressor cells were induced in the mice before primary skin cancers were evident. The suppressor cells prevented the rejection of all UV-induced tumors, even though these tumors exhibited individually specific transplantation antigens [1]. These suppressor lymphocytes appeared to be specific for UV-induced cancers, however, because exposure to UV radiation did not impair the rejection of transplanted allogeneic tumors or syngeneic tumors induced by other carcinogens [7].

Suppressor T lymphocytes also seemed to be important for the development of primary UV-induced tumors. When normal mice injected with T lymphocytes from UV-irradiated donors were exposed to UV radiation, the latent period for the development of primary tumors was reduced by about one half [8]. Additional studies demonstrated that the systemic effect induced by UV irradiation of one site markedly accelerated the induction of skin cancers by subsequent UV irradiation of a second site [9,10]. The finding that UV irradiation of the skin caused a specific, systemic immunosuppression that seemed to play an important role in UV carcinogenesis suggested that there might be close connections between skin and the immune system.

CUTANEOUS IMMUNE CELLS

Another line of evidence implicating skin as an immunologic organ stemmed from the discovery of unique populations of lymphoid cells within the epidermis. Although many immune cells such as lymphocytes, mast cells, granulocytes, and macrophages have been known for many years to participate in cutaneous immune reactions, the extent of the resident immune cells in the skin is only now being recognized. Epidermal Langerhans cells originate from the bone marrow [11] and have a dendritic morphology, forming an interconnecting network throughout the epidermis. Although these cells had been thought to play an immunologic role since 1973 [12,13], their definitive identification as members of the immune system resulted from studies employing monoclonal antibodies against cell surface markers of lymphoid cells. The cells express class II histocompatibility antigens, which function as recognition molecules among cells of the immune system [14,15]. Investigation of the function of these cells indicated that they serve as cutaneous antigen presenting cells [16], and thus are similar in origin, surface markers, and function to cells of the macrophage-monocyte-histiocyte lineage [17].

A second population of cutaneous immune cells has been identified recently in murine skin [18,19]. These cells are also dendritic in appearance, but they express the T lymphocyte surface marker, Thy-1. Because these cells do not express other surface markers generally found on mature T lymphocytes, and because they do express some markers found on natural killer cells, there has been speculation that the Thy-1^+ dendritic epidermal cell represents a cutaneous NK cell that serves an immune surveillance function [18,19]. Alternatively, there is evidence suggesting that these cells might participate in activation of the suppressor pathway of the immune response [20].

Recently, these cells have been shown to contain rearranged T cell receptor genes and to express gamma-delta heterodimers that appear to constitute a functional T cell receptor [21]. This finding suggests that the cells belong to the category of immature T lymphocytes, rather than to that of NK cells or macrophages. The equivalent of this cell in human skin may have been identified recently [22]. What biological role the Thy-1+ cells play in the skin is unclear. The assignment of a function to these cells and an assessment of their significance in cutaneous immunology, physiology, and pathology remain topics of active investigation.

Another unexpected finding made in recent years is that keratinocytes can produce a variety of immunologic effector molecules and can express class II antigens under certain conditions [23]. Thus, there is considerable evidence that the skin has a unique relationship to the immune system. Although the details of this relationship are still being elucidated, the implications for certain cutaneous reactions are quite apparent. One of the most interesting examples of interaction between skin and the immune system comes from studies of the effects of UV radiation on contact hypersensitivity reactions.

SUPPRESSION OF CONTACT HYPERSENSITIVITY BY UV RADIATION

Exposing mice to UV radiation interferes with the induction of contact hypersensitivity (CHS) and leads to the induction of hapten-specific suppressor T lymphocytes. This suppression can occur by means of both local and systemic effects of UV radiation. In the local suppression model, mice are exposed to several very low doses of UV radiation (~ 1 kJ/m^2) and then sensitized with the hapten through the UV-irradiated skin. The CHS reaction is markedly reduced in these animals, and T lymphocytes that suppress the induction of CHS can be found in their spleen [24,25]. Exposure of the skin to this regimen of UV irradiation also produces morphological and biochemical changes in epidermal Langerhans cells [24] but seems not to affect the Thy-1$^+$ dendritic epidermal cells [26]. These findings have led to the hypothesis that damage to the antigen presenting Langerhans cells by UV radiation is somehow responsible for activation of the suppressor cell pathway. Several different approaches have suggested that there is a second cell involved in activation of the suppressor cell pathway. Granstein et al. [27] coupled a hapten to epidermal cells and exposed them to UV radiation in vitro. Injection of these cells into normal mice resulted in the induction of suppressor cells, and treatment of the cells with anti-I-J antibody and complement before injection eliminated their suppressor-inducing activity. These results suggest that an I-J$^+$ cell in UV-irradiated epidermis is involved in activation of suppressor cells. Sullivan et al. [28] used a fluorescence activated cell sorter to isolate pure populations of Ia$^+$ Langerhans cells and Thy-1$^+$ dendritic cells from murine epidermis. These cell populations were conjugated with hapten and injected into normal mice. The Langerhans cells induced CHS, but the Thy-1$^+$ cells induced suppression, again suggesting the participation of two cells in the regulation of CHS: one responsible for activation, and one for suppression [20]. Recently, our group has studied the activity of lymph node cells draining the site of hapten application [26]. When injected into the footpad of normal mice, antigen presenting cells within the lymph node cell population induce CHS in the recipients. However, draining lymph node cells from UV-irradiated donors induced suppressor lymphocytes. The CHS-inducing cells were Ia$^+$, Thy-1$^-$, and radioresistant, whereas the suppressor-inducing cells were Ia$^-$, Thy-1$^+$, and radiosensitive. These results also suggest the participation of a Thy-1$^+$ cell in activation of the suppressor cell pathway, but whether this is the Thy-1^+ dendritic epidermal cell or a lymph node cell is not yet clear. Collectively, these data suggest that UV radiation damages Langerhans cells in the skin, impairing their antigen presenting function and resulting in suppressor cell activation by means of a second cell. It is not yet certain whether the second cell is a T suppressor-inducer cell that is stimulated directly by antigen, or an antigen presenting cell that specifically activates the suppressor cell pathway.

In the systemic suppression model, mice are exposed to a much higher dose of UV radiation (~ 50 kJ/m^2), and the hapten is applied 3 to 7 days later on unexposed skin. This protocol also results in a depressed CHS response and the appearance of hapten-specific suppressor T lymphocytes that prevent the induction of all immune responses to the hapten [29,30]. How UV irradiation alters the immune response to haptens applied at a site distant from the irradiation is not yet clear. However, recent evidence suggests that a soluble mediator released from UV-irradiated keratinocytes may be involved [31]. Both of these models of suppression of CHS could explain the generation of the suppressor cells in UV-irradiated mice that inhibit tumor rejection. Furthermore, they illustrate the intimate connections between the skin and the immune system.

CONCLUSIONS

The significance of these findings for human skin cancers and cutaneous metastases is not known. What is known, however, is that the Langerhans cells in human skin are altered morphologically by UV radiation [32] and that immune responses are perturbed in people exposed to sunlight and tanning salons [33,34]. Also, severe immunosuppression is associated with a greatly increased risk of developing cancers on sun-exposed skin [35,36]. The very recent realization of the extensive involvement of the immune system with the skin is now providing the impetus for many investigations on the role of cutaneous immunity in a variety of skin disorders, including skin cancers. Because of the great immunologic potential of the skin, it should be possible to mobilize cutaneous immunity and direct it against cutaneous malignancies.

REFERENCES

1. Kripke ML: J Natl Cancer Inst 53:1333–1336, 1974.
2. Kripke ML, Fishers MS: J Natl Cancer Inst 57:211–215, 1976.
3. Kripke ML, Fidler IJ: Cancer Res 40:625–629, 1980.
4. Fisher MS, Kripke ML: Proc Natl Acad Sci USA 74:1688–1692, 1977.
5. Fisher MS, Kripke ML: J Immunol 121:1139–1144, 1978
6. Daynes RA, Spellman CW: Cell Immunol 31:182–187, 1977.
7. Kripke ML, Thorn RM, Lill PH, Civin CI, Fisher MS, Pazmino NH: Transplantation 28:212–217, 1979.
8. Fisher MS, Kripke ML: Science 216:1133-1134, 1982.
9. DeGruiji FR, van der Leun JC: Photochem Photobiol 35:379–383, 1982.
10. Strickland PT, Creasia D, Kripke ML: J Natl Cancer Inst 74:1129–1134, 1985.
11. Katz SI, Tamaki K, Sachs DH: Nature 282:324–326, 1979.
12. Silberberg I: Acta Derm Venereol 55:112, 1973.
13. Silberberg I, Baer RL, Rosenthal SA: J Invest Dermatol 66:210–217, 1976.
14. Klareskog L, Tjernlund UM, Forsum U, Peterson PA: Nature 268:248–250, 1977.
15. Rowden G, Lewis MG, Sullivan AK: Nature 268:247–248, 1977.
16. Stingl G, Katz SI, Clement L, Green I, Shevach EM: J Immunol 121:2005–2013,1978.
17. Stingl G, Katz SI, Shevach EM, Rosenthal AS, Green I: J Invest Dermatol 71:59–64, 1978.

18. Bergstresser PR, Tigelaar RE, Dees JH, Streilein JW: J Invest Dermatol 81:286–288, 1983.
19. Tschachler E, Schuler G, Hutterer J, Leibl H, Wolff K, Stingl G: J Invest Dermatol 81:282–285, 1983.
20. Sullivan S, Bergstresser PR, Tigelaar RE, Streilein JW: J Immunol 137:2460–2467, 1986.
21. Koning F, Stingl G, Yokoyama WM, Yamada H, Maloy WL, Tschachler E, Shevach EM, Coligan JE: Science 236:834–837, 1987
22. Groh V, Yokozeki H, Binder A, Stingl G: J Invest Dermatol (Abst) 88:492, 1987.
23. Choi KL, Sauder DN: J Leukocyte Biol 39:343–358, 1986.
24. Toews GB, Bergstresser PR, Streilein JW: J Immunol 124:445–453, 1980.
25. Elmets CA, Bergstresser PR, Tigelaar RE, Wood PJ, Streilein JW: J Exp Med 158:781–794, 1983.
26. Okamoto H, Kripke ML: Proc Natl Acad Sci USA 84:3841–3845, 1987.
27. Granstein RD, Lowy A, Greene MI: J Immunol 132:563–565, 1984.
28. Sullivan S, Bergstresser PR, Tigelaar RE, Streilein JW: J Invest Dermatol 84:491–495, 1985.
29. Noonan FP, DeFabo EC, Kripke ML: Photochem Photobiol 34:683–689, 1981.
30. Ullrich SE, Azizi E, Kripke ML: Photochem Photobiol 43:633–638, 1986.
31. Swartz T, Urbanska A, Gschnait F, Luger TA: J Invest Dermatol 87:289–291, 1986.
32. Aberer E, Schuler G, Stingl G, Honigsmann H, Wolff K: J Invest Dermatol 76:202–210, 1981.
33. Hersey P, Haran G, Hasic E, Edwards A: J Immunol 131:171–174, 1983.
34. Hersey P, Hasic E, Edwards A, Bradley M, Haran G, McCarthy WH: Lancet, March 12, 545–548, 1983.
35. Penn I: Transplant Proc 7:323–326, 1975.
36. Hymes KB, Greene JB, Marcus A: Lancet, September 19, 598–600, 1981.

DNA Methylation Patterns and Tumor Heterogeneity

Peter A. Jones, Lois A. Chandler, Hamid Ghazi, Thomas Ahlering, and Louis Dubeau

Urological Cancer Research Laboratory, USC Cancer Center, Los Angeles, California 90033

DNA methylation is one important component of a multilevel control system for gene expression in vertebrate cells. Methylation patterns are copied with a high but not absolute degree of fidelity, thus allowing for diversity of patterns and cellular phenotypes. Chemical carcinogens interfere with this information coding system and might therefore alter gene expression by changing patterns of gene methylation. Methyltransferase levels are increased in tumorigenic cells, which may lead to a decreased stringency of methylation control. Analysis of methylation patterns in tumorigenic cells shows strikingly heterogeneous, clone-specific methylation patterns which even extend to the level of individual gene alleles. Methylation of the c-Ha-*ras* gene changes during tumor growth and metastasis in the nude mouse providing additional evidence that alterations in 5-methylcytosine distribution might play a role in the generation of tumor heterogeneity.

Key words: DNA methylation, heterogeneity, metastasis, nude mouse

The inappropriate expression of normal or mutated cellular genes leads to altered cellular phenotypes which are presumably responsible for the aberrant biological behavior of neoplasms. Neoplastic cells are often highly heterogeneous at the cellular and biochemical levels and it is this inherent heterogeneity and capacity to generate further heterogeneity during tumor evolution, which ultimately limits our ability to control cancer. Understanding the molecular mechanisms responsible for phenotypic evolution is therefore the long-term goal of this and many other laboratories.

Our hypothesis is that aberrant control of DNA methylation is responsible, in part, for the emergence of biochemical and cellular heterogeneity. The methylation of specific cytosine residues in DNA is thought to be one part of a mechanism for suppressing gene activity in eukaryotic cells [1,2]. Methylation patterns are tissue specific and undermethylation is often associated with the active expression of specific gene sequences. Drugs which interfere with the methylation of cytosine residues in DNA are highly potent inducers of gene expression [3], providing additional evidence that this postsynthetic modification is relevant to gene control. DNA methylation patterns are not as

Received April 30, 1987.

© 1988 Alan R. Liss, Inc.

rigorously copied as the DNA base sequence itself to allow for alteration of methylation patterns during cellular differentiation and development. This inherent capacity for alteration might also be important in the generation of cellular diversity which is a hallmark of cancer.

INFLUENCE OF CHEMICAL CARCINOGENS ON DNA METHYLATION

Since specific methylation patterns are associated with the control of gene expression in normal cells, it follows that alterations in these patterns could give rise to the aberrant gene expression observed in neoplastic cells. Several investigators have shown that DNAs treated with chemical carcinogens such as dimethylsulfate [4] or acetoxyacetylamino fluorene [5] have a decreased ability to accept methyl groups from S-adenosylmethionine in the presence of crude preparations of methyltransferase enzymes. We confirmed these studies using hemimethylated DNA substrates extracted from cells treated with low doses of 5-azacytidine (5-aza-CR) and showed that a diverse range of ultimate chemical carcinogens could inhibit the transfer of methyl groups to hemimethylated DNA [6]. The formation of alkali-labile sites in the DNA also lessened its ability to accept methyl groups in vitro but the methylation reaction was less sensitive to thymine dimers or double strand breaks. Carcinogenic agents may therefore be able to cause heritable changes in DNA methylation patterns in certain cell types by a variety of mechanisms including adduct formation, induction of apurinic sites, single stranded breaks, and direct inhibition of the methyltransferase enzyme.

The genomic level of cytosine methylation can also be significantly diminished in dividing 3T3 cells treated with several aromatic hydrocarbon carcinogens [7]. All chemical carcinogens that were tested and were known to transform 3T3 cells initiated significant reductions in 5-methylcytosine (5mCyt) content by 48 hr after carcinogen treatment. However, 5- to 50-fold higher concentrations of some noncarcinogens which did not transform 3T3 cells also induced significant reductions in DNA cytosine methylation. Thus the inhibition of DNA methylation may be an important step in the initiation of oncogenic transformation of 3T3 cells, but decreases in DNA 5mCyt levels alone could not account for the onset of this multistep process.

The fact that carcinogens can induce hypomethylation would suggest that they should be capable of activating genes because of the known association of hypermethylation with gene inactivity. Indeed, two recent studies show that this is the case for HeLa cells containing a suppressed hypoxanthine phosphoribosyltransferase gene [8] or Chinese hamster cells containing an inactive thymidine kinase gene [9]. This new information provides convincing evidence that carcinogens can react directly with the DNA methylation system for controlling vertebrate gene expression.

DNA METHYLATION LEVELS IN HUMAN TUMORS

There have been conflicting results regarding the levels of methylation in human tumors. Decreased, increased, or unchanged levels of 5mCyt have been reported in human and animal tumors and also in tumor cell lines [10]. We measured the overall 5mCyt levels in human tumor cell lines and freshly explanted pediatric tumors and could detect no generalized decrease in the levels of methylation within the tumors relative to normal cells [11]. On the other hand, Goelz et al. [12] have provided evidence that demethylation of certain genes might occur early in the development of colonic tumors in humans. The methylation patterns within specific genes might therefore be more relevant to altered cellular behavior than the overall levels of 5mCyt in the genome.

Since methylation patterns within cells are controlled, to some extent, by the levels of active DNA methyltransferase enzyme, we measured the levels of extractable methyltransferase in nuclei from nine tumorigenic and nine nontumorigenic cell lines [13]. In all but two cases, the extractable methyltransferase activity was considerably higher in tumorigenic than in nontumorigenic cells. The results were confirmed by an independent technique in which the amount of 5-aza-CR which had to be incorporated into DNA to inhibit the methylation of newly incorporated cytosine residues was measured. Tumorigenic cells required larger doses of the drug to inhibit DNA methylation to the same extent as their nontumorigenic counterparts. Thus it was shown, by two separate approaches, that tumorigenic cells contained higher methylating capacity than nontumorigenic cells. The overabundance of methyltransferase activity might contribute to less rigorous control of the methylation reaction and alter DNA methylation patterns, thus affecting phenotypic stability. Studies with isolated nuclei have indicated that the methyltransferase is a nuclear matrix associated enzyme and rapidly modifies newly synthesized DNA [14]. Since the enzyme appears to be reversibly associated with the matrix in a cell cycle dependent way [15], it could well be that variations in the amount and possibly location of methyltransferase in tumor cells are responsible for decreased methylation fidelity.

PATTERNS OF DNA METHYLATION IN HUMAN TUMOR CELLS

We extended our studies on DNA methylation within human tumor cell lines to a determination of the methylation status of collagen, c-Ha-*ras* and thymidine kinase genes [16]. The DNA of each cell line generated a unique banding pattern for each gene examined when digested with the methylation sensitive enzymes HpaII or HhaI. No generalized trend of gene hypomethylation or decrease in overall 5mCyt contents were observed in tumor cell lines when compared to fibroblasts. The striking finding was that the cell lines were extremely heterogeneous for the methylation patterns of individual genes. This observation, coupled to our earlier findings that tumorigenic cells might have altered levels of DNA methyltransferase enzymes, suggests that methylation patterns are not rigorously copied and controlled in tumorigenic cells.

In more recent experiments we have taken advantage of the fact that the human c-Ha-*ras* gene contains a polymorphic tandem repeating unit in the 3' region of the gene [17] to examine the methylation status of individual c-Ha-*ras* gene alleles within normal and tumorigenic cells [18]. These results have shown conclusively that individual alleles of autosomal genes can contain different methylation patterns. Subclones of the human osteogenic sarcoma cell line TE85 and a derivative obtained after MNNG treatment had particularly striking methylation patterns. Each subclone had a unique and distinct methylation pattern of individual c-Ha-*ras* gene alleles.

These results therefore provided conclusive and striking evidence for extensive molecular heterogeneity within human cancer cell lines and demonstrated allelic variations of methylation patterns. In view of the known association between methylation and gene expression, it might be anticipated that this heterogeneity could result in an altered phenotype within each subclone. The methylation patterns observed may therefore be a molecular manifestation of tumor heterogeneity and have important implications in the generation of phenotypic diversity in vivo.

ALTERED DNA METHYLATION PATTERNS DURING METASTASIS IN THE NUDE MOUSE

The nude mouse has been extensively used for studies on the tumorigenicity of human cells, but the model has not proven very useful in terms of metastasis and invasion. Most tumor cells grow as encapsulated or pseudoencapsulated masses when injected subcutaneously, which appears to decrease metastasis from subcutaneous sites. Recently, Fidler [19] has focused attention on the fact that the site at which human tumors are implanted into the nude mouse can have profound effects on invasive and metastatic activity. We therefore modified a technique described by Soloway et al. [20] and injected human bladder cancer cells transurethally into nude mouse urinary bladders [21].

Two long-term bladder cancer cell lines, RT4 and EJ, were tumorigenic when injected subcutaneously into nude mice but had little potential to invade locally or metastasize before the animals succumbed to tumor burden. On the other hand, the cell lines recapitulated their behavior in the human patients from which they were derived when implanted transurethally into the urinary bladders of nude mice. The RT4 cells, which were originally derived from a papillary tumor, were noninvasive in this model and did not establish metastases at distant organ sites. However, the EJ carcinoma cell line, which was obtained from a patient with invasive cancer, metastasized and established colonies in the lungs and the lymph nodes of inoculated animals. Thus this nude mouse model allows us to investigate the possible relevance of DNA methylation changes to metastasis.

The methylation pattern of the c-Ha-*ras* gene in individual subclones of EJ cells and in tumors and metastasis derived following inoculation into nude mouse urinary bladders was determined. The results showed a striking clone-specific methylation pattern of the *ras* gene and demonstrated an apparent progressive demethylation of the gene during the process of tumorigenic growth and metastasis to the lungs of inoculated animals. It was not possible from these experiments to determine whether the demethylation event occurred as a result of selection of cells with decreased methylation of the gene or whether the gene became demethylated as a result of tumorigenic growth within the animal.

We are encouraged to proceed and further define the potential role of *ras* gene methylation in this system because the human gene was originally isolated from the EJ carcinoma cell line, and recent studies by Borrello et al. [22] have shown that methylation of the gene can result in its inactivity following transfection into NIH 3T3 cells. There is, therefore, reason to believe that this gene might be important in the tumorigenic behavior of this particular cell line and also that methylation may be important in its control. We have no evidence that the *ras* gene plays a role in metastasis as opposed to tumorigenicity; however, this experimental approach may allow us to obtain more information on the potential importance of DNA methylation in tumorigenesis and metastasis in human cancer.

A suggested role for altered methylation patterns in tumor behavior and metastasis also comes from experiments in which the metastatic phenotype has been profoundly altered by 5-aza-CR treatment [23]. Numerous studies have shown that the metastatic phenotype can be changed either positively or negatively by brief exposure to the hypomethylating agent [24–26]. Taken together with our findings of the instability of methylation patterns in tumorigenic cells, these results strongly support the idea that variation in the 5mCyt patterns imprinted on DNA can contribute to phenotypic instability.

CONCLUSIONS

There is convincing evidence that DNA methylation is important in the regulation of some, but not all, vertebrate genes. Chemical carcinogens can interfere with this information coding system and induce the expression of suppressed genetic information in some systems. Methylation patterns are not inherited with great fidelity in tumorigenic cells, and this instability may contribute to phenotypic variability. This hypothesis is supported by experiments in which it has been shown that interference with DNA methylation by 5-aza-CR treatment profoundly alters metastatic capability. Studies with human tumors metastasizing in nude mice may allow us to determine the exact relationship between DNA methylation and phenotypic diversity.

ACKNOWLEDGMENTS

This study was supported by grant CA40422 from the National Cancer Institute.

REFERENCES

1. Doerfler W: Ann Rev Biochem 52:93, 1983.
2. Riggs AD, Jones PA: Adv Cancer Res 40:1, 1983.
3. Jones PA: Cell 40:485, 1985.
4. Drahovsky D, Morris NR: Biochim Biophys Acta 277:245, 1972.
5. Salas CE, Pfohl-Leskowicz A, Lang MC, Dirheimer G: Nature 278:71, 1979.
6. Wilson VL, Jones PA: Cell 32:239, 1983.
7. Wilson VL, Jones PA: Carcinogenesis 5:1027, 1984.
8. Ivarie R, Morris JA: Mol Cell Biol 6:97, 1986.
9. Barr FG, Rajagopalan S, MacArthur CA, Lieberman MW: Mol Cell Biol 6:3023, 1986.
10. Jones PA: Cancer Res 46:461, 1986.
11. Flatau E, Bogenmann E, Jones PA: Cancer Res 43:4901, 1983.
12. Goelz SE, Vogelstein B, Hamilton SR, Feinberg AP: Science 228:187, 1985.
13. Kautiainen TL, Jones PA: J Biol Chem 261:1594, 1986.
14. Kautiainen TL, Jones PA: Biochemistry 24:5575, 1985.
15. Tubo RA, Berezney R: J Biol Chem 262:1148, 1987.
16. Chandler LA, DeClerck YA, Bogenmann E, Jones PA: Cancer Res 46:2944, 1986.
17. Krontiris TG, DiMartino NA, Colb M, Parkinson DR: Nature 313:369, 1985.
18. Chandler LA, Ghazi H, Jones PA, Boukamp P, Fusenig NE: Cell 50:711, 1987.
19. Fidler IJ: Cancer Met Rev 5:29, 1986.
20. Soloway MS, Nissenkorn I, McCallum L: Urology 21:159, 1983.
21. Ahlering TE, Dubeau L, Jones PA: Cancer Res 47:6660, 1987.
22. Borrello MG, Pierotti MA, Bongarzone I, Donghi R, Mondellini P, Porta GD: Cancer Res 47:75, 1987.
23. Frost P, Kerbel RS: Cancer Met Rev 2:375, 1983.
24. Kerbel RS, Frost P, Liteplo R, Carlow D, Elliot BE: J Cell Physiol Suppl 3:87, 1984.
25. Olsson L, Forchhammer J: Proc Natl Acad Sci USA 81:3389, 1984.
26. Trainer DL, Kline T, Mallon F, Greig R, Poste G: Cancer Res 45:6124, 1985.

Spontaneous and Oncogene-Mediated Acquisition of the Invasive Phenotype by Cells in Culture

Marc Mareel, Peter Coopman, Chris Dragonetti, Walter Fiers, Jin Gao, Ludwine Messiaen, and Frans Van Roy

Laboratory of Experimental Cancerology, Department of Radiotherapy and Nuclear Medicine, University Hospital (M.M., P.C., C.D., L.M.), and Laboratory of Molecular Biology (W.F., F.V.R.), State University Ghent, B-9000 Ghent, Belgium; and Chinese Academy of Basic Medical Sciences, Beijing, China (J.G.).

Transfection of known gene sequences was used to convert noninvasive (I^- phenotype) cell populations into invasive (I^+ phenotype) ones. The I phenotype was scored histologically in confronting chick heart cultures in vitro and in syngeneic animals or nude mice in vivo. We review here our results obtained with different cell lines. Apparently spontaneous conversion toward the I^+ phenotype during passage in vitro occured with mouse lens epithelial and Fischer rat fibroblastic cell lines. The following immortalized cell lines remained noninvasive or showed a low I^+ background: C127 mouse cells; a thymidine kinase deficient derivative (Rat2) from a Fischer rat cell line; a cell line (LTRAT1) established from a primary embryonic rat cell culture after transfection with the polyoma large-T gene; well-differentiated canine kidney epithelial cells (MDCK); murine mammary gland cells (NMuMG). With these cell types induction or enhancement of the I^+ phenotype was found after transfection with the following oncogenes: a BamHI/HindIII 69% fragment of BPV-1; the complete BPV-1 genome; the polyoma early region and origin of replication; mutated c-Ha-*ras*-1; a FBR v-*gag-fos-fox* fusion gene; polyoma middle-T. The I^+ phenotype sometimes also emerged after transfection with the following nononcogenes: a bacterial neomycin resistance gene; a herpes simplex virus I thymidine kinase gene. Induction or enhancement of the I^+ phenotype was consistently seen after passage of parental cells in vivo. The fact that these cell populations acquire the I^+ phenotype in diverse ways with or without oncogene transfections hampers interpretation of invasion at the molecular level.

Key words: invasion, oncogenes, cell lines, spontaneous conversion

Emergence of the invasive (I^+) phenotype is a key event in the progression of a neoplasia toward malignancy. The I^+ phenotype might appear before or together with or after growth transformation (G^+ phenotype). There are arguments to presume that

Received June 10, 1987.

© 1988 Alan R. Liss, Inc.

the transition from the noninvasive (I^-) toward the I^+ phenotype implicates molecular events that are different from those implicated in the transition from controlled growth (G^- phenotype) to the G^+ phenotype [discussed in ref. 1]. For example, the following combinations of these phenotypes can be observed in man: G^+, I^- (benign tumors); G^+, I^+ (malignant tumors); G^-, I^+ (trophoblast).

A number of oncogenes have been implicated in growth transformation [for review see ref. 2]. Transfection of genes into G^- cell populations followed by selection for the G^+ phenotype (dense focus formation or growth in soft agar in vitro; tumor formation in vivo) has proved to be a powerful technique for the demonstration of this role of oncogenes. We have examined whether DNA transfection could also be used to detect and isolate gene sequences implicated in the acquisition of the I^+ phenotype. Therefore, I^- cell populations had to be transfected with a variety of genes followed by selection of I^+ cells. Reliable methods to perform the latter type of selection are, however, not available [3]. So far, we have restricted ourselves to the question if known gene sequences are able to turn an I^- cell population into an I^+ one. To score for the I^+ phenotype in vivo, cell populations in different organisations were inoculated into syngeneic animals or into nude mice at various sites: s.c. injection of cell suspensions (1×10^5 to 5×10^6 cells) in the flank or in the intrascapular region; i.p. injection of similar cell suspensions; s.c. implantation of cellular aggregates (1×10^4 to 1×10^5 cells) into the tail; implantation of cellular aggregates under the renal capsule [4]. To score for the I^+ phenotype in vitro, cells were confronted with fragments of embryonic chick heart in organ culture [5] (for grading see footnote to Table II). In all these assays, invasion was evaluated through histology. For the assays in vivo, the G^+ phenotype (tumorigenicity) is a prerequisite to detect the I^+ phenotype, whereas the assay in vitro can demonstrate the I^+ phenotype in G^- cell populations as well.

We review here our gene transfection experiments with a number of cell types, part of which has been published earlier [1,6,7]. Plasmids mentioned in the present paper are listed in Table I.

TABLE I. Plasmids Used for Transfection of Various Cell Lines

Code	Gene of interest	Reference
pV69	BamHI/HindIII 69% fragment of BPV-1 plus neo^r	24
BPV-1[a]	Complete BPV-1 genome	25
pM69	BamHI/HindIII 69% fragment of BPV-1	26
pPyB1	Polyoma early region and origin of replication	27
pHSG272[b]	Neo^r	28
pHSV-Q	Herpes simplex virus I thymidine kinase gene	29
pT24	Mutated c-Ha-*ras*-1 from human cell line T24	30
pMOL 503	FBR v-*gag-fos-fox* fusion gene	31
pPyMT1	Exclusively polyoma middle-T[c]	32
pLT214	Exclusively NH$_2$-terminal 40% of polyoma large-T[c]	33
pPyLT1	Exclusively polyoma large-T[c]	33

[a] Complete genome derived from virions; [b] Cosmid; [c] Due to appropriate genome deletions. Neo^r: Bacterial neomycin resistance gene.

ACQUISITION OF INVASIVENESS DURING PASSAGE IN VITRO

Conversion from the G$^-$ to the G$^+$ phenotype during culture is a known phenomenon [review in ref. 8]. The I$^+$ phenotype also may be acquired in an apparently spontaneous way during routine passage of cell lines in vitro. In a previous set of experiments repeated over a period of 10 years we could show that this occurred at different passages ($\sim$ 40 to $\sim$ 90) for the same type of immortalized embryonic C3H mouse cells [9] (unpublished results in collaboration with M. Bracke and M. Rabaey). In the present work we found two striking examples of spontaneous conversion to the I$^+$ phenotype. Epithelial as well as fibroblastic cell lines were involved.

MLE Cells

The MLE cell line was established from C3H mouse lens epithelium and found to be I$^-$ in vitro and G$^-$ in vivo at passage 11. The cell population was expanded for transfection with a number of gene sequences including mock transfection with calcium phosphate. This was followed by further expansion up to passage 21 before examination of the I phenotype in the battery of tests mentioned above. At that time all transfectants as well as the untransfected cells produced I$^+$ tumors with a very similar histology (Fig. 1).

FR3T3C Cells

Parental immortalized Fischer rat FR3T3 cells were obtained from F. Cuzin (University of Nice, France) and were coined FR3T3C. The same source also supplied

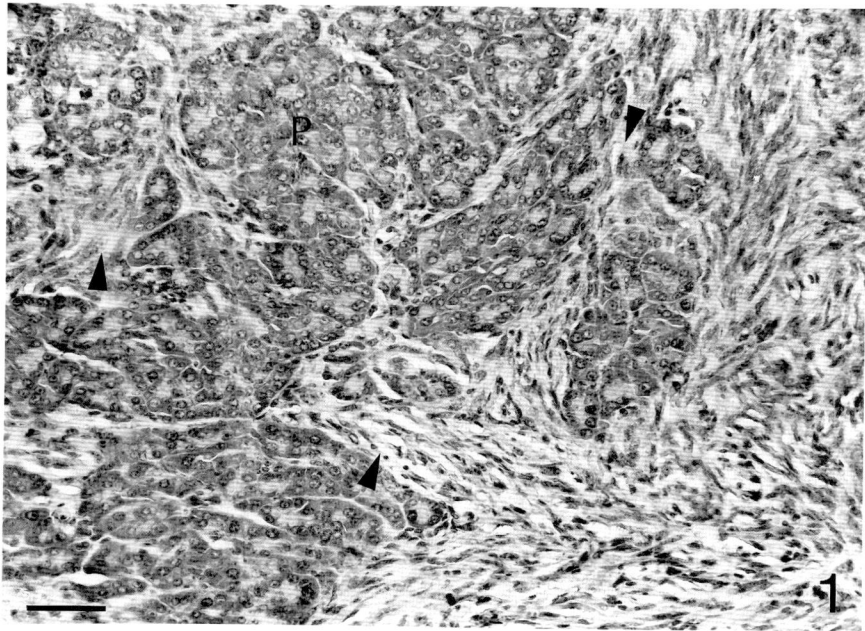

Fig. 1. Photomicrograph of a histological section from the pancreas (P) of a C3H mouse 11 weeks after i.p. injection of 5 × 10^6 untransfected MLE cells (passage 21); staining with hematoxylin-eosin. MLE cells (arrowheads) invade into the pancreas. Scale bar = 50 μm.

FR3T3C cells transfected either with the complete bovine papilloma virus type 1 (BPV-1) genome or with a plasmid containing 69% of the BPV-1 genome plus bacterial sequences (pV69). The cell lines were tested at passages 8 to 13 (FR3T3C), 5 to 18 (BPV-1-transfectants), and 8 to 19 (pV69-transfectants). All cell types were found to be I^+ in vitro and to produce I^+ tumors in vivo (P. Coopman, F. Van Roy, C. Dragonetti, J. Gao, W. Fiers, G. Meneguzzi, and M. Mareel. Invasiveness and metastatic capability of FR3T3 rat cells transfected with bovine papilloma virus type 1 DNA. Manuscript in preparation.). Most transfectants produced tumors with shorter latency periods than the parental cells but the histology of all the tumors was similar. A similar short latency period was also found with cell lines derived from tumors that were formed after s.c. injection of untransfected FR3T3C cells. Here, as in most other cases, the I^+ phenotype was acquired together with tumorigenicity.

We can only speculate about the mechanisms of apparently spontaneous emergence of the I^+ phenotype in cell populations passaged in vitro. One hypothesis is that cells in the intact organism are positionally controlled by signals from the extracellular matrix. Long-term deprivation from such signals during culture on artificial substrata might lead to some kind of downregulation of the perceptivity of the cells for these signals [10].

TRANSFECTION OF LOW- OR NONINVASIVE CELLS
C127 Cells

C127 mouse cells (obtained from F. Cuzin) [for origin of cell line see ref. 11] were tested for invasiveness in vitro before and after transfection with pV69, with another vector containing the 69% BPV-1 fragment (pM69), or with a plasmid containing the polyoma virus early region (pPyB1). Since the parental cells showed only a low background of invasiveness, we were able to demonstrate enhanced expression of the I^+ phenotype (Table II). This occurred after transfection with all types of plasmids used (Fig. 2). Transfection with pPyB1 conveyed upon these cells the capacity to grow in confrontations with chick heart in organ culture. It was, therefore, not clear from the present experiments whether progression from grade III to grade IV observed with the latter derivative reflected an increased inherent invasiveness or an increase in the number of I^+ cells through proliferation during the assay.

Rat2 Cells

The Rat2 cell line was selected by Topp [12] from an immortalized embryonic Fischer rat cell line (Rat1C) on the basis of flat morphotype, high transfectability, and thymidine kinase (tk) deficiency (resistance to bromodeoxy-uridine). Rat2 cells were I^- in vitro and produced I^+ tumors with long latency periods (about 20 weeks) after s.c. injection into syngeneic rats [7]. Testing of three Rat2 subclones in vitro revealed a low background of invasiveness (1 culture with grade III out of 17 cultures evaluated after 7 or 14 days). After transfection with a neomycine resistance (neo^r) gene (pHSG272) and selection in medium containing G418, 17 subclones were tested in vitro and 14 cultures out of 39 were found to be I^+ (grade III). After transfection with a tk gene (pHSV-Q) followed by selection in HAT-medium, or with mutated c-Ha-*ras* (pT24) or v-*fos* (pMOL 503) genes and selection through dense focus formation, all Rat2 derivatives were I^+ in vitro. Progression from grade III to grade IV was found with c-Ha-*ras* and v-*fos* but not with tk transfectants. The I^+ phenotype (grade III progressing to grade IV)

TABLE II. Invasiveness In Vitro of Parental and Transfected C127 Mouse Cells

Cell type[a]	Grading[b] after			Growth[c]
	4 days	7 days	14 days	
C127	II(3),III(1)	II(4)	II(2),III(1)	−
+pV69→MV694	II(4)	II(2),III(1)	III(4)	−
+pV69→MV695[d]	II(2),III(2)	II(1),III(3)	III(4)	−
MV695TD1	III(1),IV(2)	III(1),IV(2)	IV(3)	−
+pM69→S69	II(1),III(3)	II(1),III(2),IV(1)	III(1),IV(1)	−
+pPyB1→SCOP-C1	III(4)	III(4)	IV(2)	+

[a]Plasmids are described in Table I; the origin of the cell lines has been described in refs. 24 (MV694; MV695), 26 (S69), 27 (SCOP-C1).
[b]Grading according to ref. 34 : grade II : when confronting cells surrounded the cardiac muscle; (no invasion); grade III and IV : when confronting cells invaded less than (III) or more than (IV) half of the heart fragment.
[c]Increase in volume of the confronting pair present (+) or absent (−).
[d]The G$^+$ phenotype (focus formation; anchorage-independence; colony-forming efficiency) is more expressed in MV695 than in MV694 cells (24; P. Coopman, unpublished results).

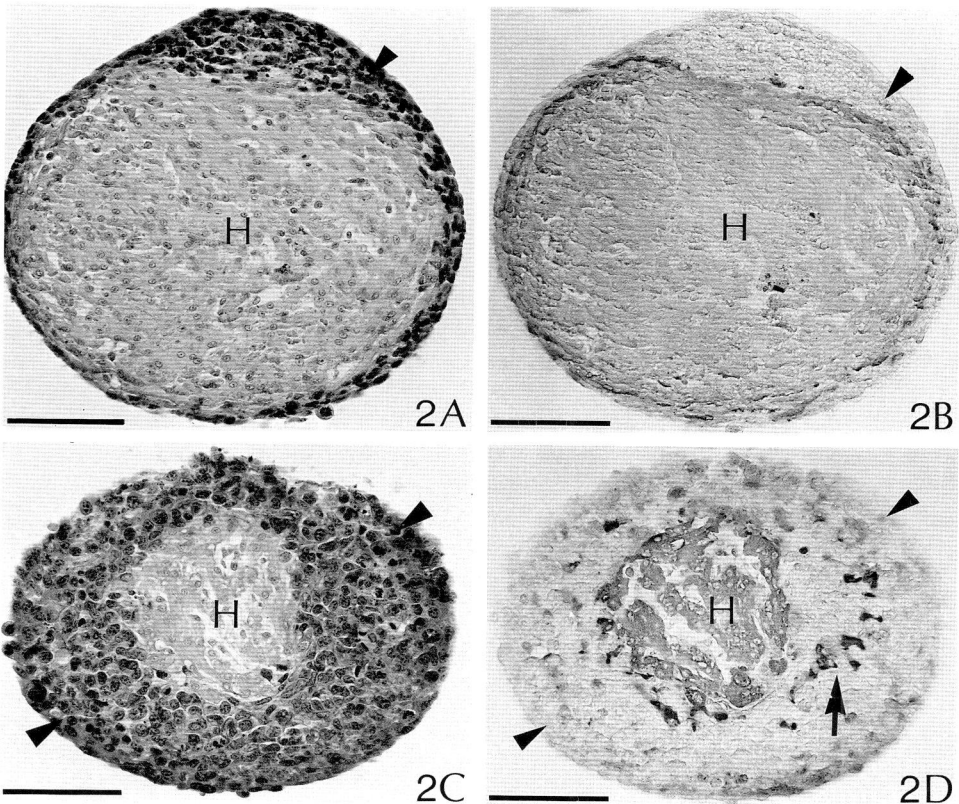

Fig. 2. Photomicrographs of histological sections from confronting cultures of C127 cells (**2A** and **2B**) and of SCOP-C1 cells (**2C** and **2D**) with embryonic chick heart (H) in organ culture; fixation after 3 days (2A and 2B) and after 7 days (2C and 2D); staining with hematoxylin-eosin (2A and 2C) and with an antiserum against chick heart (2B and 2D). C127 cells (arrowhead) do not invade (grade II, see Table II); SCOP-C1 cells (arrowheads) do invade (grade III); arrows indicate residual heart. Scale bars = 100 µm.

was also found with cell lines derived from a flank tumor or from a lung colony that were produced several months after s.c. or i.v. injection of parental Rat2 cells in syngeneic rats. Invasion was not found with a cell line established from a collagen sponge retrieved from a rat 3 days after injection of 2×10^6 Rat2 cells into the s.c. implanted sponge. This suggests that acquisition of the I^+ phenotype is dependent upon development of a tumor, more than on mere survival of cells after injection. All syngeneic rats injected s.c. or i.p. with Rat2 cells or their derivatives produced I^+ tumors in vivo that could not be distinguished from each other by histology. S.c. tumors formed by parental Rat2 cells or Rat2 subclones had a longer latency period (7 to 25 weeks) than their oncogene-bearing transfectants (1 to 2 weeks).

The experiments were repeated with one Rat2 subclone (Rat22) as the latter had a flat morphology. Here, induction or enhancement of the I^+ phenotype occurred after transfection with neo^r (pHSG272), mutated c-Ha-*ras* (pT24), neo^r plus mutated c-Ha-*ras* (pHSG272 + pT24), v-*fos* (pMOL 503), polyoma middle-T (pPyMT1), or neo^r plus polyoma middle-T (pHSG272 + pPyMT1) genes, followed by selection in G418 or through dense focus formation. Progression from grade III to grade IV was found for all transfectants except the one expressing only the neo^r gene.

As described with Rat2 cells, Rat22 cells derived from a s.c. tumor were found to be I^+ in vitro.

LTRAT1 Cells

The LTRAT1 cell line (obtained from F. Cuzin) was derived from a primary embryonic Fischer rat culture after transfection with a plasmid encoding the polyoma large-T antigen (pPyLT1). No background invasiveness in vitro was found with this cell type in repeated experiments and tumor formation was rare (1 out of 22 rats) with a latency period longer than 1 year. Transfection with the neo^r gene alone did not alter this very low tumorigenicity. Simultaneous acquisition of tumorigenicity and the full I^+ phenotype in vitro and in vivo was achieved after transfection with gene combinations such as neo^r plus mutated c-Ha-*ras* (pHSG272 + pT24), polyoma middle-T (pPyMT1), and neo^r plus polyoma large-T plus polyoma middle-T (pHSG272 + pLT214 + pPyMT1).

The experiments with noninvasive or low-invasive cell lines indicate that the I^+ phenotype could be induced or enhanced through transfection with a variety of plasmids containing different oncogenes. Transfection of some recipient cells with apparently nonrelated DNA sequences (selection genes) could to some extent induce the I^+ phenotype as well. Passage in vivo also was able to induce or enhance the I^+ phenotype.

CELL LINES PRODUCING BENIGN TUMORS

All cell lines discussed above were either nontumorigenic (G^-) or produced tumors that were invasive (G^+, I^+). So far, we found only two immortalized cell lines that produced benign tumors (G^+, I^-) after s.c. injection into nude mice.

MDCK Cells

The MDCK cell line (obtained from J. Leighton, Cancer Bioassay Laboratory, Medical College of Pennsylvania, PA) was established from canine kidney epithelium and remained well differentiated during long-term passage in vitro. In the present experiments these MDCK cells were I^- in vitro without any background, in agreement with previous observations [13]. Injection s.c. into nude mice revealed a minor degree of growth transformation, since small nodules were formed which, later on, regressed. Histology of such nodules showed benign (I$^-$) cysts with little or no mitotic activity. Transfections of MDCK cells with a neo^r gene (pHSG272) did not alter the I$^-$ phenotype as revealed by testing both in vitro and in vivo. By contrast, after transfection with the mutated c-Ha-*ras* gene (pT24) and selection for colony formation in soft agar, MDCK cells became I$^+$ in vivo. These MDCKpT24 cell lines differed from each other by the fraction of cells expressing high amounts of human p21-*ras* oncogene product (from 0.1 to 100%) as revealed by immunocytochemistry with monoclonal antibody Y13-259 [14]. MDCKpT24 cells showed no or moderate invasion in vitro and produced I$^+$ tumors in vivo that consisted of both differentiated and undifferentiated areas. Tumor-derived cell lines were enriched in p21-*ras* expressing cells and were consistently I$^+$ in vitro.

NMuMG Cells

The NMuMG cell line (purchased at passage 9 from the American Type Culture Collection, Rockville, MD) was established from an outbred mouse mammary gland [15] (H. Smith, personal communication). After s.c. injection into nude mice, NMuMG cells produced progressively growing cysts (G$^+$, I$^-$), as shown in Figure 3A. Staining with an antiserum against laminin (obtained from L. Liotta, National Cancer Institute, Bethesda, MD) showed a continuous basement membrane lining the cysts (Fig. 3B). In vitro these cells were I$^-$, with a continuous basement membrane separating the well-differentiated mouse epithelium from the chick cardiac tissue. Transfection of NMuMG cells with a mutated c-Ha-*ras* gene (pT24), without further selection, induced the I$^+$ phenotype in vivo. Tumors produced by transfected cell populations consisted of benign (I$^-$) cysts and of areas of undifferentiated carcinoma invading into various organs (Figs. 3C and 3D). Transfection with a neo^r gene (pHSG272) followed or not by G418 selection did not induce the I$^+$ phenotype in vivo.

The experiments with both MDCK and NMuMG cells show that transfection with the mutated c-Ha-*ras* gene is able to turn an I$^-$ cell population into an I$^+$ one, confirming results obtained by others [16–18].

INTERPRETATION OF TRANSFECTION EXPERIMENTS

The present experiments show that the I$^+$ phenotype can be acquired by cultured cells in various ways: 1) passage in vitro; 2) passage in vivo; 3) transfection with various gene sequences.

Apparently spontaneous acquisition of the I$^+$ phenotype through passage in vitro hampers most experiments including DNA transfections. This was clearly demonstrated also by our experiments with MLE cells and with FR3T3C cells. Also at least somewhat sensitive to similar alterations are MDCK cells (our unpublished results) and NMuMG cells (H. Smith, personal communication; our unpublished results), which are otherwise attractive because they produce benign tumors in nude mice.

Induction or enhancement of invasiveness through passage in vivo, as observed by us and by others [19], constitutes a paradox. Why do cells progress toward the I$^+$ phenotype when they are put back in an environment that was close to their natural environment? The following two observations indicate selection in vivo of preexisting subpopulations. 1) Parental cells produced tumors with long latency periods suggesting a high TD50 (number of tumor cells giving rise to tumors in 50% of injected animals) and by implication a low proportion of tumorigenic cells. 2) Enhancement of cells

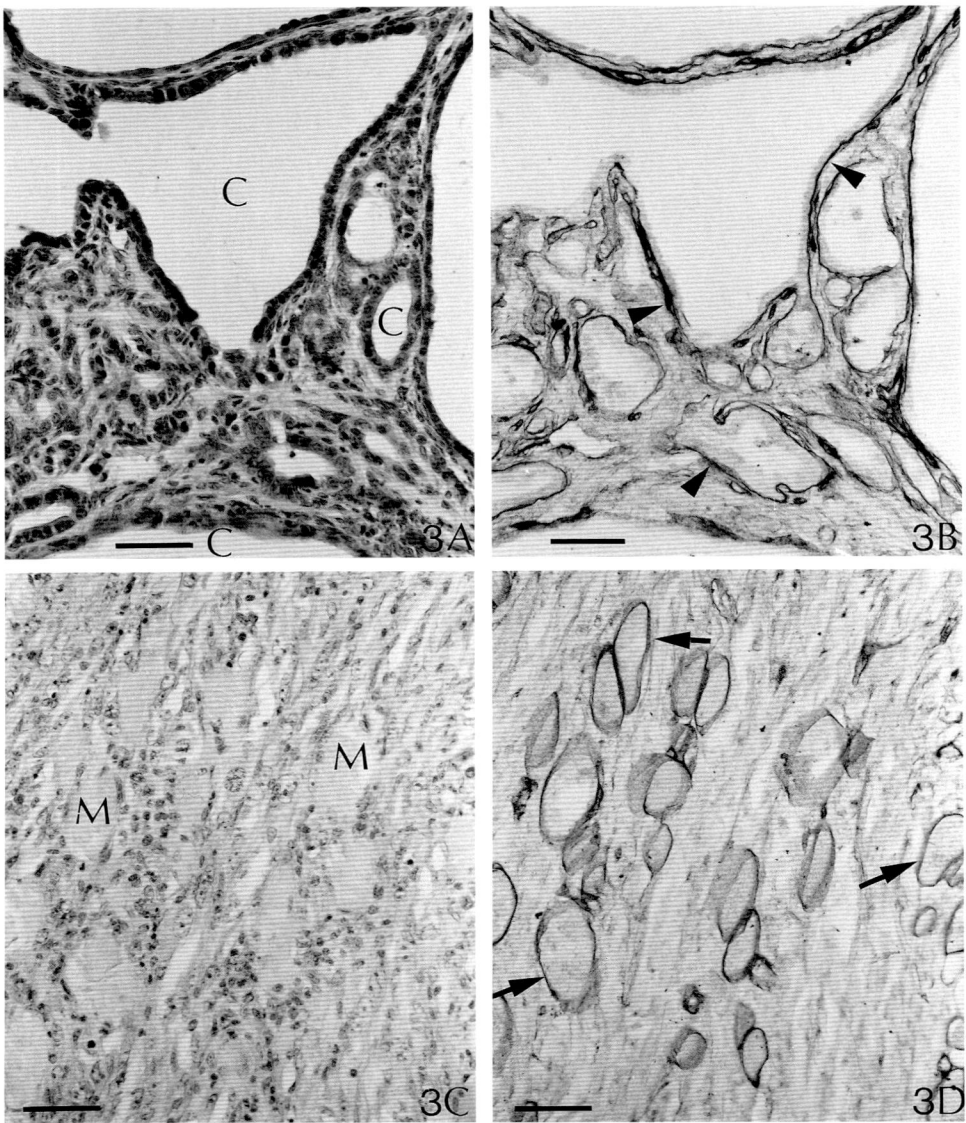

Fig. 3. Photomicrographs of histological sections from s.c. tumors produced in nude mice after injection of parental NMuMG cells (**3A** and **3B**) and of NMuMG cells after cotransfection with plasmids (pHSG272 and pT24) encoding neo^r and the mutated *ras*-protein (**3C** and **3D**); staining with hematoxylin-eosin (3A and 3C), and with an antiserum against laminin (3B and 3D). Parental cells formed a cystic (C) tumor, with continuous basement membrane (arrowheads) lining the cysts. Transfected cells formed an undifferentiated carcinoma invading into muscle (M) and skin (not shown); basal lamina around muscle (arrows). Scale bars = 50 μm.

expressing high levels of p21 was found in MDCK cell lines derived from primary tumors in nude mice.

It is nevertheless suggested by our results that transfection with presumptive oncogenes is an efficient and rapid way to induce the I^+ phenotype. This might be achieved in various ways that need not be mutually exclusive. 1) Transfection and/or selection procedures might exert a selection pressure favoring a minor preexisting I^+ subpopulation. Such a background of I^+ cells was shown in most Fischer rat fibroblastic cell lines or their derivatives and in mouse C127 cells, but less so in LTRAT1 cells, MDCK cells, and NMuMG cells. However, it should be noticed that the latter cell types were less extensively tested for background invasiveness. Acquisition of metastatic capability, and by implication the I^+ phenotype, through the transfection procedure per se, was also described by others [20]. 2) Insertion of novel gene sequences into the host cell genome might activate unknown host genes that are implicated in invasion. This can be achieved, for example, by oncogene-mediated cellular enhancer activation [21] or by insertional mutation [2]. The fact that transfection with a variety of plasmids containing different oncogenes yielded similar results with regard to conversion toward the I^+ phenotype favors the idea of host gene activation. However, the high frequency observed in most cases for this conversion contradicts fortuitous activation of a single host invasion gene by promoter/enhancer insertion. 3) Uncontrolled expression of transfected gene products or expression of mutated gene products might be responsible for invasiveness. For most oncogene products a mechanistic role in invasion is not obvious. The c-Ha-*ras* protein family constitutes an attractive candidate for such a role because of its similarities to GTP binding proteins (G-proteins) known to be involved in transducing signals from the cell surface [22].

In conclusion, it becomes increasingly obvious that the transfected *ras* oncogene especially is able to convey, in addition to the G^+ phenotype, the I^+ phenotype (present data) and even the metastatic phenotype [review in ref. 23] upon more or less appropriate recipient cells. What cautions against premature conclusions and extrapolations is 1) the ease with which these malignant phenotypes often can also be induced or enhanced by other oncogenes, non oncogenes, or even mere manipulations; and 2) the widely differing ability with which, for instance, the *ras* oncogene induces the I^+ phenotype in diverse cell systems. Despite these difficulties, continued study at the molecular level of invasion as a key step in the development of malignancy is warranted.

ACKNOWLEDGMENTS

Research in the authors' laboratories is supported by grants from the A.S.L.K. Kankerfonds, the F.G.W.O. (39.0009.83; 3.0005.84), and the Sport Vereniging tegen de Kanker, Brussels, Belgium. P.C. and L.M. are recipients of a fellowship from the I.W.O.N.L.; F.V.R. is Research Associate of the N.F.W.O., Belgium. The authors thank L. Baeke, B. Buysse, A. De Schepper, F. Van Houtte, and A. Verspeelt for technical assistance, J. Roels van Kerckvoorde for preparing the illustrations, and G. Matthys-De Smet for typing the manuscript. The excellent help of G. Liebaut, P. Suffys, R. Beyaert, and K. Vleminckx in different parts of the work described is greatly appreciated.

REFERENCES

1. Mareel MM, Van Roy FM: Anticancer Res 6:419–436, 1986.
2. Bishop, MJ: Science 235:305–311, 1987.
3. Mareel MM, Van Roy FM, Messiaen LM, Boghaert ER, Bruyneel EA: J Cell Sci Suppl 8:141–163, 1987.
4. Boghaert ER, Distelmans W, Van Ginckel R, Mareel MM: Invasion Metastasis 7:230–241, 1987.
5. Mareel M, Kint J, Meyvisch C: Virchows Arch B Cell Pathol 30:95–111, 1979.
6. Gao J, Van Roy F, Messiaen L, Cosaert J, Liebaut G, Coopman P, Fiers W, Mareel M: Pathol Res Pract 182:48–57, 1987.
7. Van Roy FM, Messiaen L, Liebaut G, Jin G, Dragonetti CH, Fiers WC, Mareel MM: Cancer Res 46:4787–4795, 1986.
8. Pontén J: Biochim Biophys Acta 458:397–422, 1976.
9. Mareel M, de Ridder L, De Brabander M, Vakaet L: J Natl Cancer Inst 54:923–929, 1975.
10. Bracke ME, Van Cauwenberge RML, Storme GA, Coopman P, Van Larebeke N, Mareel M: Anticancer Res 6:1273–1278, 1986.
11. Lowy DR, Dvoretzky I, Shober R, Law M-F, Engel L, Howley PM: Nature 287:72–74, 1980.
12. Topp WC: Virology 113:408–411, 1981.
13. Schroyens W, Bruyneel R, Tchao R, Leighton C, Dragonetti C, Mareel M: Invasion Metastasis 4:160–170, 1984.
14. Furth ME, Davis LJ, Fleurdelys B, Scolnick EM: J Virol 43:294–304, 1982.
15. Owens RB, Smith HS, Hackett AJ: J Natl Cancer Inst 53:261–269, 1974.
16. Hynes NE, Jaggi R, Kozma SC, Ball R, Muellener D, Wetherall NT, Davis BW, Groner B: Mol Cell Biol 5:268–272, 1985.
17. Thorgeirsson UP, Turpeenniemi-Hujanen T, Williams JE, Westin EH, Heilman CA, Talmadge JE, Liotta LA: Mol Cell Biol 5:259–262, 1985.
18. Collard JG, Schijven JF, Roos E: Cancer Res 47:754–759, 1987.
19. Walsh JW, Zimmer SG, Oeltgen J, Markesbery WR: Neurosurgery 19:185–200, 1986.
20. Kerbel RS, Waghorne MS, Man MS, Elliott B, Breitman ML: Proc Nat Acad Sci USA 84:1263–1267, 1987.
21. Wasylyk C, Imler JL, Perez-Mutul J, Wasylyk B: Cell 48:525–534, 1987.
22. Kamata T, Sullivan NF, Wooten MW: Oncogene 1:37–46, 1987.
23. Nicolson GL: Cancer Res 47:1473–1487, 1987.
24. Meneguzzi G, Binétruy B, Grisoni M, Cuzin F: EMBO J 3:365–371, 1984.
25. Grisoni M, Meneguzzi G, De Lapeyrière O, Binétruy B, Rassoulzadegan M, Cuzin F: Virology 135:406–416, 1984.
26. Binétruy B, Meneguzzi G, Breathnach R, Cuzin F: EMBO J 1:621–628, 1982.
27. Rautmann G, Glaichenhaus N, Nahgashfar Z, Breathnach R, Rassoulzadegan M: Virology 122:306–317, 1982.
28. Brady G, Jantzen HM, Bernard HU, Brown R, Schütz G, Hashimoto-Gotoh T: Gene 27:223–232, 1984.
29. Post LE, Conley AJ, Mocarski ES, Roizman B: Proc Natl Acad Sci USA 77:4201–4205, 1980.
30. Fasano O, Taparowsky E, Fiddes J, Wigler M, Goldfarb M: J Mol Appl Genet 2:173–180, 1983.
31. Michiels L, Van Roy F, de Saint-Georges L, Merregaert J: Virus Res 5:11–26, 1986.
32. Treisman R, Novak U, Favaloro J, Kamen R: Nature 292:595–600, 1981.
33. Rassoulzadegan M, Naghashfar Z, Cowie A, Carr A, Grisoni M, Kamen R, Cuzin F: Proc Natl Acad Sci USA 89:4354–4358, 1983.
34. Bracke ME, Van Cauwenberge RM-L, Mareel MM: Clin Exp Metastasis 2:161–170, 1984.

Prostate Cancer and the Invasive Phenotype: Application of New In Vivo and In Vitro Approaches

James M. Kozlowski, Robert McEwan, Harold Keer, Julia Sensibar, Edward R. Sherwood III, Chung Lee, John T. Grayhack, Adriana Albini, and George R. Martin

Department of Urology, Northwestern University Medical School, Chicago, Illinois 60611 (J.M.K., H.K., J.S., E.R.S., C.L., J.T.G.); The Upjohn Company, Molecular Biology Research, Kalamazoo, Michigan 49001 (R.M.); Laboratory of Developmental Biology and Anomalies, National Institute of Dental Research, National Institutes of Health, Bethesda, Maryland 20892 (A.A., G.R.M.)

> The development of more effective treatment stratagems for locally invasive (stage C) or metastatic (stage D) prostate cancer will require a sophisticated understanding of these biologically aggressive tumor systems. Such studies have been hindered by the scarcity of biologically relevant human prostate tumor material amenable to in vivo propagation in nude mice and subsequent in vitro analysis. The present study was directed at these perceived needs and demonstrates 1) the establishment of libraries of invasive and metastatic tumor cell variants following the intrasplenic injection of human prostate cancer cell lines PC-3 and DU-145 into athymic nude mice; 2) the utility of EJ-ras oncogene transfection of DU-145 (low metastatic) with respect to the production of highly metastatic transfectants; 3) the ability of diethylstilbestrol to up-regulate the metastatic potential of cell line PC-3; 4) the feasibility of detailed in vitro analysis of fresh benign/malignant human prostate systems following isolation of epithelial/stromal fractions using a discontinuous Percoll gradient, serum-free media, and essential growth factors; 5) the application of two-dimensional gel electrophoresis to establish discriminating protein profiles on these cellular populations; and 6) the use of basement membrane biomatrix (MATRIGEL) in a 5-hr chemoinvasion assay (modified Boyden chamber) to assess the invasive capacity of previously established and freshly derived human prostate tumors.

> Key words: Boyden chamber, extracellular matrix, two-dimensional gel electrophoresis, Percoll gradient, serum-free media, diethylstilbestrol (DES), transfection, metastatic variants, intrasplenic injection, nude mouse

Adenocarcinoma of the prostate is the second most common cancer among American men with recent estimates suggesting that it will account for 19% (90,000 cases) of newly diagnosed cancer in that population. Furthermore, prostate cancer is currently

Received August 19, 1987.

© 1988 Alan R. Liss, Inc.

responsible for 10% (26,100 cases) of male cancer deaths and is rapidly approaching parity with colorectal cancer as the second most common cause of male cancer death within the United States [1]. Unfortunately, between 40% and 80% of patients will present with advanced stage disease at the time of initial diagnosis [2]. Curative therapy is not available for these patients, and the vast majority will succumb to disease progression typified by early involvement of the regional pelvic lymph nodes (obturator-hypogastric) with synchronous or metachronous dissemination to the skeletal system [3–6].

These rather ominous statistics have stimulated the investigation of numerous approaches designed to enhance our perception of the biological potential of individual prostate cancers. These include 1) tumor grade [7–10]; 2) the Gleason histotype [11,12]; 3) tumor volume [13]; 4) nuclear roundness [14,15]; 5) DNA content and ploidy [16–21]; 6) nucleolar size [22]; 7) nuclear androgen receptor content [23]; and 8) the level of expression of the Harvey-ras oncogene [24]. Although these approaches have contributed to our understanding of the disease process, current perceptions regarding those features of this neoplasm that may distinguish biologically indolent from aggressive tumor systems are still primitive and lack biopredictive ability when applied to individual patients.

It appears that most malignant neoplasms are biologically heterogeneous and consist of a diverse array of cellular subpopulations differing from one another in a wide variety of phenotypes, including that of invasiveness and metastatic capacity. This phenotypic diversity, which permits selected variants to develop from the primary tumor, accounts for the differences frequently noted between the parental tumor and its metastases [25]. Isaacs and Coffey have recently demonstrated the existence of androgen-dependent and androgen-resistant subpopulations existing within the Dunning R-3327-H rodent prostatic adenocarcinoma [26]. Their documentation of heterogeneity within this system lends credence to the long-standing clinical impression of cellular diversity existing within human prostate cancers. Useful information has also been derived from investigations performed using the other rodent models for prostate adenocarcinoma, which include the Noble [27], ACI [28], and Pollard [29,30] tumors.

Despite their obvious importance, such investigations cannot substitute for an in-depth analysis of human prostate cancer as assessed following successful xenografting in athymic nude mice or serial propagation in vitro. Unfortunately, heterotransplantation of human prostatic tumors into immune-deficient animals has proven to be an exceedingly difficult task, with only one out of 100 tumor specimens exhibiting a capacity for successful xenografting [31,32]. As a result, there is a scarcity of well-characterized, in vivo transplantable human prostatic tumor lines, such as the androgen-dependent tumor systems designated PC-82 [33] and HONDA [34]. Similar methodologic frustrations have been encountered in the attempt to cultivate and serially passage human prostate cancer cells in tissue culture. Again, these difficulties readily explain the paucity of well-characterized, immortalized cell lines derived from patients with adenocarcinoma of the prostate such as PC-3 [35], DU-145 [36], and LNCaP [37]. To date, only a limited number of studies have been designed to expand the pool of biologically aggressive cell variants existing within these established tumor systems [38,39].

It has been our belief that a legitimate scientific and clinical need exists to expand the existing pool of biologically relevant human prostate tumor systems available for detailed in vitro analysis and in vivo propagation in the nude mouse model. The establishment of cell libraries containing well-characterized and biologically diverse tumor systems should greatly facilitate investigation of the invasive phenotype as it applies to prostate cancer and may well shed light on the equally critical issue of organ-specific patterns of metastasis. The information contained within this paper details the approaches utilized and the results obtained by our laboratory over the past several years in the pursuit of these goals.

UTILITY OF THE NUDE MOUSE MODEL FOR THE STUDY OF HUMAN PROSTATE CANCER

In 1969 Rygaard and Povlsen reported the successful xenografting of human tumors using athymic nude mice as recipients [40]. Since that time, there have been numerous published reports that have confirmed the usefulness of the nude mouse model for the propagation and expansion of human neoplasms [41–46]. This in vivo approach is most attractive since the majority of successfully xenografted human tumors maintain those morphological and biochemical characteristics typical of the neoplasm growing within the natural host [47,48]. Furthermore, the response of these xenografts to cytotoxic agents is often predictive of the actual clinical response [49–51]. Despite its demonstrated utility, several problems became readily apparent that appeared to diminish the efficacy of the nude mouse model with respect to the study of human neoplasms. First, successful xenografting of a diverse array of human tumors proved difficult. Despite the rather routine nature in which melanomas, carcinomas of soft tissues, and sarcomas can be successfully xenografted, carcinomas of the breast, prostate, and stomach have proved quite refractory to routine propagation in the nude mouse [52,53]. Second, the nude mouse model did not appear to permit full conservation of the metastatic capacity exhibited by clinically aggressive human tumors. In fact, a number of studies suggested that metastasis of human tumors in nude mice was an exceedingly rare event [54,55]. A few recent studies have been at variance with this view and have suggested that certain human tumor cell lines will metastasize following injection into nude mice [56–58]. However, such observations have been in the minority, and the common perception has been maintained that the overall incidence of metastasis as demonstrated in nude mice is low despite the xenografting of clinically "malignant" human tumors. Finally, the apparent inadequacy of the nude mouse model made it difficult to demonstrate convincingly the existence within human tumors of cellular populations possessing different capacities for invasion and metastasis, despite previous investigations using rodent tumors that confirmed such phenotypic diversity [58–61].

More recent observations have revealed that the metastasis of human tumor cell lines implanted into nude mice is not a rare event, and, in fact, this animal model can be used with great success to select out metastatic subpopulations existing within heterogeneous, unselected "parental" tumor systems [62–63]. Indeed, the successful propagation, expansion, and in vivo selection of many human tumors (including prostate cancer) is now possible and has been greatly facilitated by a more sophisticated awareness of certain critical host-related and tumor-related factors. With respect to the former, although athymic nude mice lack functionally mature T-lymphocytes, they are capable of generating a significant immunologic response to foreign antigens, including 1) a normal response to T-cell-independent antigens with the generation of natural antibodies reactive with tumor cells [64]; 2) macrophages capable of tumoricidal activity following in vivo stimulation with bacterial adjuvants [65]; and 3) high levels of natural killer cell (NK) activity [66,67]. The latter observation is of particular relevance in light of recent information suggesting a primary role for NK cells in the destruction of circulating tumor emboli [64,66]. Moreover, it is now well established that an inverse correlation exists between levels of NK cell activity and the incidence of experimental (intravenous) metastasis of rodent and human tumor systems in nude mice [68]. It appears that the successful xenografting and subsequent metastasis of human tumors in athymic nude mice is more likely to occur in animals with low levels of NK cell activity, the latter being contingent on such variables as 1) age (less than 3 weeks old); 2) strain (Balb/c or beige variant mice); and 3) absence of immunogenic stimulation (healthy animals maintained in specific pathogen-free conditions) [69]. Consistent with these observations, a number of studies have demonstrated enhancement of pulmonary and extrapulmonary metastases in nude mice following the in vivo depletion of NK cells by pretreatment with cyclophosphamide, beta-estradiol, and antiasialo GM1 [70–72].

Despite the importance of the NK system, recent studies have suggested that the status of NK cell activity in the modulation of human tumor spread in nude mice may not be as critical a factor for many human neoplasms as it appears to be in the metastasis of transplantable rodent tumors [62]. It is now apparent that a variety of tumor cell-related and methodology-related factors affect the ability to assess the metastatic capacity of human tumor systems in nude mice [62,63]. With respect to tumor cell properties, a number of recent studies have validated the earlier impressions of Sharkey and Fogh, who stressed that the intrinsic biological characteristics of the human tumor cell line in question constituted the major determinant in regulating metastatic spread in the nude mouse model [73]. Other important considerations stem from the observation that the majority of human tumors have slower growth rates than most rodent or murine neoplasms [62]. This finding coupled with the need to utilize a xenogeneic system suggests the wisdom of certain modifications in experimental design, including 1) the use of increased tumor dose (10^6–10^7 cells); 2) prolonged experimental duration (8–12 weeks); and 3) the supplementation of gross examination of organs with a systematic examination of appropriate histological sections in order to detect subclinical metastatic foci [62].

In addition to these admittedly important considerations regarding host and tumor cell properties, recent attention has been appropriately directed at those simple methodologic manipulations that can be performed in order to permit human tumors full expression of their invasive and metastatic capacity as assessed in nude mice. One consideration of great importance is ascertaining that the route of tumor injection adheres to the precepts of the cranial-caudal growth gradient [74–77]. This primitive morphogenetic gradient has been shown to influence dynamically the regional differences in growth of normal and neoplastic cells (Table I). Kyriazis and associates demonstrated that implantation of human tumors in a subcutaneous site overlying the anterior aspect of the lateral thoracic wall (craniad site) resulted in a higher incidence of metastasis than did injection of the same tumor dose deposited into the caudal flank region [78]. Recent studies have reinforced the validity of these observations and suggest that the apparent inability of human tumor xenografts to metastasize in nude mice may simply reflect the choice of a suboptimal site for tumor deposition (Table II) [62].

A major methodologic advance resulted from the realization that conventional routes of tumor inoculation may significantly underestimate the metastatic potential of a particular human tumor undergoing evaluation in nude mice [62]. For example, a distinctive fibrous sheath or pseudocapsule frequently envelops subcutaneously xenografted human tumors, impairs vascularization of the tumor mass, and presents a for-

TABLE I. Regional Differences Reflected Within the Cranial-Caudal Growth Gradient*

	Cranial	Caudal
DNA synthesis	>	<
Susceptibility to carcinogens	>	<
Tumor growth rate	>	<
"Take" of skin graft	>	<
Temperature	>	<
Microvascularity	>	<
Metabolic rate of oxygen consumption (MRO$_2$)	>	<
Wound tensile strength	>	<
Immune response	<	>

*Adapted from Auerbach and Auerbach [75].

midable barrier to invasion of the body wall [79]. The latter event was cited by Sharkey and Fogh as a major determining factor with respect to the development of spontaneous metastases (following subcutaneous injection) of human tumors in nude mice [73]. The intrasplenic (i.s.) route of injection was chosen in order to circumvent this restrictive barrier and to provide the injected tumor cells with a "favorable microenvironment" conducive to enhanced survival, multiple sites of implantation, and subsequent metastasis [62]. This approach seemed worthwhile in light of previous observations documenting the efficacy of intraperitoneal injection for the dissemination of human tumor cells coupled with the finding of Witte and Ber who noted improved growth of hybridoma cells injected into the spleens of recipient mice [80,81]. Since the intrasplenic injection assay permitted maximum expression of the metastatic phenotype of human prostate cancer cell lines PC-3 and DU-145, a brief description of the technique is warranted.

TABLE II. Spontaneous Metastasis of Human Prostate Cancer Cell Lines Following Subcutaneous (s.c.) Injection Into Nude Mice*

Cell line	No. of animals with microscopic pulmonary metastasis from[a]	
	Cranial s.c. site[b]	Hindlimb footpad[c]
DU-145	0/15 (no take)	0/15 (no take)
PC-3	1/10[e]	2/10[e]
PC-3LM[d]	8/10[e]	3/10[e]

*Four-week-old female Balb/c nude mice obtained from the animal production area of the NCI—Frederick Cancer Research Facility served as recipients.
[a]Serial sections from lungs of each animal were examined for presence of microscopic parenchymal metastases 8 weeks following tumor injection.
[b]1×10^6 viable cells in 0.2 ml HBSS.
[c]5×10^5 viable cells in 0.05 ml HBSS.
[d]Liver metastasis-derived variant line developed from grossly apparent liver nodules that resulted from the direct i.s. injection of PC-3 cells 6 weeks previously.
[e]100% tumor take.

Intrasplenic Injection Assay

Groups of 4-week-old Balb/c nude mice were briefly anesthetized with methoxyfluorane (Metofane) and placed in the right lateral decubitus position. A transverse incision was made in the left flank region traversing the skin and peritoneum. The medial splenic tip was identified, and its position was stabilized by gentle traction on the tail of the pancreas. Each animal received 1×10^6 tumor cells (PC-3 or DU-145) suspended in 0.1 ml of Hanks balanced salt solution (HBSS) by injection into the medial splenic tip using a 27-gauge needle attached to a 1-cc tuberculin syringe. An ideal injection resulted with the creation of a visible "pale" wheal, the latter being indicative of adequate disruption of the splenic parenchyma and propagation of the injected material via the splenic vein into the portal venous system. The spleens were then returned to the abdominal cavity, and the wound was closed in one layer with surgical clips. The animals were observed daily while being maintained under specific pathogen-free conditions. Sterile necropsy was performed 8–12 weeks following injection or upon the development of large local tumors and/or ascites.

The intrasplenic injection of human prostate cancer lines PC-3 and DU-145 provided a number of interesting results. Although highly tumorigenic in nude mice, cell line PC-3 demonstrated minimal capacity for spontaneous (subcutaneous injection) metastasis even with tumor deposition in the craniad position (Table II). Furthermore, no significant evidence of experimental metastasis was observed following tail vein injection of the unselected, heterogeneous parental tumor in 3-week-old nude mice (Table III). Following intrasplenic injection, the majority of animals demonstrated impressive tumor burdens [Table IV], including prominent intrasplenic tumors with invasion of the body wall and subadjacent diaphragm (Fig. 1), capsular and/or invasive liver metastases (Fig. 2), prominent metastases to foregut and hindgut lymphatics (Fig. 3), metastases to the pulmonary parenchyma and mediastinal lymph nodes (Figs. 4, 5), and tumor-rich ascites (Fig. 6). These organ-related metastatic foci could be easily harvested at the time of sterile necropsy and established as sublines. Following confirmation of human origin by karyotype analysis, these variant lines together with the unselected parental tumor were designated the PC-3 family (Table V).

Of great interest is the fact that the majority of these metastasis-derived variants exhibited significantly greater capacity for experimental metastasis when injected in parallel with the heterogeneous, unselected parental tumor (Table VI). In fact, many of these sublines produced multiple, gross tumor nodules following injection in 3-week-

TABLE III. Experimental Metastasis of Human Prostate Cancer Cell Lines After i.v. Injection Into Nude Mice*

Cell line	Median no. (range) of grossly apparent lung tumor nodules[a]	No. animals with microscopic metastases in lungs[b]
DU-145	0	1/15
PC-3	0	1/15
PC-3LM[c]	38 (0–>250)	13/15

*Three-week-old female Balb/c nude mice received i.v. injections of 1×10^6 cells in 0.2 ml HBSS; animals were killed 8 weeks later and autopsied.
[a]No. of grossly apparent tumor foci on lung surface obtained with the aid of a dissecting microscope.
[b]Five-micron-thick serial sections from lungs of each animal were examined for presence of microscopic parenchymal metastases.
[c]See legend, Table II for description.

TABLE IV. Metastasis of Human Prostate Cancer Cell Lines in Nude Mice After Intrasplenic Injection of Tumor Cells

Cell line	No. animals with metastasis to			No. animals with tumor ascites
	Lung	Regional lymph nodes[a]	Liver	
DU-145[b]	4/30	1/30	1/30	1/30
PC-3	16/20	17/20	20/20	13/20

[a]Omental, mesenteric, and mediastinal lymph nodes were fixed, stained, and sectioned for determination of tumor involvement.
[b]All splenic tissue was examined and were found to contain subcapsular and/or intraparenchymal microscopic foci of the injected tumor cell line. The PC-3 line produced grossly apparent local tumor "take" in every instance.

TABLE V. The PC-3 Family

PC-3 parental cell line (P)
PC-3 liver metastasis (LM)
PC-3 lymph node metastasis (LNM)
PC-3 ascites (ASC)
PC-3 lung metastases (LGM)
PC-3 intrasplenic (ISP)
PC-3 muscle invasive (MI)
PC-3 met mix (MM)[a]

[a]Established by pooling equal aliquots of cell lines PC-3LM, PC-3ASC, PC-3LGM, and PC-3LNM.

TABLE VI. Experimental Metastasis of a Human Hormone-Resistant Adenocarcinoma Cell Line (PC-3) and Its In Vivo-Derived Metastatic Variants*

Cell line	No. of grossly apparent lung tumor nodules[a]	No. of animals with microscopic lung metastases[b]
PC-3	0, 0, 0, 0, 0 0, 0, 0, 0, 0 0, 0, 0, 0, 0	1/5
PC-3 liver metastasis	>250, >250, >250, >250, >250 38, 33, 26, 14, 12 6, 5, 4, 0, 0	13/15
PC-3 ascites	>250, >250, >250, 30, 20 12, 6, 3, 1, 0	10/10
PC-3 lung metastasis	>250, >250, >250, >250, 53 27, 20, 12, 8, 3	9/10

*Three-week-old Balb/c nude mice received tail vein injections of 1×10^6 tumor cells (in 0.2 ml of HBSS). Eight weeks later the animals were killed and autopsied.
[a]After 24 hr of fixation in Bouin's solution, the lungs were examined with a dissecting microscope, and the number of gross, peripheral lung tumor nodules were counted.
[b]Examination of five stepwise serial sections (5 μm thick) from lungs of each animal.

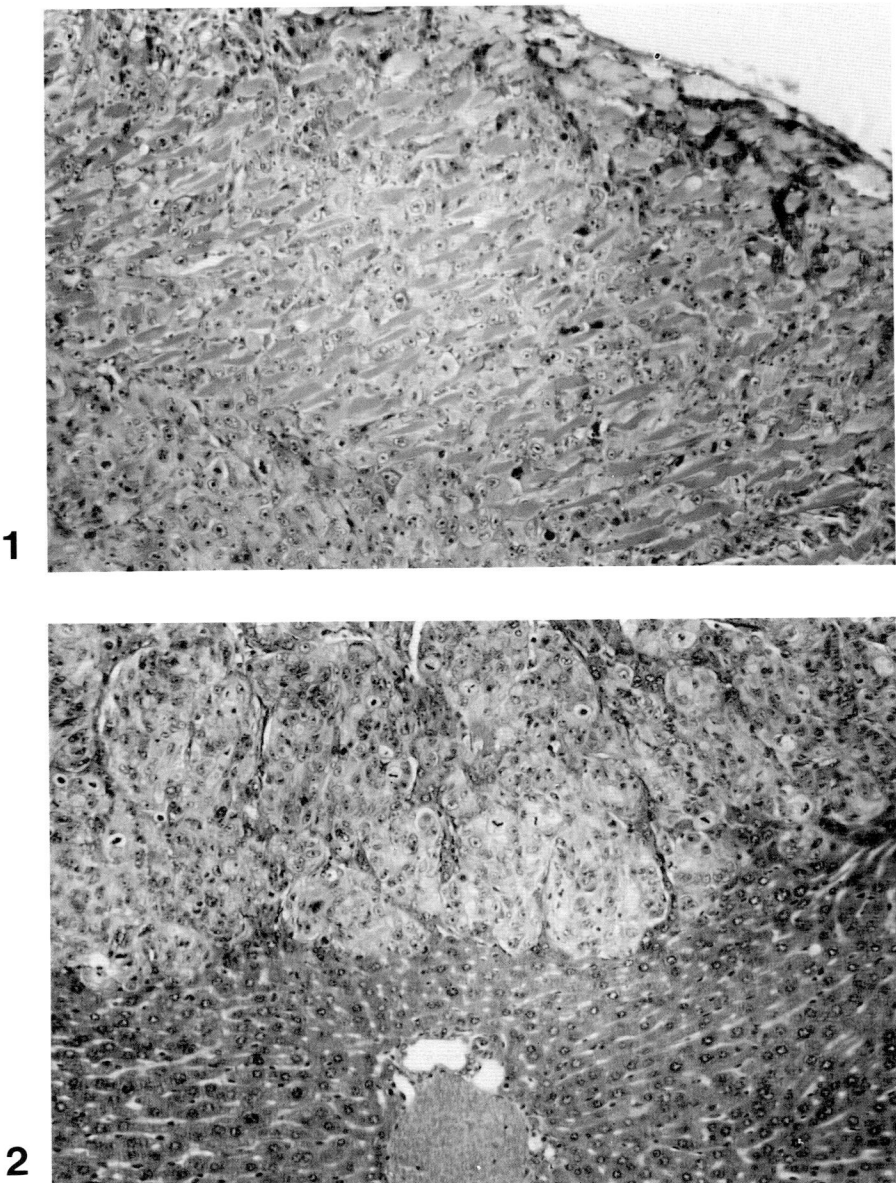

Fig. 1. PC-3 8 weeks following intrasplenic injection demonstrating diffuse infiltration of the muscular component of the left hemidiaphragm. Variant cell line PC-3MI was derived from a similar muscle-invasive tumor. H&E, ×200.

Fig. 2. Intraparenchymal hepatic metastasis noted after intrasplenic injection of PC-3. Note progression toward the central vein and presence of numerous mitotic figures. PC-3LM was derived from a similar invasive hepatic metastasis. H&E, ×200.

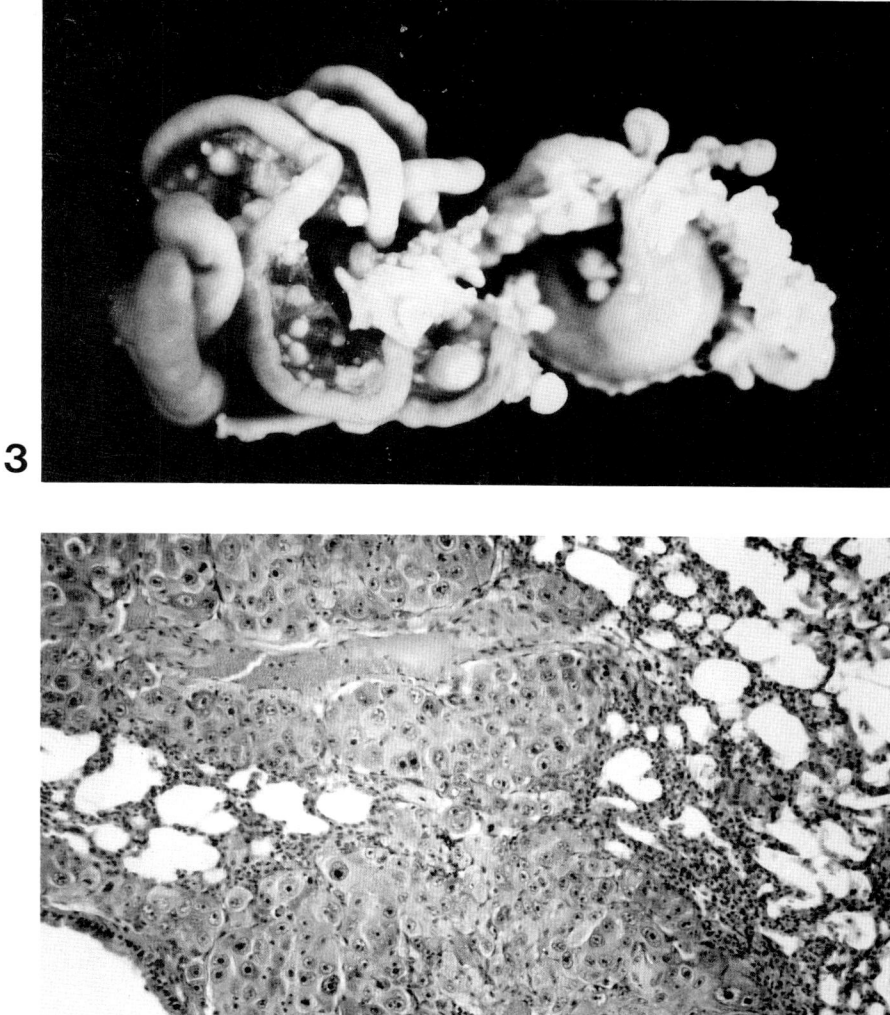

Fig. 3. Extensive, multifocal involvement of omental and mesenteric lymph nodes following intrasplenic injection of PC-3. Cell line PC-3LNM was established by harvesting several of the large tumor-filled lymph nodes depicted in this photograph (tissues were fixed in Bouin's solution for 24 hr prior to photography).

Fig. 4. The development of extensive pulmonary micrometastases following the intrasplenic injection of PC-3. Note the presence of nuclear and nucleolar pleomorphism and the typical distribution around the pulmonary capillary bed. Cell line PC-3LGM was derived from a synchronous, grossly apparent lung tumor nodule. H&E, ×200.

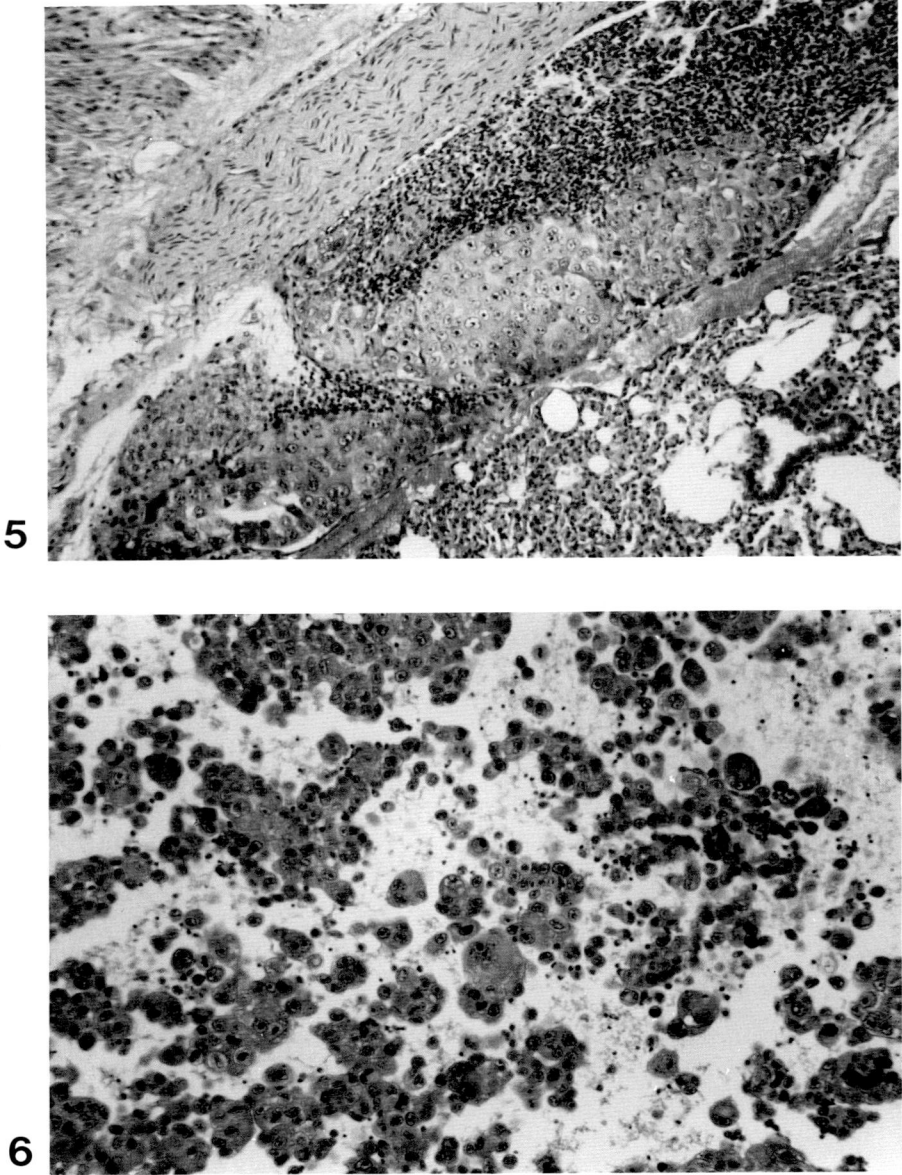

Fig. 5. Mediastinal lymph node metastasis that developed 8 weeks following the i.s. injection of PC-3. The node has been substantially replaced by tumor cells. Note its location between uninvolved lung parenchyma (**below**) and nerve sheath (**above**). H&E, ×200.

Fig. 6. Tumor-rich ascites that developed following i.s. injection of PC-3. Note the presence of prominent nucleoli and frequent mitotic figures. Sterile aspiration of a similar ascites-bearing animal permitted the establishment of cell line PC-3ASC. H&E, ×300.

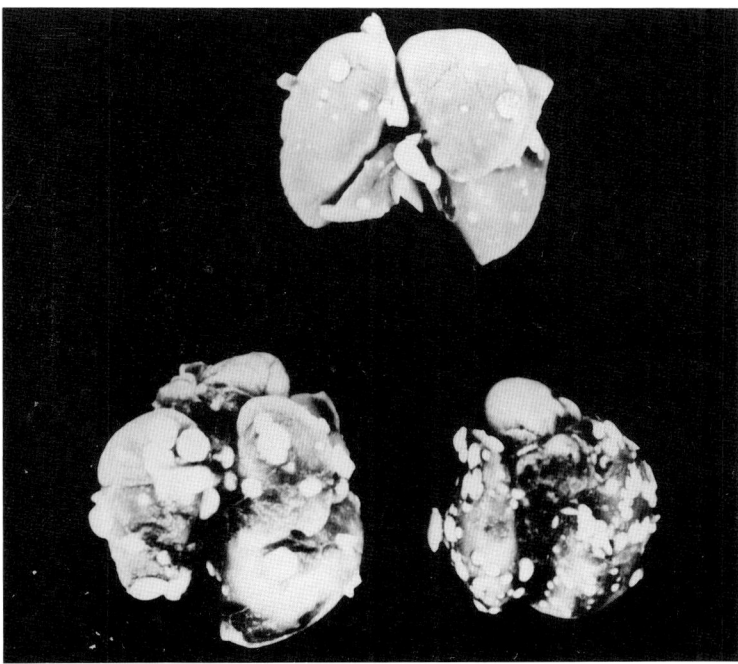

Fig. 7. Multifocal, macroscopic pulmonary metastases noted 8 weeks after the i.v. injection of PC-3ASC into 3-week-old nude mice. The parental, unselected cell line PC-3 failed to produce such visible tumor burdens despite repetitive injection.

old nude mice (Fig. 7). In this respect, the ascites-derived variant (PC-3ASC) is of particular interest. It demonstrated a markedly amplified metastatic capacity when compared to the unselected parental line coupled with prominent changes in its Giemsa-banded karyotype. This cell line exhibited a large number of minute and double-minute chromosomes that were not apparent in the karyotype profile of the parental tumor (Figs. 8, 9). In virtually all other respects, the karyotypes were identical and consistent with previously reported studies [35]. Whether such differences are associated with changes in oncogene expression is unclear at this point, but it is a subject of ongoing investigation. Thus, it appears that the intrasplenic injection of PC-3 permits the expression of an aggressive phenotype not appreciated using conventional metastasis assays. Moreover, the technique permits the isolation and expansion of organ-related variant sublines, which differ markedly from the parental tumor with respect to metastatic capacity.

In distinction, cell line DU-145 demonstrated minimal subcutaneous or intrasplenic tumorigenicity given the 2-month time constraints of the experimental design (Table II). Not unexpectedly, this cell line demonstrated a biologically indolent phenotype, with little evidence of metastatic capacity in experimental (Table III), spontaneous (Table II), and intrasplenic metastasis assays (Table IV). With respect to the latter, repetitive attempts at intrasplenic injection resulted in one animal demonstrating prominent local tumor growth associated with invasive liver metastases (Fig. 10), metastases to mesenteric lymph nodes, and ascites. These organ-related variants were expanded in vitro, and their human origin was verified in a manner similar to that described for the PC-3 family.

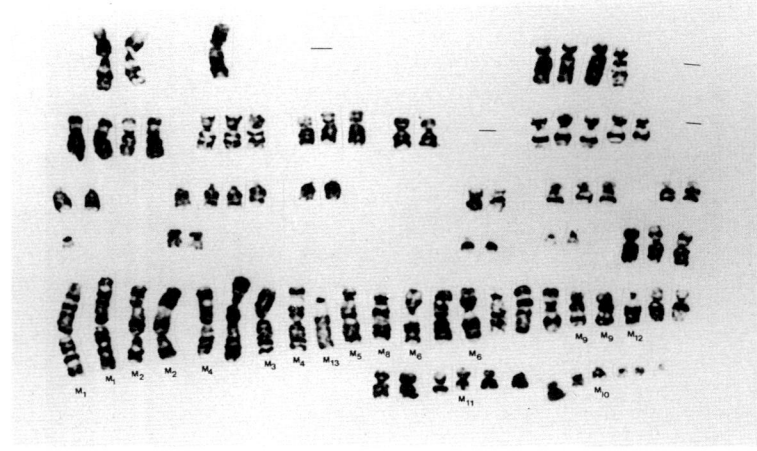

Fig. 8. Giemsa-banded karyotype cell line PC-3. Marker and unassignable chromosomes are grouped together at the bottom. M13 represents a new marker derived in part from chromosome 19. (Photograph courtesy of Dr. M. E. Kaighn.)

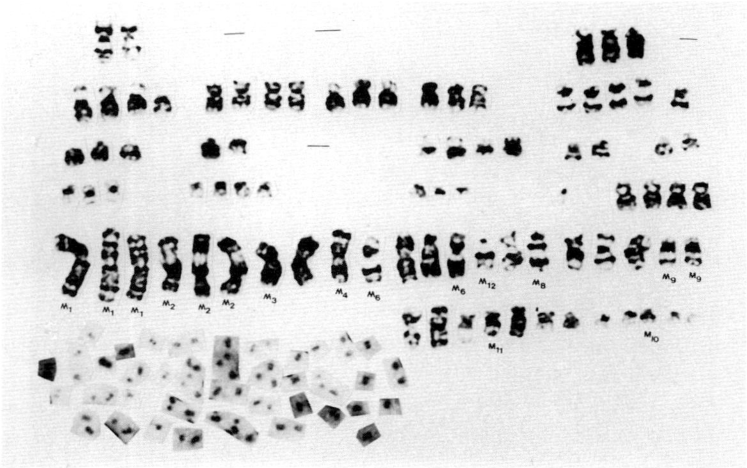

Fig. 9. Giemsa-banded karyotype of PC-3ASC passage 5. Note the large number of minute and double-minute chromosomes at the lower left. (Photograph courtesy of Dr. M.E. Kaighn.)

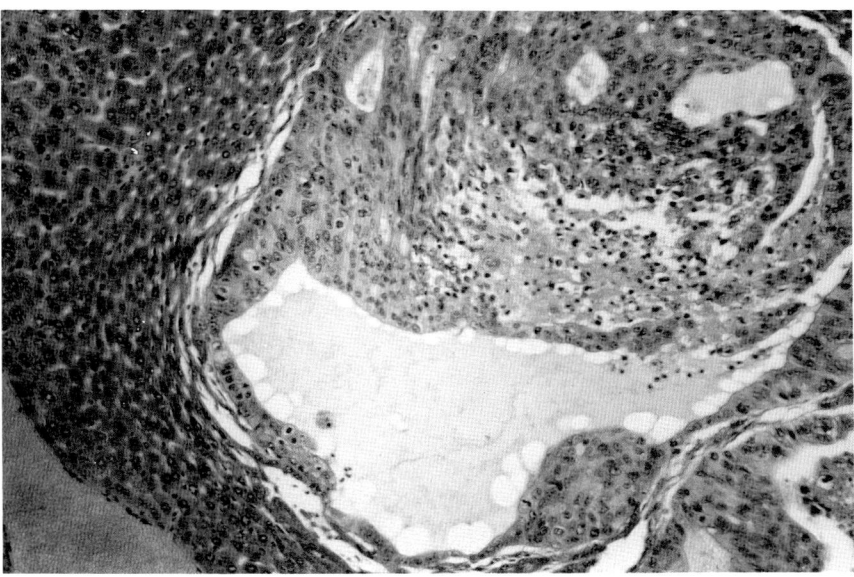

Fig. 10. Invasive, cavitating liver metastasis produced following the i.s. injection of DU-145P. Numerous mitotic figures together with prominent amount of nuclear pleomorphism can be appreciated. Aggressive cell line DU-145LM was derived from such a focus. H&E, ×200.

Parallel comparison of the aggressive liver metastasis (DU-145LM) with the unselected parental line (DU-145P) revealed a marked discordance of tumorigenicity and metastatic capacity (Table VII). Of interest, the metastatic phenotype of cell line DU-145LM was only demonstrable following intrasplenic injection (data not shown) suggesting that a microenvironmental selection process may have occurred. Nonetheless, this variant along with the other in vivo selected members of the DU-145 family (Table VIII) constitute a useful library of sublines, the majority of which possess invasive/metastatic phenotypes distinctly different from the parental line of origin.

A number of factors appear to be responsible for the demonstrated efficacy of the intrasplenic metastasis assay (Table IX). The tumors are devoid of a restrictive fibrous

TABLE VII. Comparison of DU-145P With Its In Vivo-Derived Variant DU-145LM in the Intrasplenic Metastasis Assay

Cell line	Behavior following intrasplenic injection in nude mice	
	Local tumors[a]	Visceral metastases[b]
DU-145P	1/30	1/30
DU-145LM[c]	9/10	9/10

[a]Intrasplenic tumor formation. Unlike DU-145P, variant cell line DU-145LM resulted in tumor formation within 2 months of craniad s.c. inoculation in 4/10 animals tested.
[b]Gross and microscopic evidence of metastases in liver, mesenteric lymph nodes, and lung.
[c]Derived from invasive liver metastasis that developed following i.s. injection of DU-145P.

TABLE VIII. The DU-145 Family*

DU-145 intrasplenic (ISP)
DU-145 LM intrasplenic (ISP)
DU-145 liver metastasis (LM)
DU-145 LM ascites (ASC)
DU-145 LM lymph node metastasis (LNM)
DU-145 LM muscle invasive (MI)

*The production of metastatic foci following i.s. injection of DU-145 LM resulted in this establishment of variant lines: DU-145 LM (ASC), DU-145 LM (LMN), DU-145 LM (MI), and DU-145 LM (ISP).

sheath, exhibit excellent vascularity, and demonstrate minimal, if any, tumor necrosis. A time-course distribution study performed using I-125-labeled tumor cells readily demonstrates that intrasplenic injection provides direct and immediate access to the portal venous system with predominant distribution to the liver and foregut/hindgut lymphatics. Of particular interest, nearly one-third of the input dose is still retained in the liver at 24 hr (Table X). These results contrast sharply to earlier observations made following the systemic intravenous injection of radiolabeled tumor cells. The latter studies revealed less than 1% of the input dose still retained in the pulmonary parenchyma [82]. The efficacy of intrasplenic injection may, in part, reflect prolonged cell survival within a relatively nonturbulent portal venous system. Following portal venous injection, it is likely that spontaneous metastases develop from locally growing tumors, invasive body wall/diaphragmatic variants, and multifocal sites of tumor deposition including the omentum, hepatic capsule and liver bed, and mesenteric lymphatics. Pulmonary (parenchymal) and mediastinal lymph node metastases are relatively common events (Table IV) and may be related to diaphragmatic invasion and persistent ''seeding'' from smaller metastatic foci in the abdomen. Ascites probably develops as a result of lymphatic obstruction and transudation of tumor cells from the serosal surface of the mesentary and hepatic capsule. The precepts of the cranial/caudal growth gradient may also apply to tumor cells injected intraperitoneally [76]. The intrasplenic injection technique, thus, adheres in principle to the growth gradient concept. Finally, this approach may permit exposure of certain tumor cells to a favorable ''microenvironment'' conducive to further growth and metastasis.

Despite its apparent utility in the evaluation of these established prostate cancer cell lines, the intrasplenic injection assay proved less helpful in the in vivo cultivation, expansion, and metastasis of fresh prostate cancer. Only 1 of 7 evaluated tumors demonstrated local intrasplenic growth and metastasis. The tumor was designated TH-1018 and was derived from a prostatic adenocarcinoma treated by radical retropubic prostatectomy. The permanent hematoxylin and eosin (H&E) sections of the primary tumor

TABLE IX. Advantages Inherent in the Intrasplenic Injection Assay

1. No restrictive ''pseudocapsule''
2. Minimal tumor necrosis because of enhanced vascularity as for intraperitoneal injection
3. Enhanced tumor cell survival compared to systemic i.v. injection
4. Access to portal vein parallels experimental metastatic assay
5. Multifocal secondary metastases parallel spontaneous metastasis assay
6. Adheres to rationale of cranial-caudal gradient

TABLE X. Organ Distribution of I-125-Labeled B16-BL6 Melanoma Cells Following Intrasplenic Injection*

Time of death	Percent viable cells[a]							
	Blood[b]	Heart	Lung	Liver	Spleen	Foregut[c]	Hindgut[c]	(R) kidney
5 min	0.10	0.05	0.06	77.10	21.58	0.74	0.37	0.46
15 min	0.50	0.05	0.14	74.87	20.20	3.45	0.74	0.07
30 min	0.56	0.06	0.10	71.96	19.29	1.87	0.39	0.07
1 hr	0.75	0.04	0.08	70.24	16.24	2.65	1.00	0.06
2 hr	0.29	0.05	0.07	64.58	23.46	3.23	1.13	0.10
6 hr	0.09	0.04	0.05	38.08	12.71	1.55	0.58	0.05
8 hr	0.17	0.04	0.05	56.72	8.76	0.89	1.18	0.06
1 day	0.07	0.04	0.04	28.61	13.84	1.71	1.40	0.33

*Recipient animals were 6-week-old Balb/c nude mice (5 mice/time interval).
[a]Each animal received 500,000 I-125-labeled cells in 0.2 ml HBSS via intrasplenic injection.
[b]0.2 ml of blood.
[c]Stomach and small intestine.
[d]Large intestine.

revealed it to be moderately well differentiated, possessing a Gleason score of 7. Of interest, this tumor produced prominent, multifocal pulmonary metastases following intrasplenic injection.

It appears likely that further modifications in the nude mouse model will be required in order to enhance the utility of this system for the assessment of fresh prostate cancers. Previous reports have alluded to the utility of further immune suppression by pretreatment with anti-gamma interferon antibodies, suggesting that a more profound inhibition of macrophage and natural killer cell function may prove beneficial in this regard [83,84]. More recent observations have emphasized the importance of the favorable "microenvironment" with respect to the deposition, growth, and subsequent metastasis of fresh human colon and renal cell cancers [85,86]. Injection of colorectal carcinomas into the portal venous system via intrasplenic injection and the subrenal capsule injection of human renal cell cancers permitted frequent growth and metastasis. Of importance, both tumor systems manifested patterns of metastasis similar to those demonstrated in man. It seems likely that similar refinements will be required for the routine evaluation of fresh human prostate cancer in the immune-deficient animal. A number of such approaches are currently under investigation in our laboratory, including 1) the feasibility of periprostatic or intravesical injection of prostate cancer cells in athymic nude mice providing access to the urogenital sinus "milieu"; 2) direct injection of fresh prostate cancer cells into the ventral prostate of nude rats; 3) the efficacy of androgen "boosting" using silastic implants and minipumps containing dihydrotestosterone; and 4) probing additional means of immune suppression, such as irradiation therapy and the injection of methylpalmitate to provide additional macrophage inhibition.

ESTABLISHMENT OF BIOLOGICALLY AGGRESSIVE DU-145 VARIANTS BY DNA TRANSFECTION

Recent studies have demonstrated a correlation between the levels of expression of the Harvey-ras oncogene and the presence of biologically aggressive human colon, bladder, and prostate carcinomas [24]. With respect to the latter, Viola and associates assessed the level of expression of the p-21 protein product of the cellular Harvey-ras oncogene in prostate tissues derived from normal subjects, patients with benign prostatic hyperplasia (BPH), and in patients with varying grades of prostate cancer. This assessment was performed in a semiquantitative manner by employing the RAP-5 monoclonal antibody in an avidin-biotin-complex immunoperoxidase assay. Stromal and epithelial cells from normal controls and patients with BPH showed no evidence for p-21 antigen expression. In contrast, one-third of the prostate specimens with grade 1 carcinoma, two-thirds with grade 2 cancers, and all patients with higher-grade cancers demonstrated significant levels of p-21 expression. Although preliminary, these observations do suggest a possible direct relationship between H-ras oncogene expression and escalating levels of biologically aggressive prostate cancer.

These recent insights provided the stimulus for our laboratory to assess the impact of Harvey-ras oncogene transfection on the biological behavior of cell line DU-145. The latter seemed ideally suited to serve as a transfection recipient for a variety of reasons, including 1) it is a tranformed hormone-resistant prostate cancer cell line of human origin; 2) tumorigenicity is marginal following subcutaneous and intrasplenic injection within the constraints of a 2-month experimental duration; and 3) there is little evidence of invasive or metastatic potential in the unselected parental cell line [62]. Thus, any transfection-associated "up regulation" of the aggressive phenotype would be easily demonstrable.

The essential components of the transfection procedure employed include 1) the plasmid vector pBR 322; 2) C57BL6 mouse embryo carrier DNA; 3) selective markers for G418 (neo) resistance; and 4) the mutated EJ-ras oncogene derived from the T-24 bladder carcinoma cell line along with its normal EC-ras [allele]. The transfection protocol involves a modification of the gene transfer procedure designed by Korsaro and Pearson [87] and can be summarized as follows.

DNA Transfection of Cell Line DU-145

Twenty-four hours prior to gene transfer, DU-145 tumor cells were plated at a density of 5×10^5 cells/100-mm petri dish in Dulbecco's minimum essential medium (MEM) containing high glucose (4,500 mg/liter), 10% fetal bovine serum (FBS), and nonessential amino acids. Mouse embryo carrier DNA (10 µg/dish) and plasmid DNA (5 µg/dish) were mixed with distilled water and 2× Hank's balanced salt solution (HBSS); 2× calcium chloride was added dropwise with gentle agitation followed by vortexing. The DNA:calcium phosphate mix was incubated at room temperature for 30 min. The resulting precipitate was vortexed gently, and 1 ml was added dropwise over 100-ml petri dishes containing DU-145 tumor cells and evenly distributed by gentle agitation. The DNA was incubated with the tumor cells for 6 hr and then removed. The cells were refed with DMEM, 10% fetal bovine serum, and nonessential amino acids. Cells were cultivated for 48 hr without in vitro selection (G 418) and then split 1 to 4 and replated in media containing DMEM, 10% fetal bovine serum, nonessential amino acids, and G 418 (200 µg/ml). The cells were grown in the presence of drug until foci were formed and then split again into fresh media containing G 418 until the cells formed a confluent monolayer. Prior to nude mouse injection, G 418 was removed from the media in order to permit expansion of the populations. In vitro documentation of successful transfection was provided by dot blot analysis (data not shown).

This technique was used to establish a family of tumor cell variants designated the DU-145 transfectants (Table XI). Cell lines DU-1, DU-EJ7, and DU-EJ8 resulted

TABLE XI. DU-145 Transfectants

Cell line	Transfected DNA
DU-1	EJ-ras
DU-EJ7	EJ-ras
DU-EJ8	EJ-ras
DU-1 ascites(ASC)[a]	EJ-ras
DU-4	neo(G 418)
DU-2	EC-ras

[a]Established from tumor-rich ascites that developed following i.s. injection of DU-1.

from the transfection of the mutated EJ-ras oncogene. Cell line DU-1 ascites (ASC) is an in vivo selected variant established from the tumor-rich ascites produced by DU-1 following intrasplenic injection. DU-4 and DU-2 represent control transfectants. The former was transfected with a marker providing neomycin (G 418) resistance. The latter represents the transfection of the normal EC-ras allele.

The in vivo behavior of these transfected cells is depicted in Table XII. As expected, the biological behavior of cell line DU-4 parallels that of the nontransfected parental cell line DU-145. Both cell lines demonstrate minimal tumorigenic potential following both subcutaneous and intrasplenic injection. Furthermore, their metastatic potential is negligible. Of interest, transfection with the EC-ras allele (DU-2) markedly enhanced local tumor formation following intrasplenic injection. This was not observed following injection of the same transfectant in the craniad subcutaneous position. Not unexpectedly, EC-ras transfection made but a modest impact upon the metastatic capacity of this otherwise biologically indolent system. With respect to the in vitro derived EJ-ras transfectants (DU-1, DU-EJ7, DU-EJ8), they all demonstrated markedly enhanced intrasplenic tumorigenicity. As was true of the DU-2 transfectant, enhanced tumor formation following intrasplenic injection was not associated with a similar ability to form local tumors following deposition in the craniad subcutaneous position. Only the in vivo-derived transfectant (DU-1ASC) demonstrated enhanced tumorigenic potential following tumor deposition in either site. Consistent with previous observations, EJ-ras transfection markedly amplified the metastatic capacity of the involved cell lines, with the exception of the EJ-8 variant. The complexity of this process is further highlighted by the observation that as with tumorigenicity, the metastatic potential of the various EJ-ras transfectants

TABLE XII. Effect of H-ras Transfection Upon the Metastatic Phenotype of Cell Line DU 145-P

Cell line	DNA transfected	Behavior following intrasplenic injection in nude mice		Local tumors following craniad s.c. injections
		Local tumors[a]	Visceral metastasis[b]	
DU-1	EJ-ras	9/10	7/10	0/10
DU-1ASC	EJ-ras	10/10	9/10	8/10
DU-EJ7	EJ-ras	9/10	8/10	0/10
DU-EJ8	EJ-ras	8/10	2/10	1/10
DU-4	neo	0/10	0/10	0/10
DU-2	EC-ras	8/10	2/10	0/10

[a]Intrasplenic growth.
[b]Gross and microscopic involvement of liver, mesenteric lymph nodes, and lungs.

could only be assessed following intrasplenic injection. That technique permitted the demonstration of multifocal, gross visceral metastases. Similar analysis using conventional experimental and spontaneous metastases assays failed to define these rather dramatic changes in biological behavior (data not shown).

Several points deserve emphasis as a result of these observations. First, cell line DU-145 is a biologically useful system in which to assess the impact of oncogene transfection. Second, transfection with a mutated allele of the H-ras oncogene was associated with a markedly amplified tumorigenic and metastatic potential in this otherwise indolent human prostate cancer cell line. Third, these dramatic shifts in biological behavior could only be appreciated following intrasplenic injection. The latter observation suggests the need to critically examine any given in vivo model used to assess the biological impact of DNA transfection when performed in human systems. Conventional metastasis assays did not reveal the significant biological changes produced by DNA transfection in this tumor system. It is likely that future in vivo studies regarding the impact of genomic perturbation on fresh and established human prostate cancers will require that serious consideration be given to both the integrity of the animal model utilized and the site of tumor deposition.

THE EFFECT OF DIETHYLSTILBESTROL (DES) UPON THE BIOLOGICAL BEHAVIOR OF CELL LINES PC-3 AND DU-145 IN THE NUDE MOUSE MODEL

DES is a synthetic estrogen that is frequently and successfully utilized in the treatment of metastatic androgen-responsive carcinoma of the prostate. Its efficacy has been attributed to a number of factors, including 1) a disruption of the hypothalamic-pituitary-testicular axis by inhibiting the release of luteinizing hormone (LH) from the pituitary; 2) an increase in sex hormone-binding globulin resulting in a decrease in free, physiologically active serum testosterone; and 3) a partial suppression of testosterone biosynthesis by the interstitial cells of Leydig [88]. In addition, at supraphysiologic doses DES has been shown to inhibit the conversion of testosterone to its physiologically active moiety, 5-dihydrotestosterone and to decrease DNA polymerase activity in prostate cancer cells in tissue culture [88,89].

Despite its beneficial impact in a majority of patients with disseminated, hormone-responsive prostate cancer, DES has well-recognized clinical side effects [88,89]. The most noteworthy among the latter are its predisposition to arterial and venous thrombosis, fluid retention, and hypertension [90,91]. Although of questionable significance within this clinical context, experimental studies have documented a number of other deleterious features of diethylstilbestrol, including its mutagenic and immunosuppressive potential. The mutagenicity of DES in animals and man has been attributed to a number of features, including 1) its promotion of sister-chromatid exchanges, 2) the enhancement of non disjunction and/or loss of chromosomes, and 3) the presence of prominent colchicine-like properties [92–96]. With respect to its impact on the immune system, DES has been shown to decrease antibody production, inhibit the release of and response to interleukin-1 (IL-1) and interleukin-2 (IL-2), impair macrophage and T-cell function, and decrease the pool of NK-cell precursors [97–104].

The inhibitory effect of DES upon NK-cell-mediated cytotoxicity seemed worthy of further investigation for several reasons. First, earlier studies had shown that nude mice pretreated with intraperitoneal silastic implants containing beta-estradiol demonstrated markedly reduced NK-cell activity, which appeared to increase the susceptibility of these animals to the experimental and spontaneous metastasis of cell lines of DU-145 and PC-3 [105]. Of interest, the tumorigenic potential of DU-145 was also significantly increased in the presence of beta-estradiol [105]. On the basis of these data, it seemed logical to expect a similar impact of the synthetic estrogen, diethystilbestrol. Second, the effect of DES upon the biological activity of hormone-resistant prostate cancer is a clinically relevant concern. Although 80% of patients with metastatic prostate cancer will respond to androgen-ablation (including DES administration), the majority of such patients will ultimately relapse with androgen-resistant disease within 1–2 years [106]. Although DES has demonstrated effectiveness in those patients with androgen-responsive tumors, its impact upon the biology of predominantly hormone-resistant prostate cancer seems to warrant further clarification. For these reasons, a series of experiments were performed in order to assess the impact of DES upon NK-cell activity in the nude mouse and to assess the susceptibility of animals so treated to the growth and metastasis of cell lines DU-145 and PC-3. The methodologic approaches can be briefly summarized as follows.

Suppression of NK-Cell Activity With Diethylstilbestrol

The technique employed was similar to that reported by Kozlowski and associates using beta-estradiol to suppress murine NK-cell activity [105]. Briefly, silastic tubes (Dow-Corning, Midland, MI) were filled with 5 mg of DES powder (Sigma Chemical Co., St. Louis). Such segments were placed in HBSS containing Gentamycin (0.5 mg/ml) for 24 hr prior to their implantation into the peritoneal cavity of 4-week-old Balb/c nude mice. The animals were anesthetized with methoxyfluorane (Metofane, Pitman-Moore, Inc, Washington Crossing, NJ). The implants were placed into the abdominal cavity following the creation of a 10-mm incision through the skin and peritoneum. The wound was closed in one layer with several wound clips (Autoclip; Clay-Adams, Parsippany, NJ). Control animals received empty (sham) implants.

Assay for NK-Cell Mediated Cytotoxicity

Twenty-four hours prior to the conduct of each assay, maximal NK-cell activation was initiated by the intravenous (i.v.) administration of polyinosinic-polycytidylic (Poly I:C) acid (50 μg/mouse). Nonadherent spleen effector cells were tested for in vitro NK-cell-mediated cytotoxicity using the standard chromium 51 release assay [107]. These cells were added to radiolabeled YAC-1 lymphoma target cells at effector/target ratios of 50:1, 25:1, 12:1, and 6:1 in Linbro U-shaped wells of 96-well microtiter plates (Flow Laboratories, Inc., McLean, VA). The percentage of killing was defined as:

$$\% \text{ cytotoxicity} = \frac{E - C}{T} \times 100$$

where E represents cpm released into supernatant in the presence of effector cells, C is cpm released by target cells in the absence of effectors, and T is total input in cpm/well. Samples were run in triplicate, and the experimental error for each group was 5% or less. In addition to using the YAC-1 lymphoma target, cell lines DU-145, PC-3, and PC-3LM were radiolabeled with tritiated ^{3}H-proline and used as target cells in a 24-hr release assay [108].

Experimental and Spontaneous Metastasis Assays

DU-145, PC-3, and PC-3LM tumor cells were harvested by overlaying subconfluent monolayer tissue cultures with 0.25% trypsin:0.02% ethylenediamine tetraacetic acid (EDTA) for about 1 min. Following dislodgement, the cells were washed in RPMI-1640 plus 10% fetal bovine serum and resuspended in HBSS. Only tumor cell suspensions with greater than 95% viability (trypan blue exclusion) were used for in vivo studies. For the conduct of experimental pulmonary metastasis, each mouse received 1×10^6 tumor cells suspended in 0.2 ml via lateral tail vein injection. Spontaneous metastasis was assessed following injection of 1×10^6 cells in 0.2 ml subcutaneously in the anterior aspect of the lateral thoracic region. Eight weeks was allowed to elapse prior to determination of each assay at which point the mice were killed, and their lungs were removed, rinsed in sterile water, and fixed in Bouin's solution. Evidence of gross pulmonary involvement was determined by manually counting the number of peripheral lung tumor nodules under a dissecting microscope after 24 hr of organ fixation. Detailed histologic examination was also performed using tissue paraffin blocks, which were cut 5 μm thick and stained with H & E.

The impact of diethylstilbestrol upon murine NK-cell activity directed against the standard YAC-1 lymphoma target cell is illustrated in Table XIII. Virtually complete suppression is noted 8 weeks following intraperitoneal implantation of DES-containing Silastic implants. These results are consistent with previously reported observations regarding the impact of beta-estradiol using identical methodologic approaches [105]. Table XIV illustrates that cell lines DU-145, PC-3, and PC-3LM are also sensitive targets to NK-cell-mediated cytotoxicity. Pretreatment for 8 weeks with DES resulted in a marked suppression of poly I:C-stimulated NK-cell cytotoxicity directed against these cell lines. Thus, pretreatment with DES inhibited the NK-cell-mediated cytotoxicity of both YAC-1 lymphoma and human prostate cancer cell targets. These in vitro observations may partially account for the impact of DES upon the in vivo behavior of the prostate cancer cell lines under study. These results are summarized in Table XV. It can be seen that nude mice pretreated with DES-containing implants were more susceptible to both experimental and spontaneous metastasis when compared to the control (sham implant) group. This finding was noted in all cell lines tested. Moreover, a DES-

TABLE XIII. Effect of Treatment With Diethylstilbestrol on NK-Cell-Mediated Cytotoxicity Against YAC-1 Lymphoma Target Cells

Weeks postimplant[a]	Group	Percent cytotoxicity at effector:target ratio[b]			
		50:1	25:1	12:1	6:1
2	Sham	71.6	54.3	36.3	24.7
	DES	73.8	61.7	41.2	25.8
4	Sham[c]	41.5	30.0	25.6	18.7
	DES[c]	16.3	13.8	9.2	8.8
6	Sham[c]	79.2	65.3	52.5	37.4
	DES[c]	30.6	17.3	12.5	10.3
8	Sham[c]	45.5	34.4	23.6	15.3
	DES[c]	9.3	5.1	2.0	3.7

[a]Four-week-old BALB/c nude mice received i.p. silastic implants containing DES or empty SHAM controls.
[b]All animals received Poly I:C (50 μg i.v.) 24 hr prior to the assay.
[c]$P \leq .001$ compared to controls.

TABLE XIV. Effect of Diethylstilbestrol on NK-Cell-Mediated Cytotoxicity Against Human Prostate Adenocarcinoma Targets Labeled With ^{3}H-Proline*

Cell line	Group	Percent cytotoxicity at effector:target ratio			
		100:1	50:1	25:1	12:1
DU-145	Sham	92.7	69.3	44.4	28.8
	DES	72.9	36.2	22.5	33.6
PC-3	Sham	50.5	20.7	0.6	9.2
	DES	22.5	0	0	5.6
PC-3LM	Sham	41.0	14.7	1.5	11.2
	DES	29.3	13.1	12.0	18.7

*Implants were initiated 8 weeks before the in vitro assay in 4-week-old BALB/c nude mice. All animals received Poly I:C (50 μg i.v.) 24 hr prior to the assay.

TABLE XV. Effect of Treatment With Diethylstilbestrol on Experimental and Spontaneous Metastasis of Human Prostate Adenocarcinoma Cell Lines in Nude Mice

Cell lines	Treatment[a]	Experimental pulmonary metastasis[b]	Spontaneous pulmonary metastasis[c]
DU 145	Sham	0/5	0/5[d]
	DES	2/5	3/5[e]
PC3-P	Sham	0/5	1/5
	DES	3/5	4/5
PC3-LM	Sham	0/5	1/5
	DES	3/5	5/5

[a]Recipient animals were 8 weeks following insertion of i.p. silastic implants containing DES or empty SHAM controls.
[b]1×10^6 tumor cells injected i.v. via a lateral tail vein.
[c]1×10^6 tumor cells injected s.c. in the lateral aspect of anterior thoracic wall.
[d]No local tumor take.
[e]80% local tumor take.

enriched milieu was associated with a marked enhancement in tumorigenicity for cell line DU-145 and is consistent with previous observations regarding the impact of beta-estradiol upon local tumor formation in this biologically indolent tumor system [105]. Figure 11 depicts a typical in vivo growth curve highlighting the impact of DES upon the "take" and growth rate of cell line DU-145 injected in the craniad subcutaneous position.

The in vitro data documenting DES-induced NK-cell inhibition and the in vivo results demonstrating amplification of experimental and spontaneous pulmonary metastasis in the presence of a DES-enriched environment are certainly consistent and imply a causal relationship. However, the enhanced tumorigenicity noted for cell line DU-145 in the presence of DES cannot be easily explained on the basis of NK-cell inhibition. Consequently, an experiment was designed to assess the potential impact of a DES-enriched milieu upon the metastatic phenotype of locally growing neoplasms. Cell line PC-3 was chosen because of its highly tumorigenic potential coupled with the absence of gross and microscopic pulmonary metastases following intravenous injection. Tumor cells (1×10^6) were injected into the craniad subcutaneous position of Balb/c nude mice that had received either DES-containing or sham silastic implants 1 week previously.

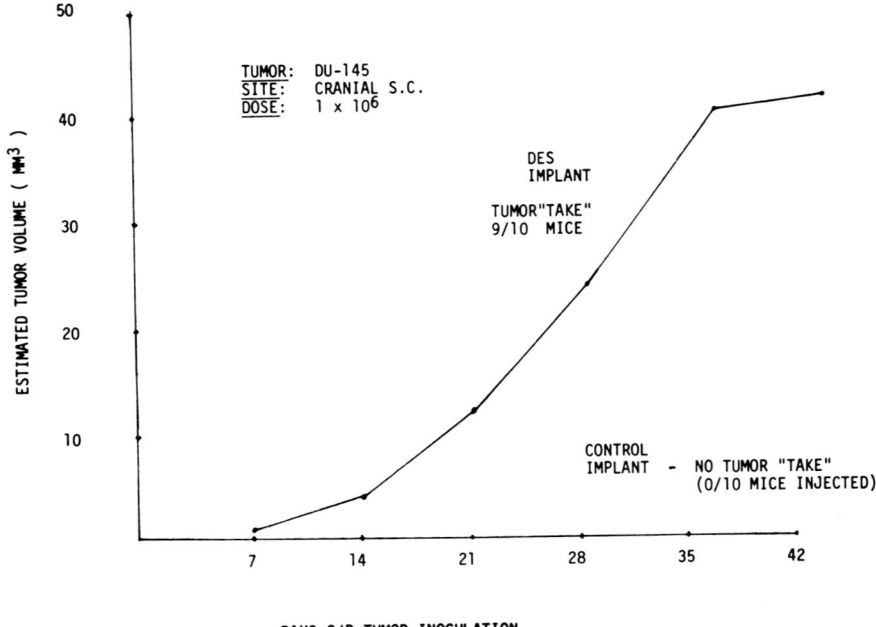

Fig. 11. In vivo growth curves of cell line DU-145. Once local growth was discernible, tumor measurements were performed three times per week using Vernier calibers. The average tumor volume was calculated according to the equation of volume equals $0.4 \times A \times B^2$, in which A is the larger diameter, and B is the smaller [109]. Within the time constraints (35–42 days) of this experiment, local tumors were noted in 90% of the DES-treated animals. No visible tumor growth was noted in any of the control animals.

Local tumors were noted in all animals studied (data not shown). These expanding neoplasms were allowed to grow in their respective environments for 8 weeks. At that time, the local tumor xenografts were harvested, mechanically/enzymatically dissociated, and established in monolayer tissue culture. Again, verification of human origin was ascertained by simple karyotype analysis. The variant line, designated PC-3DES, was expanded in vitro so as to generate adequate numbers of cells for a small-scale animal study. Table XVI illustrates the results of an experimental metastasis assay performed using PC-3 tumor cells cultivated in the presence of sham or DES-containing implants. It is readily apparent that a marked change in metastatic potential has occurred in cell line PC-3DES with 90% of the mice demonstrating gross pulmonary metastasis (Fig. 12). The control group demonstrates negligible metastatic capacity following tail vein injection. These results are consistent with previously published data regarding the in vitro established cell line PC-3 [105]. This rather dramatic amplification of metastatic phenotype in cell line PC-3DES suggests that other mechanisms be invoked besides inhibition of host effector response. A direct impact of DES upon the involved tumor cell is certainly tenable and warrants further evaluation.

In conclusion, DES shares with beta-estradiol the ability to significantly inhibit NK-cell mediated cytotoxicity in nude mice. This deleterious impact on host immune effector response may account for the observed enhancement of experimental and spon-

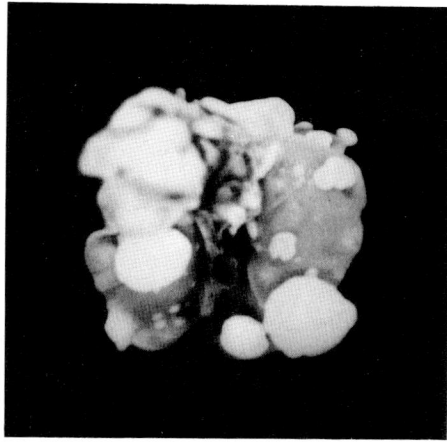

Fig. 12. Multifocal lung tumor nodules that developed 8 weeks following the intravenous injection of PC-3DES into 3-week-old nude mice. Grossly demonstrable tumor burdens were not seen in any of the control animals.

taneous pulmonary metastases of the human hormone-resistant prostate cancer cell lines evaluated in this model system. However, a direct impact of DES upon cell lines DU-145 and PC-3 is suggested by the enhancement in tumorigenicity noted in the former and marked amplification in the metastatic phenotype observed in the latter, in the presence of a DES-enriched environment. It is unclear whether the human host with metastatic, hormone-resistant prostate can be similarly effected by concomitant DES administration. Certainly, the observations generated from the admittedly limited in vitro and in vivo studies depicted above suggest the need for further investigation in this area.

TABLE XVI. Effect of In Vivo Exposure to Diethylstilbestrol Upon Experimental Pulmonary Metastasis of Human Prostate Adenocarcinoma Cell Line PC-3*

Cell line[a]	Dose (i.v.)	No. of grossly apparent lung tumor nodules[b]	Animals with microscopic metastasis in the lungs[c]
PC-3 PARENT	1×10^6	0, 0, 0, 0, 0, 0, 0, 0, 0, 0, 0, 0, 0, 0, 0	1/15
PC-3 DES	1×10^6	0, 1, 16, 95, 100, >250, >250, >250, >250, >250	9/10

*Cell line PC-3 DES was derived by enzymatic dissociation of s.c. tumor (PC-3) grown in BALB/c nude mice containing i.p. silastic implants of DES. The duration of in vivo exposure to DES was 8 weeks.
[a]Three-week-old nude mice received i.v. injections; animals were killed 8 weeks later and autopsied.
[b]No. of grossly apparent tumor foci on lung surface obtained with the aid of a dissecting microscope.
[c]Serial sections from lungs of each animal were examined for the presence of microscopic pulmonary metastasis.

THE ESTABLISHMENT OF EPITHELIAL CELL CULTURES FROM FRESH HUMAN PROSTATE TISSUES USING 1) DISCONTINUOUS PERCOLL GRADIENT CENTRIFUGATION TO SEPARATE STROMAL/EPITHELIAL FRACTIONS, 2) SERUM-FREE MEDIA, AND 3) ESSENTIAL GROWTH FACTORS

Our understanding of the biology of human prostate cancer and benign prostatic hyperplasia (BPH) has been significantly hindered by the inability to maintain human prostatic epithelial cells in a tissue culture environment [110]. This flaw in our scientific armamentarium is primarily responsible for the paucity of available prostate cancer cell lines amenable to repetitive, detailed analysis. Many obstacles to the successful propagation of the stromal and epithelial components of human prostatic tissues have been overcome as a result of such innovations as 1) the separation of stromal and epithelial elements with a high degree of purity using Percoll gradient centrifugation; (2) the development of serum-free media, which permits the propagation and expansion of prostatic epithelial cells in finite tissue culture; 3) a better understanding of those essential growth factors required to maintain normal prostatic "epitheliality"; and 4) a more sophisticated perception of those tissue culture prerequisites for the successful passage of prostate epithelial cells. Each of these issues will be briefly discussed in the following paragraphs.

The normal human prostate may contain up to 30% stromal elements [111]. Efficient segregation of these cellular constituents is desirable for a variety of reasons. First, effective elimination of this stromal component would facilitate the propagation, expansion, and analysis of the epithelial populations that make up benign and malignant prostates. Second, isolation of these glandular and stromal elements with a high degree of purity would permit the investigation of the dynamics attendant to glandular-stromal interaction. The latter is thought to play an integral role in the modulation of prostatic growth and function [112]. The development of a five-step discontinuous Percoll gradient technique was an important methodologic advance that permitted the separation of stromal elements from distinct epithelial subsets within the rat ventral prostate [113]. We have employed a modification of this procedure in order to separate these cellular elements from fresh benign and malignant human prostate glands. A summary of the technique is described below.

Five-Step Discontinuous Percoll Gradient Centrifugation

Fresh prostatic tissue is placed in a 100 × 20-mm petri dish and minced into fragments measuring 1 mm^3. These tissue fragments are then transferred to dissociating flasks to which will be added 15 ml of dissociating solution. The latter consists of 200 units/ml of collagenase type 1 (Sigma) plus 250 µg/ml of DNA-ase type 1 (Sigma) dissolved in RPMI 1640 medium with 10% fetal calf serum. The cells are dissociated for 18 hr at 37°C with gentle shaking. The freed cells are transferred to Percoll gradients aafter washing (× 2) and resuspension in phosphate-buffered saline (PBS).

Percoll (Pharmacia) is diluted with PBS to establish a 20% solution. Using 1 × PBS, dilutions are made to establish 15%, 10%, 7.5%, and 5% Percoll solutions. These are layered at 2 ml/layer from 20% to 5% in 15-ml conical tubes while marking each interface. The dissociated cells are gently layered on top, and the tubes are spun at 2,000g for 1/2 hr at 25°C. This technique generally results in the formation of very homogeneous bands (Fig. 13). The top interface at the media/5% is primarily the stromal component (Fig. 14). The 5%/7.5% interface consists of very-cuboidal-appearing epithelial cells, which probably represent secretory elements (Fig. 15), while the 7.5%/10% interface often reveals a second epithelial population characterized by more elongated cells, probably constituting the basal cell compartment (Fig. 16). The 10%/15% and 15%/20% interface represents debris and dead cells.

Following elution and washing ($\times$ 2) of the representative bands, the cells are plated overnight in phenol red-free RPMI 1640 plus 10% fetal bovine serum in order to promote attachment. These cells are refed the following morning with phenol red-free RPMI 1640 plus 10% fetal bovine serum for the stromal component and serum-free media plus growth factors for the epithelial fractions.

The development of serum-free media that is capable of supporting the growth of prostatic epithelial cells represents another major advance in tissue culture methodology. The use of serum-containing media is undesirable for a variety of reasons, including 1) its variability in growth-promoting activity when one lot of serum is compared to another; 2) toxicity, especially when high serum concentrations are employed; 3) its recognized interference with specialized cellular functions; 4) the ever-present potential for contamination by a variety of infectious agents; and 5) the ability of serum in the culture media to act as a selection factor that favors the proliferation of one cell type over another [114]. Recently, several new serum-free media formulations have been constructed specifically for the cultivation of benign and malignant human prostatic epithelial cells and include media preparations designated PFMR-4 [114] and WAJC-404 [115]. Each has evolved along slightly different lines from Ham's F-12 media. We

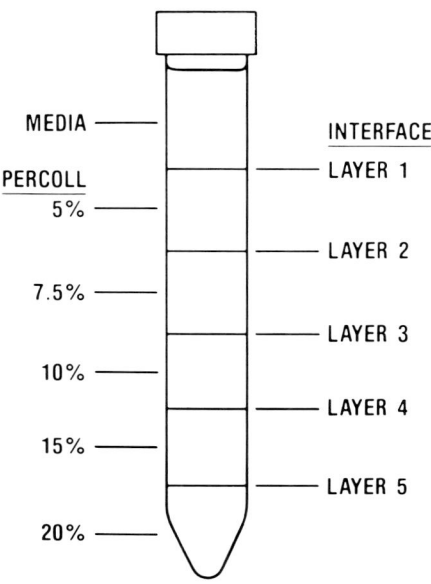

Fig. 13. Illustration of banding layers obtained following discontinuous Percoll gradient centrifugation. Layer 1 contains predominantly stromal elements representing various mixtures of mesenchymal and smooth muscle cells. Layers 2 and 3 represent discrete epithelial cell bands thought to contain secretory and basal cell elements, respectively.

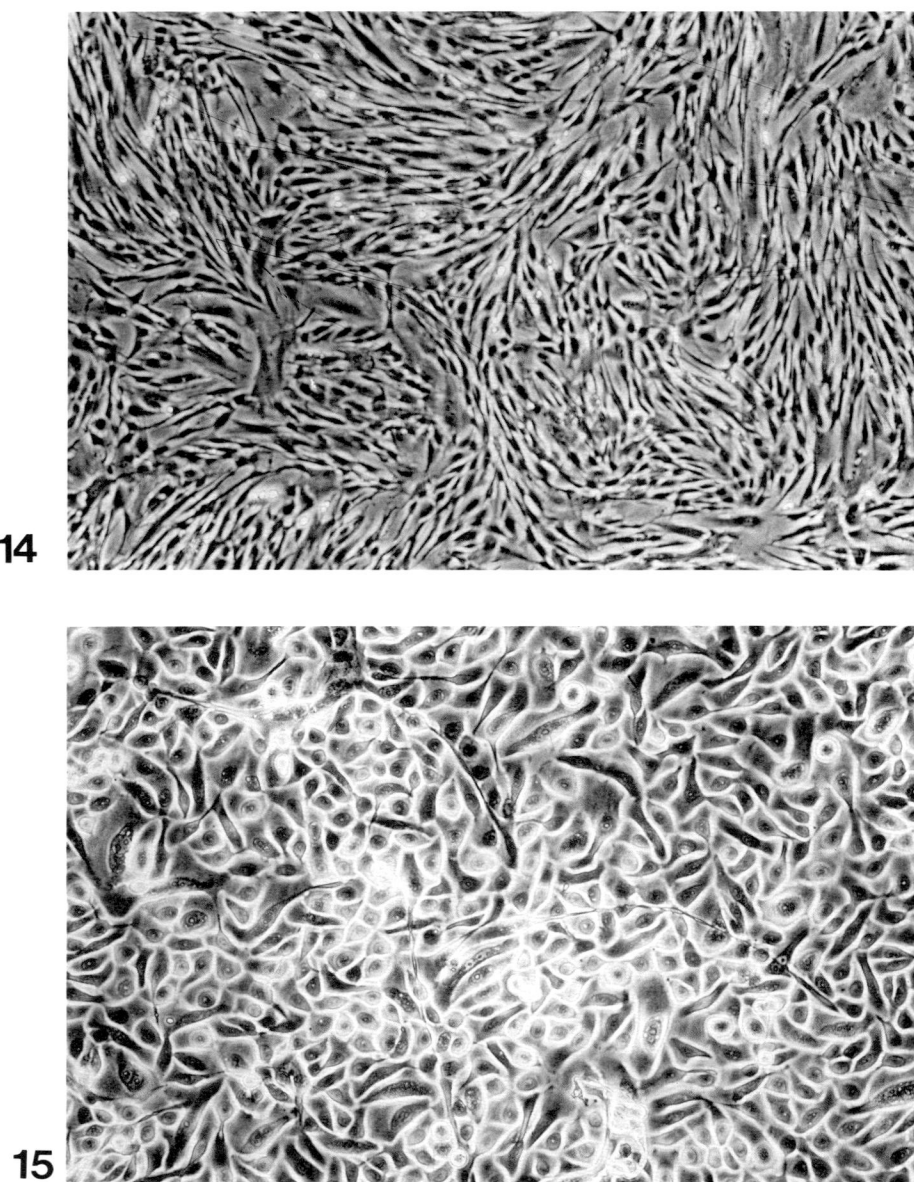

Fig. 14. Representative example of prostatic stromal cells isolated from layer 1. ×200.

Fig. 15. Epithelial cells derived from the 5%/7.5% interface (layer 2) consisting predominantly of cuboidal-appearing cells possibly representing secretory elements. ×200.

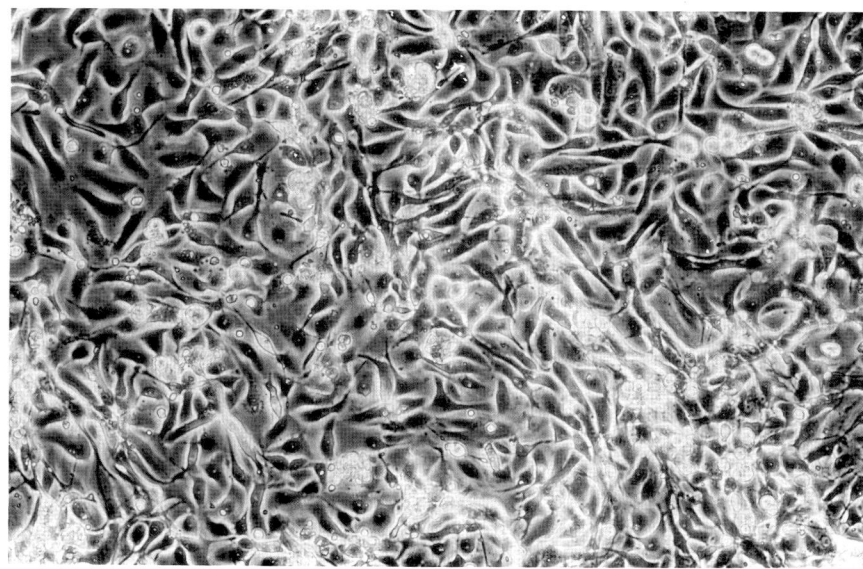

Fig. 16. Epithelial cell populations aspirated from the 7.5%/10% interface (layer 3) demonstrating a more elongated morphology possibly reflecting their origin from the basal cell compartment. ×200.

have used WAJC-404 almost exclusively. An important constituent of this basic nutrient media is a relatively low ionic calcium concentration (0.13 mM calcium). The latter has been shown to be essential for the establishment of single cell suspensions, for normal cell attachment to a plastic substratum, and for the detachment of the cellular monolayer into single cells and small aggregates following treatment with collagenase [116].

The removal of serum from such media preparations mandates the selective addition of essential growth factors to permit the cultivation of benign and malignant human prostatic epithelial cells in tissue culture. For example, several studies have suggested that cholera toxin is a potent mitogen for prostatic epithelial cells [117]. It appears to act by increasing levels of intracellular cyclic AMP by catalyzing the ADP ribosylation of the GTP-binding regulatory component of adenylate cyclase. In addition, bovine pituitary extract appears to supply not only prolactin but also a yet-uncharacterized essential epithelial cell growth factor that is present within this neural tissue [116]. The media composition employed in our studies is summarized below.

Preparation of Serum-Free Media

The nutrient stock medium is WAJC-404 (Irvine Scientific). Growth factors are added to this basic stock solution and include 1) a combination of insulin-transferrin-selenium, bovine serum albumin (BSA), and linoleic acid also designated CR-ITS+ (Collaborative Research). Five milliliters of this mixture is added to every 500 cc of basic medium; 2) bovine pituitary extract also designated CR-BPE (Collaborative Research) 50 µg/ml; 3) prolactin (L7135-Sigma) 2 µg/ml; 4) epidermal growth factor also designated CR-EGF (Collaborative Research) 10 ng/ml; 5) cholera toxin (C-3012-Sigma) 10 ng/ml; and 6) polyvinyl pyrrolidone (PVP-40, Sigma) 2 mg/ml.

It has recently been reported that the prerequisites for successful finite serial culture of prostate epithelial cells include 1) low ionic calcium concentration; 2) presence of bovine hypothalamus extract; 3) the use of collagenase to promote cellular detachment from the established monolayer; and 4) splitting of the cells before they reach a critical density of 6,000 cells/m^2 [116]. Such an approach routinely permits epithelial cells to proliferate at an exponential rate through three to four serial passages. The details of cell maintainence and passage can be briefly summarized:

Maintenance and Passage of Prostatic Epithelial Cells

All media is changed or cells are split two times per week. The approach to the latter consists of 1) the stromal component will be split with 0.25% trypsin/EDTA (Irvine Scientific) warmed to 37°C and then inactivated with RPMI + 10% fetal bovine serum. These cells are split 1 to 4 and replated in phenol red-free RPMI 1640 + 10% fetal bovine serum. 2) Epithelial cells are detached from the monolayer with 675 units/ ml of collagenase type 1 (Worthington) in HBSS with rotation at 37°C for 20 min to 1 hr followed by inactivation with RPM 1640 + 10% FBS. These epithelial cells are placed in a 1:1 mixture of previous conditioned media and fresh media on an overnight basis. The latter is followed by conversion to fresh serum-free media + essential growth factors the following morning. The cells are split 1 to 2 and generally have slow doubling times. Cryopreservation in liquid nitrogen can be performed by sequential freezing of 10^6 cells/ ml in 10% dimethylsulfoxide (DMSO) with RPMI 1640 + 5% fetal bovine serum.

Over the past 18 months, we have utilized the above-mentioned cell separation and tissue culture approaches in order to generate an expanded library of epithelial and stromal fractions from benign and malignant human prostates. The purity of separation and the maintenance of prostatic "epitheliality" was confirmed by histochemical staining of Cytospin (Shandon Inc., Pittsburgh) preparations following elution of the bands from the Percoll gradient. Such preparations were probed for the expression of prostatic acid phosphatase, prostate specific antigen, and cytokeratin expression. In general, separation and serial passage resulted in stromal and epithelial cell cultures of greater than 95% purity. Table XVII represents a list of fresh prostate cancer and BPH specimens from which stromal and epithelial components have been separated, passaged, and cryopreserved.

An attempt was made to further characterize some of these fresh prostate systems tabulated above. As stated previously, of the fresh prostate cancers only TH-1018 demonstrated local intrasplenic tumor growth and subsequent metastasis in the nude mouse model. In addition to this in vivo assessment, representative examples of these benign and malignant systems were further characterized using two-dimensional gel electrophoresis and with respect to their ability to invade basement membrane matrix. A summary of these studies constitutes the concluding two segments of this paper.

ANALYSIS OF THE PROTEIN COMPOSITION OF EPITHELIAL/STROMAL CELLS CONSTITUTING BENIGN AND MALIGNANT HUMAN PROSTATES

Available evidence suggests that multiple phenotypic differences exist that serve to distinguish invasive and metastatic cancer cells from their biologically indolent counterparts [118]. One of the best studied of these parameters is that of increased or altered protein production on the part of biologically aggressive tumor cells [119]. For example, truly "malignant" tumor systems have been associated with increases in laminin receptor

TABLE XVII. Prostate Cancer Specimens and BPH Specimens From Which Stromal and Epithelial Components Have Been Separated, Passaged, and Cryopreserved

Prostate cancer specimens	BPH specimens
KH-1227	JC-1024
RR-1004	JK-0219
JK-1012	ES-201
TH-1018	MS-327
CT-402	HG-411
DV-430	HP-418
JC-220	BC-730
	SF-807
	HZ-807
	HM-821
	LD-905
	BE-1119
	HM-1031
	JG-0106
	LK-317
	WF-318
	JC-415

content coupled with enhanced production and secretion of various protein moieties, including type 4 collagenase, heparinase, plasminogen activator, cathepsin B, and autocrine motility factor [120–122]. It seems likely that additional investigation will reveal a number of unique differences in protein constitution serving to characterize metastatic cancer cells. In fact, it is entirely conceivable that some of these differences may prove to be subtle and specific to the tumor system under study.

In order to probe such differences in protein composition, we have utilized the ISO-DALT system of two-dimensional (2-D) gel electrophoresis that was developed by Anderson and Anderson [123,124] following a series of modifications of the original technique described by O'Farrel [125]. The first dimension (the ISO system) is designed to separate a mixture of solubilized protein in acrylamide gels on the basis of ISO-electric points (pI) of each protein. The DALT system is the second dimension electrophoresis, which separates the proteins on the basis of their molecular weight (MW). We have elected to apply this relatively new technology toward the establishment of detailed maps of secretory, cell surface, and total cell proteins that make up stromal and epithelial isolates of benign and malignant human prostate systems. Since proteins are products of cellular phenotypic expression and since each cell type produces a characteristic profile of proteins, detection of abnormal protein distribution patterns could signify important changes in phenotypic expression. The entire procedure has been described in detail by Tollaksen and associates [126]. A brief description of the methodology is contained in the following paragraphs.

Specimen Preparation

Cells destined for 2-D electrophoresis are solubilized in 9 M urea, 2% dithiothreitol, 4% Nonidet P40, and 4% LKB ampholyte, pH 3.5–10. The protein content of the resultant mixture is analyzed by the Bradford method [127]. An aliquot of 100 μg of protein is generally used for electrophoresis. The remainder of the prepared sample is stored at −80°C until further analysis is required.

The ISO-DALT System

In the first dimension the gels are cast in elongated glass tubing (17.8 cm long and 1.5 mm in diameter) containing 9 M urea, 5% acrylamide, and ampholyte whose pH ranges from 3 to 10. Prefocusing is carried out for 1 hr at 200 volts. Approximately 30 µl of the sample (equivalent to 100 µ of protein) is loaded onto each tube. The ISO electric focusing is carried out at a constant voltage overnight for 14,000 volt-hr. At the end of each isoelectric focusing, the gels are extruded from the glass tube and equilibrated in a Tris buffer containing glycerol, (SDS) sodium dodecyl sulfate and a small amount of Bromophenol blue, pH 6.8. The second dimension is conducted in slab gels (17.8 × 17.8 cm^2, 1.5 mm thick) consisting of a 9–18% gradient of acrylamide. The ISO gel is carefully loaded onto the top of the DALT gel. The DALT tank contains a buffer that consists of Tris, glycine, and SDS. The electrophoresis is carried out at a constant voltage of 100–150 volts for a convenient overnight run of about 16 hr. The slab gels can then be removed for silver staining using a procedure adopted from the method described by Guevara and associates [128]. For permanent record-keeping, images of completed ISO-DALT gels are transferred to positive black and white Kodak X-Omat duplicating film according to the procedure of Harrison [129,130]. With this procedure, protein spots are imaged black regardless of their color in the silver-staining gels.

Figure 17 provides a comparison of 2-D gel slabs performed on epithelial cell-enriched (insert A) and stromal cell-enriched (insert B) populations derived following the passage of BPH tissue over a discontinuous Percoll gradient. Upon comparison of the profiles of proteins in these gels, a protein (MW 40,000; pI 5.8) equivalent to that of cytokeratin was consistently present at higher concentrations in the gel slabs containing proteins from epithelial cells as compared to those from stromal cells. The intensity of this protein spot was analyzed and equivalent to that of actin (MW 42,000; pI 6.0) by computerized densitometry. A relative intensity (RI = total intensity of the protein/total

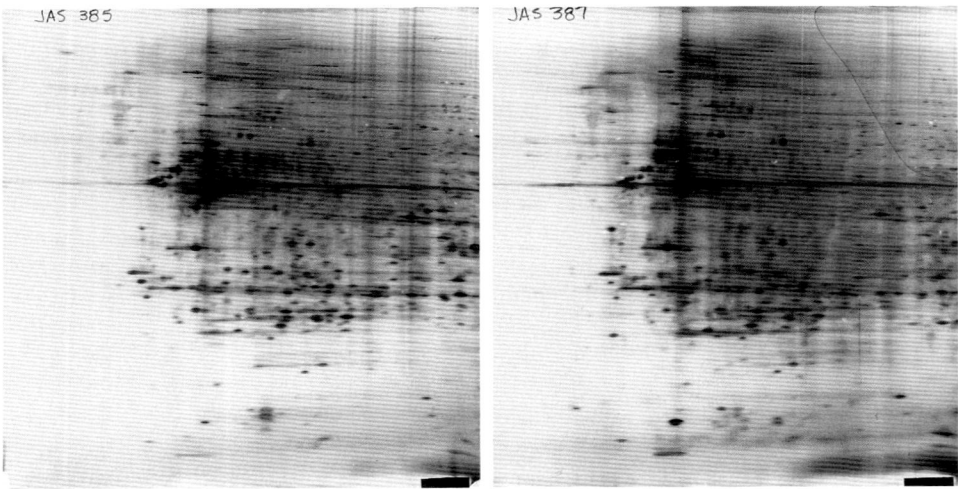

Fig. 17. Representative 2-D gels depicting the protein constitution of epithelial (**A**) and stromal (**B**) cell fractions derived from human BPH specimens and segregated using discontinuous Percoll gradient centrifugation. See text for detailed description.

intensity of actin) was then derived for each specimen. The mean RI value was 0.32 ± 0.04 (SE) for the epithelial cells and 0.11 ± 0.02 for the stromal cells. These results reflect the analysis of epithelial and stromal compartments from seven patients with BPH. This difference was statistically significant as determined by the paired Student t-test ($P < .01$). Thus, 2-D electrophoresis is a highly useful tool in identifying and discriminating microproteins that serve to distinguish epithelial from stromal compartments in the human prostate. Admittedly more challenging is the quantitative and qualitative discrimination of 2-D gels representing total cellular protein derived from prostate cancer cell lines PC-3 and DU-145, together with in vivo selected metastatic variants. Such comparisons are seen in Figure 18A–D.

Although a number of protein additions and deletions are apparent from a visual comparison of the respective gels, the large number of protein spots in such gel slabs renders a manual analysis inadequate. To overcome these significant methodologic difficulties, several computer systems have been developed by major laboratories for extracting information from such gels. The major functions of these systems include background and noise removal, protein spot identification and quantitation, and spot comparison among different gels. We are currently utilizing a software designated microcomputer based system (MBS) that was designed by Indiana Biotech, Inc. for 2-D gel analysis. The software is compatible with the IBM-AT microcomputer. The hardware of the MBS consists of an IBM-PC and 20-megabyte hard disk, an RCA video camera, a PC-EYE digitizer card, a color graphic display, a system 9 pseudo-color card, a Houston instrument plotter, and an Epson printer. This software permits routine noise reduction, background removal, peak of spot detection, peak combination and spot registration, spot shape registration, interactive routine for landmark setting, global comparison routine, and utility routine.

In conclusion, 2-D gel electrophoresis is a powerful tool capable of resolving complex mixtures of proteins in cells and in body fluid. With the addition of sophisticated computer-based image analysis, it may provide important information with respect to unique protein differences that serve to distinguish metastatic variants from the primary tumor of origin.

THE GROWTH MORPHOLOGY AND BEHAVIOR OF HUMAN PROSTATE CELLS CULTIVATED ON BASEMENT MEMBRANE MATRIX

The metastatic cascade is a descriptive term referring to a series of biological events that begins with progressive growth of the primary tumor and culminates in the development of a proliferating metastatic focus within a distant organ or site [131]. As stated previously, a substantial amount of evidence suggests that the development of metastases represents the selection from the parenteral tumor of a unique subpopulation of truly "malignant" cells, which are endowed with properties that enhance their survival through this arduous process [132–135]. A fundamental requirement for the successful completion of the metastatic cascade is the degradation of the host basement membrane. The latter represents an intricate meshwork of a unique collagen subtype (type 4), specific attachment to glycoproteins (laminin, entactin, and nidigen), and heparan sulfate proteoglycan [136,137].

A three-step hypothesis has been proposed describing the dynamics of tumor cell invasion of the basement membrane extracellular matrix [138–140]. First, metastatic cells have been shown to possess high-affinity receptors for laminin, the occupation of

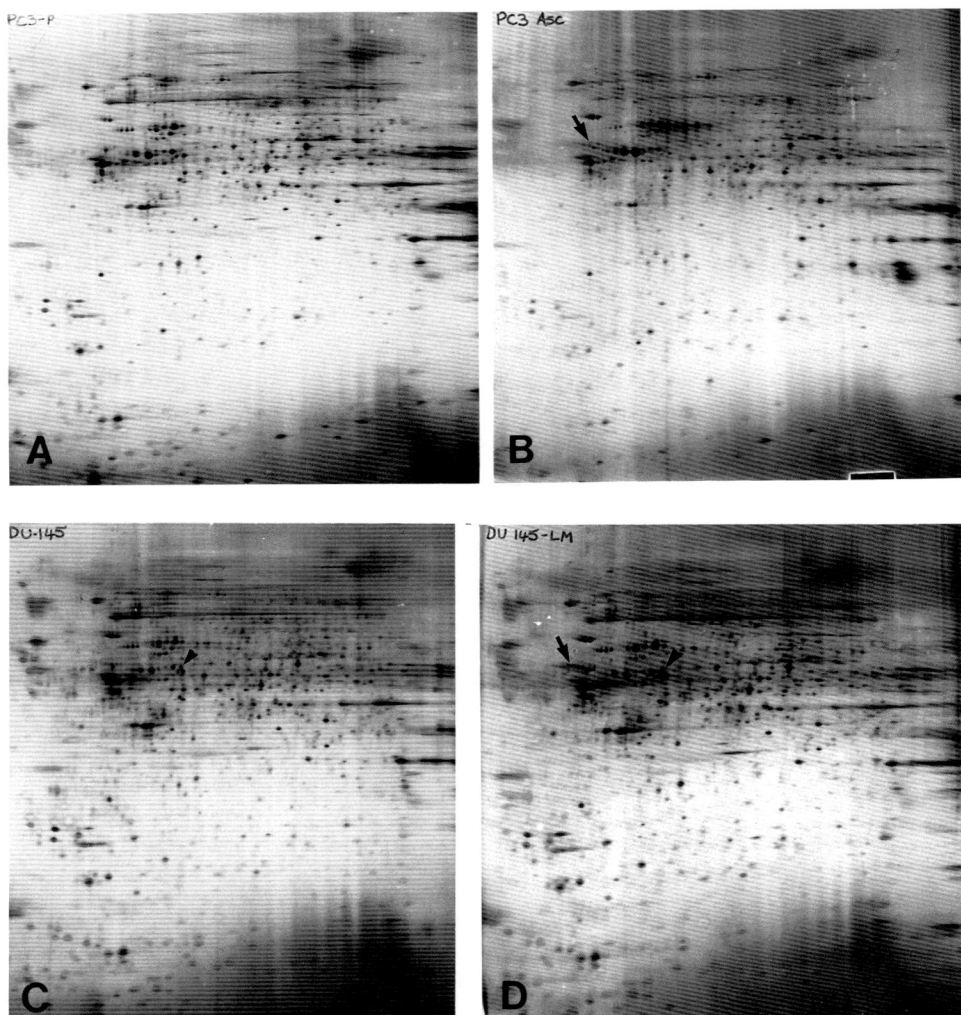

Fig. 18. Two-dimensional protein profiles of PC3-P (**A**), PC3-ASC (**B**), DU-145 (**C**), and DU-145LM (**D**). Although the profiles among the four cell lines are remarkably similar, subtle differences do exist. A comparison of the PC3 and DU-145 cell lines reveals the presence of a prominent spot (pI 6, MW 65 KD arrowhead) in the DU-145 series. This protein moiety is either absent or present at low staining intensity in the PC3 family. In addition, an increase in protein staining intensity is noted at the location of pI 5 and MW 66KD (arrow) for both metastatic subsets of PC3 and DU-145.

which forms a matrix between the cell surface laminin receptor and type 4 collagen. Second, metastatic cells thus attached are capable of elaborating large amounts of type 4 collagenase and heparinase, which results in the destruction of the collagen and proteoglycan components of the basement membrane. Third, tumor cells traverse the areas of proteolytic destruction with directed locomotion being, influenced by the elaboration of autocrine motility factor produced by the invading front of tumor cells [141].

In the majority of rodent and human systems analyzed, metastatic capacity has been shown to correlate closely with the presence of specific high-affinity receptors for laminin and with the capability of such cells to generate basement membrane degrading protease [142–148]. The strategic importance of this phase of the metastatic cascade has stimulated a great deal of interest in the construction of in vitro invasion assays which might simulate in vivo events regarding the degradation of host basement membrane [149].

Albini and associates have recently demonstrated their ability to distinguish biologically indolent from aggressive tumor systems by an analysis of their respective growth morphology and invasive potential using a reconstituted basement membrane preparation designated MATRIGEL [150]. The latter is a solubilized tissue extract of the basement membrane producing murine sarcoma designated the Englebreath-Holm-Swarm. This substance is a laminin-rich basement membrane extract that is commercially available through Collaborative Research, Inc. (Lexington, MA). The gel is stored at $-20°C$ but when warmed under physiological conditions, MATRIGEL creates a basement membrane in vitro that has been shown to promote the attachment of and support the growth and differentiation of a diverse array of benign and malignant cells [151–153].

The growth morphology exhibited by tumor cells plated on a thin layer of MATRIGEL reliably distinguishes biologically indolent neoplasms from those possessing invasive capacity [150]. The former grow as single cells, which ultimately form scattered clusters or dome-like aggregates (Fig. 19A,B). In contrast, truly "malignant" cells manifest a distinctly different growth morphology, characterized by the appearance of numerous filopodial extensions that promote the spreading and migration of such cells onto the matrix interface [Fig. 20A,B]. With time, these invasive cells may demonstrate a halo of degraded matrix around their peripheral margin, ultimately traverse the basement membrane barrier, and attach to the underlying plastic substratum. Such morphological differences are often apparent 2–3 hr after plating and are consistently observable for several days thereafter. This in vitro technique can be summarized as follows.

Morphology of Tumor Cells on MATRIGEL

Precooled 35-mm Petri dishes are routinely utilized. MATRIGEL is shipped in quantities of 10 ml/vial and stored at $-20°C$. It requires thawing on ice followed by gentle pipetting onto the tissue culture plates. In general 0.5 ml is used to coat a 35-mm Petri dish. The pipette tip is used to wet all surfaces of the plate and to distribute the MATRIGEL evenly. The plates are incubated at 37°C and 5% CO_2 in a humidified environment for approximately 60 min. The cell suspension to be tested ($1-5 \times 10^4$ cells/dish) is plated using complete media appropriate for the cell type. The culture dishes are returned to the incubator and refed every 2–3 days with photomicroscopy being performed on a daily basis in order to record the evolution of growth morphology on the gel matrix (Fig. 21).

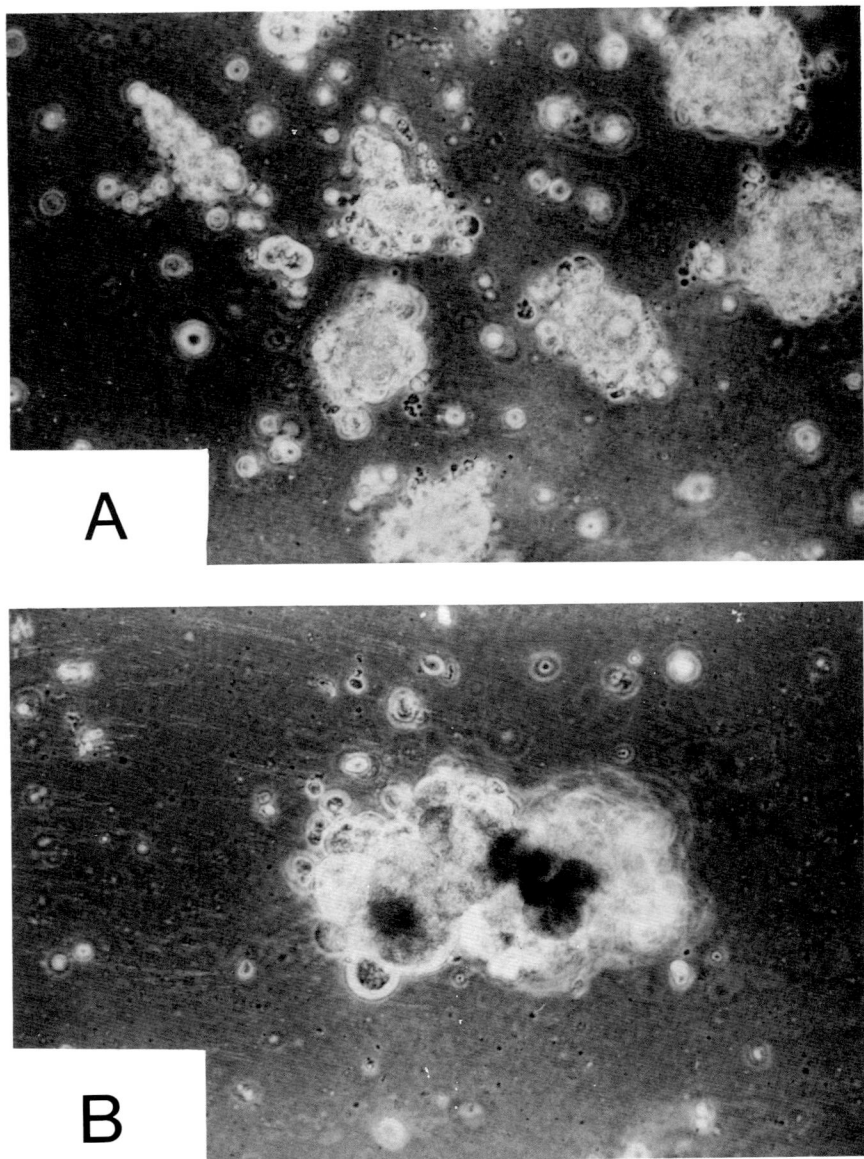

Fig. 19. Cell line DU-145 demonstrating cell clustering characteristic of biological indolent tumors **19A**. × 40. A high-power view of one of these cellular domes is depicted in **19B**. ×200. Note the absence of filopodial extensions and the intact matrix interface.

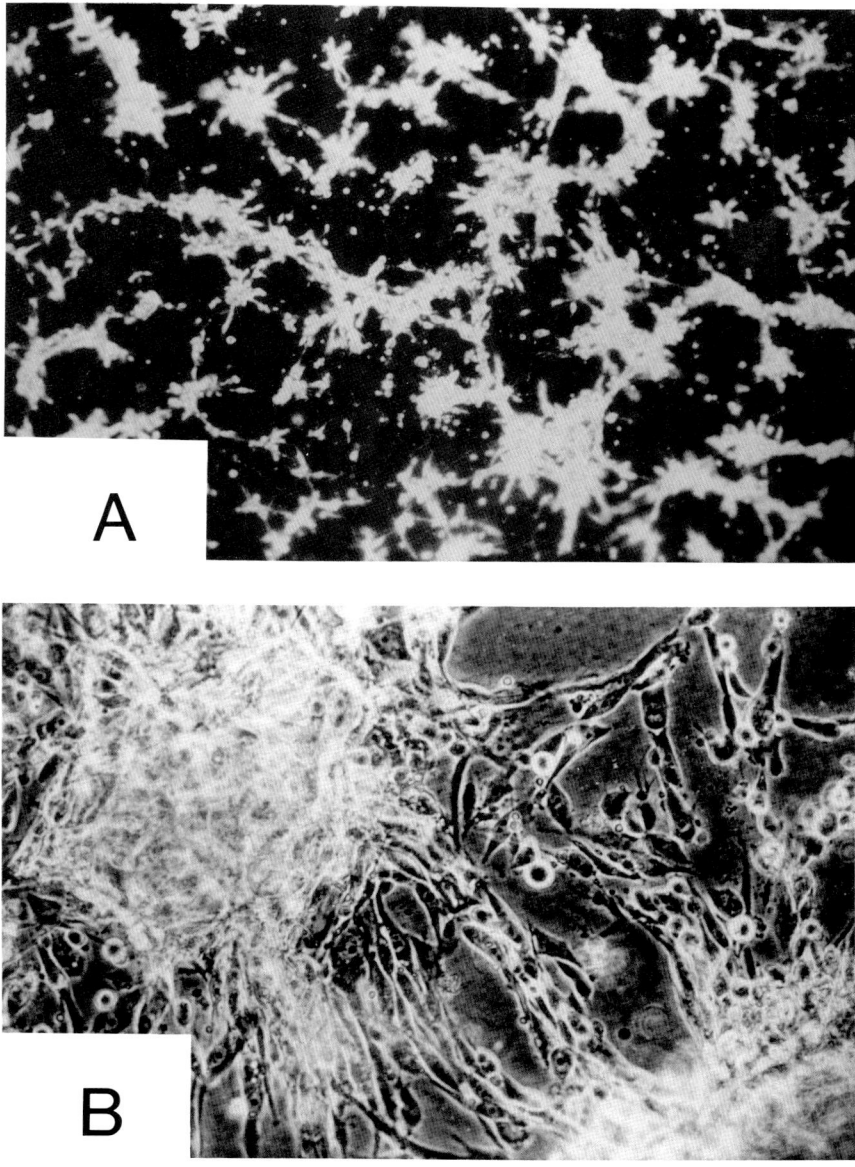

Fig. 20. Note the characteristic stellate or "starburst" appearance of cell PC-3 plated on basement membrane MATRIGEL **20A**. ×40. **20B** provides a high-power view of two adjacent cell clusters demonstrating the filopodial extensions typically seen when aggressive tumor systems are plated on basement membrane matrix. ×200.

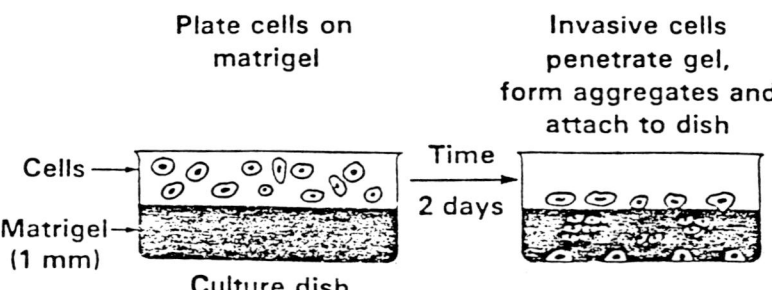

Fig. 21. Illustration representing the plating of tumor cell suspensions on MATRIGEL-coated culture dishes. The growth morphology exhibited by the tumor system under study coupled with its ability to degrade the matrix interphase provide useful information regarding its invasive potential.

This relatively simple technique has been used to assess the growth morphology of benign human prostatic epithelial cells obtained from BPH specimens following the cell isolation procedures noted previously. In each case, the plated cells form scattered dome-like aggregates so characteristic of biologically indolent systems. These features are duplicated when cell line DU-145 is plated under similar conditions (Fig. 19A,B). It should be recalled that this parental cell line is minimally tumorigenic and demonstrates a very low level of aggressiveness when assessed in the nude mouse model. In contrast, the in vivo-derived metastatic variant DU-145LM demonstrates the prompt development of filopodial extensions, which promote cell spreading along the surface of the matrix interface and subsequent matrix degradation (Fig. 22). An even more spectacular demonstration of this stellate or "starburst" appearance is noted following the cultivation of cell line PC-3 under similar conditions (Fig. 20A,B). It should be recalled that this cell line has easily demonstrable metastatic capacity when assessed via the intrasplenic injection assay. Thus, the in vitro and in vivo assessments provide complementary and corroborative information. This technique has also proven useful in the assessment of some fresh human prostate cancers. Figure 23 demonstrates an aggressive growth morphology noted following the plating of cell strain DV-430. The latter was derived following radical retropubic prostatectomy from a gland diffusely involved by prostate cancer with a Gleason histotype of 7. Of interest, only a minority of the plated cells exhibited the aggressive pattern depicted. This suggests that the aggressive component of such cancers may represent but a small subset of the overall tumor burden.

Recently, Albini and associates have developed a modified Boyden chamber chemoinvasion assay, which permits the quantitation of tumor cell invasiveness [150]. In this assay, blind well chemotaxis (Boyden) chambers are employed. The barrier interface consists of a polyvinylpyrrolidone (PVP-free) polycarbonate filter (Nuclepore, CA) measuring 13 mm in diameter and possessing pores measuring 12 μm (Fig. 24). Previous studies have determined that optimal results were obtained by coating the filter interface with 50 μg of MATRIGEL (Table XVIII) and by extending the experimental duration to 5 hr in vitro (Table XIX). The methodologic details of the MATRIGEL bioinvasion assay can be briefly summarized.

Five-Hour Chemoinvasion Assay

The MATRIGEL-coated filters (50 μ/filter) are air-dried and placed in the Boyden chambers between the chemoattractant (lower well) and the cellular compartment (upper

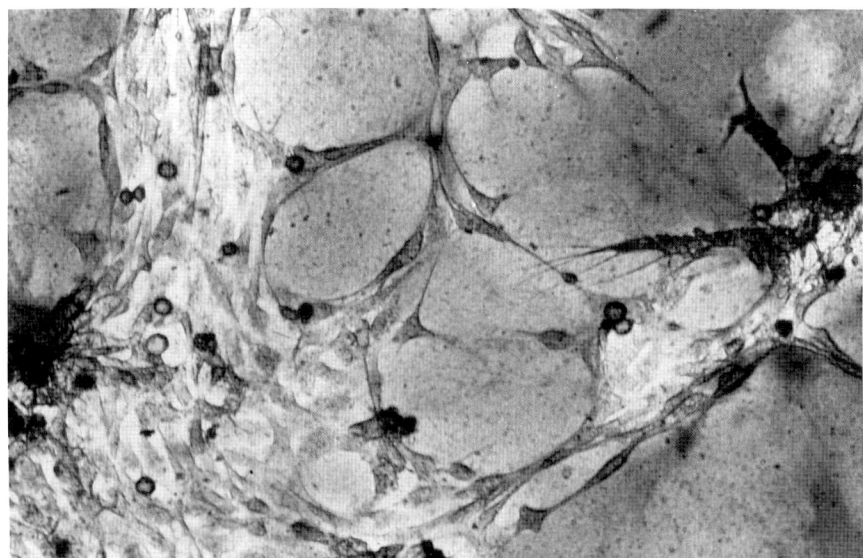

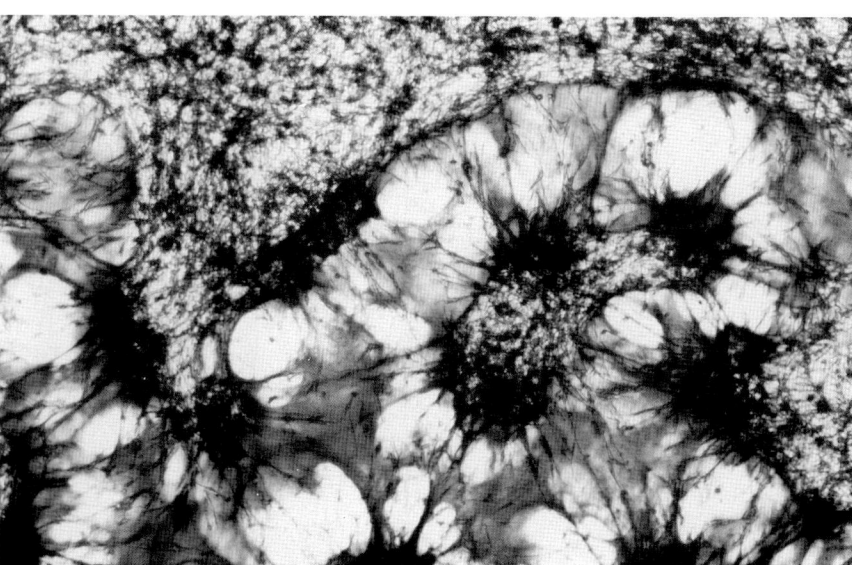

Fig. 22. Appearance of in vivo-derived metastatic variant line, DU-145LM. Note the prominent filopodial extensions demonstrated in this aggressive cell line. This feature readily distinguishes this tumor from its biologically indolent parental line of origin, DU-145 (see Fig. 19). ×200.

Fig. 23. Growth morphology on MATRIGEL exhibited by freshly derived prostate cancer designated DV-430. Note the appearance of an aggressive or "spreading" phenotype. ×200.

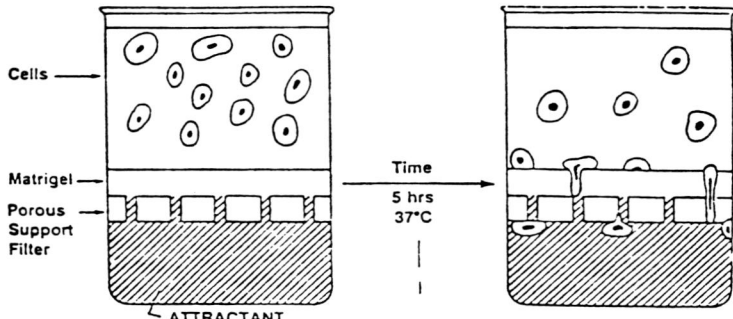

Fig. 24. Illustration of the modified Boyden chamber invasion bioassay. This system permits the use of a wide variety of chemoattractants and can be adapted to permit the sterile retrieval of invasive tumor cells for subsequent in vitro enrichment and in vivo propagation.

TABLE XVIII. Effect of Coating on the Invasion of Reconstituted Basement Membrane*

Cell line	Matrigel coating			
	100 µg	50 µg	25 µg	12.5 µg
NIH-3T3	0.0	0.46	19.0	30.0
DU-145 Par	0.0	4.0	12.0	36.0
PC-3P	2.0	11.0	25.0	45.0
DU-145 LM	0.0	34.0	37.0	>100

*Adapted from Albini et al. [150].

TABLE XIX. Time Dependence of the Invasion of Reconstituted Basement Membrane*

Cell line	1 hr	2 hr	3 hr	5 hr	6 hr
3T3	0	0	0	1	3
DU-145P	0	0	0	0	0
T24/3T3	0	0.5	1	30	75
PC3-P	0	0.8	0.4	16	43

*Adapted from Albini et al. [150].

well). With respect to the latter, $2-3 \times 10^5$ tumor cells are plated per chamber distributed as single cell suspensions in RPMI 1640 + 2% fetal bovine serum. The standard chemoattractant consists of either a dilute solution of MATRIGEL (1:50) or NIH3T3 conditioned medium. The chemoattractant is placed in the lower chamber prior to the insertion of the intervening filter. The assay chambers are incubated at 37°C at 5% CO_2 in a humidified environment for 5 hr. At the conclusion of this incubation interval, the cells on the upper surface of the filter are wiped off by gentle mechanical debridment. Those cells that have migrated to the lower surface of the filter constitute the invasive variance and are fixed in 70% methanol and stained with H&E. All assays are carried out in triplicate, and the migrated cells are counted in five microscopic fields per filter.

Table XX illustrates the close correlation noted between invasiveness as assessed

TABLE XX. Comparison of In Vitro Invasiveness and the In Vivo Metastasis of Primary and Continuous Prostate Cell Lines*

Cells	No. of cells invaded/field	No. animals developing visceral metastasis following intrasplenic injection
BPH	0.0	0/10
DU-145P	1.8	1/25
DU-145LM	31.2	9/10
PC-3P	19.6	28/30

*Adapted from Albini et al. [150].

in the 5-hr chemoinvasion assay and metastatic potential following intrasplenic tumor injection. As one would expect from nontransformed cells, BPH epithelial cells demonstrate neither invasiveness nor metastatic potential. Similarly, cell line DU-145 can be designated biologically indolent by both in vitro and in vivo criteria. This is in contrast to the behavior exhibited by its in vivo-derived metastatic variant, DU-145LM. This cell line exhibits significant invasiveness and metastatic capacity. Similar findings are noted for cell PC-3.

Thus, the 5-hr chemoinvasion assay nicely complements the intrasplenic metastasis assay with respect to providing biologically relevant information regarding the tumor systems under evaluation. Ongoing research activities are currently focused upon the viable recovery of invasive cells so as to permit in vitro enrichment of invasive variants. Similarly, the technique is being adapted to permit the evaluation of freshly derived human prostate cancers.

SUMMARY

Although in many respects prostate cancer remains a biological enigma, novel in vivo and in vitro approaches such as those described in this report may enhance our understanding of this intriguing disease. It seems imperative that such new techniques provide us with a clearer perception of those biological features that distinguish clinically aggressive from indolent prostate cancer. It is obvious that traditional approaches of proven value should not be abandoned. However, a critical need exists to employ new and promising strategies that may assist in the elucidation of those key features pertinent to the invasive and metastatic phenotype as it applies to human prostate cancer. Only with the acquisition of such biologically relevant insights can we hope to formulate new and effective treatment stratagems for this disease.

ACKNOWLEDGMENTS

These studies were supported in part by the Edwin and Lucy Kretschmer Fund of Northwestern University Medical School, the American Cancer Society, Illinois Division (grant 84-29), the Amoco Foundation, and Northwestern University Cancer Center. During the conduct of these studies the senior author (J.M.K) was a junior faculty clinical fellow of the American Cancer Society (grant 778-A). The excellent technical and scientific assistance of Livia Arvay, William Coukos, and Robert Pasciak is greatly appreciated.

REFERENCES

1. Silverberg E, Lubera JA: CA 36:9, 1986.
2. Catalona WJ: "Prostate Cancer." Orlando, FL: Grune and Stratton, Inc., 1984, p 58.
3. Whitmore WF, Jr: Cancer 32:1104, 1973.
4. Elkin M, Mueller HP: Cancer 7:1246, 1954.
5. Arnheim FK: J Urol 60:599, 1948.
6. Saitoh H, Hida M, Shimbo T, Nakamura K, Yamagata J, Saitoh T: Cancer 54:3078, 1984.
7. Harada M, Mostofi FK, Corle DK, Byar DP, Trump BF: Cancer Treat Rep 61:223, 1977.
8. Gaeta JF, Asirwatham JM, Miller G, Murphy GP: J Urol 123:689, 1980.
9. Mostofi FK: Semin Oncol 3:161, 1976.
10. Mobley TL, Frank IN: J Urol 99:321, 1968.
11. Gleason DF: In Tannenbaum M (Ed): "Urologic Pathology: The Prostate." Philadelphia: Lea and Febiger, 1977, pp 171–197.
12. Kramer SA, Spahr J, Brendler CB, Glenn JF, Paulson DF: J Urol 124:223, 1980.
13. Stamey TA: Monogr Urol 3:67, 1982.
14. Diamond DA, Berry SJ, Jewett HJ, Eggleston JC, Coffey DS: J Urol 128:729, 1982.
15. Epstein JI, Berry SJ, Eggleston JC: Cancer 54:1666, 1984.
16. Benson MC, McDougal DC, Coffey DS: The Prostate 5:27, 1984.
17. Zetterberg A, Esposti PL: Acta Cytol (Baltimore) 20:46, 1976.
18. Ronstrom L, Tribukait B, Esposti PL: The Prostate 2:79, 1981.
19. Fredericksen P, Thommesen P, Kjaer TB, Bichel P: Acta Pathol Microbiol Immunol Scand [A] 86:461, 1978.
20. Zetterberg A, Esposti PL: Scand J Urol Nephrol [Suppl] 55:53, 1980.
21. Muntzing J: Semin Urol 10 (Suppl 3):16, 1983.
22. Tannenbaum M, Tannenbaum S, Desanctis PN, Olsson CA: Urology 19:546, 1982.
23. Brendler CB, Isaacs JT, Follansbee AL, Walsh PC: J Urol 131:694, 1984.
24. Viola MV, Fromowitz F, Oravez S, Deb S, Finkel G, Lundy J, Hand T, Thor A, Schlom J: NEJM 314:133, 1986.
25. Fidler IJ, Kozlowski JM: Urology [Suppl] 23:29, 1984.
26. Isaacs JT, Coffey DS: Cancer Res 41:5070, 1981.
27. Noble RL: Cancer Res 37:1929, 1977.
28. Shain SA, McCullough B, Segaloff A: JNCI 55:177, 1975.
29. Pollard M: JNCI 51:1235, 1973.
30. Pollard M: The Prostate 1:201, 1980.
31. Reid LC, Shin S: In Fogh J, Giovanella C (eds): "Experimental and Clinical Research." New York: Academic Press, 1978, pp 315–351.
32. Reid LC, Sato G: J Cell Biol [Suppl] 70:287a, 1976.
33. Hoehn W, Schroeder FH, Riemann JF, Joebsis AC, Hermanek P: Prostate 1:95, 1980.
34. Ito YZ, Nakazato Y: J Urol 132:384, 1984.
35. Kaighn ME, Shankar N, Ohnuki Y, Lechner JF, Jones LW: Invest Urol 17:16, 1979.
36. Stone KR, Mickey DD, Wunderli H, Mickey GH, Paulsen DF: Int J Cancer 21:274, 1978.
37. Horoszewicz JS, Leong SS, Chu TM, Wajsman ZL, Friedman M, Papsidero L, Kim U, Chai LS, Kakati S, Arya SK, Sandberg AA: Prog Clin Biol Res 37:115, 1980.
38. Ware JL, Paulson DF, Mickey GH, Webb KS: J Urol 128:1064, 1982.
39. Ware JL, Lieberman AP, Webb KS, Vollmer RT: Exp Cell Biol 53:163, 1985.
40. Rygaard J, Povlsen CO: Acta Pathol Microbiol Immunol Scand [A] 77:758, 1969.
41. Shimosato Y, Kamoya T, Nagai K, Hirohashi S, Koide T, Hayashi H, Nomura T: JNCI 56:1251, 1976.
42. Sordat B, Fritsche R, Mach JP, Carrel S, Ozello L, Serotini JC: In Rygaard J, Povlsen CO (eds): "Proceedings of the First International Workshop on Nude Mice." Stuttgart: Gustave Fischer, Verlag, 1974, pp 269–277.
43. Povlsen CO, Fialkow TJ, Klein E, Klein G, Rygaard J, Weiner J: Int J Cancer 11:30, 1973.
44. Povlsen CO: Acta Pathol Microbiol Immunol Scand [A] 84:9, 1976.
45. Hanna N: In Liotta A, Hart IR (eds): "Tumor Invasion and Metastasis." The Hague: Martinus Nijoff Publishing Co., 1982, pp 43–55.
46. Fogh J, Fogh JM, Orfeo T: JNCI 59:221, 1977.

47. Povlsen CO, Jacbosen EK: Cancer Res 35:2790, 1975.
48. Sharkey FE, Fogh JM, Hajdu SI, Fitzgerald PJ, Fogh J: In Fogh J, Giovanella BC (eds): "The Nude Mouse in Clinical Research." New York: Academic Press, Inc., 1978, pp 187–214.
49. Bellet RE, Danna V, Mastrangelo MJ Berd D: JNCI 63:1185, 1979.
50. Giovanella BC, Stehlin JS, Williams LJ, Jr, Lee S, Shepard R: Cancer 42:2269, 1978.
51. Ovajera AA, Houchens DP, Barker AD: Ann Clin Lab Sci 8:50, 1978.
52. Giovanella BC, Stehlin JS, Williams LJ Jr: JNCI 52:921, 1974.
53. Reid LC, Shin SI: In Fogh J, Giovanella BC (eds): "The Nude Mouse in Experimental and Clinical Research." New York: Academic Press, 1978, p 313.
54. Sharkey FE, Fogh J.: Int J Cancer 24:733, 1979.
55. Sordat B., Fritsche R, Mach JP., Carrel S, Ozzello L, Cerotini JC: In Rygaard J, Povlsen CO (eds): "Proceedings of the First International Workshop on Nude Mice." Stuttgart: Gustave Fischer Verlag, 1974, pp 269–277.
56. Giovanella BC, Stehlin J, Williams LJ Jr: JNCI 52:921, 1974.
57. Giovanella BC, Yim SO, Morgan AC, Stehlin JS, Williams LJ: JNCI 50:1051, 1973.
58. Hanna N, Fidler IJ: Cancer Res 41:438, 1981.
59. Kyriazis AP, Kyriazis AA, McCombs WB III, Kereikis JA: Cancer Res 41:3995, 1981.
60. Hanna N: In Jamisen GA (ed): "Interaction of Platelets and Tumor Cells." New York: Alan R. Liss, Inc., 1982, pp 177–189.
61. Hanna N, Fidler I.J: Cancer Res 41:438, 1981.
62. Kozlowski JM, Fidler IJ, Campbell D, Xu Z, Kaighn ME, Hart IR: Cancer Res 44:3522, 1984.
63. Kozlowski JM, Hart IR, Fidler IJ, Hanna N: JNCI 72:913, 1984.
64. Hanna N, Davis TW, Fidler IJ: Int J Cancer 30:371, 1982.
65. Johnson WJ, Balish E: J Reticuloendothelial Soc 28:55, 1980.
66. Hanna N: Int J Cancer 26:675, 1980.
67. Herberman RB, Ninn ME, Laurin DH: Int J Cancer 16:216, 1975.
68. Fidler IJ, Kozlowski JM: Urology [Suppl] 23:29, 1984.
69. Kyriazis AP, Dipersio L, Michael G, Pesce AJ: Int J Cancer 23:402, 1979.
70. Hanna N: Int J Cancer 26:675, 1980.
71. Hanna N, Davis TW, Fidler IJ: Int J Cancer 30:371, 1982.
72. Urdal EL, Kawase I, Henney CS: Cancer Metastasis Rev 1:65, 1982.
73. Sharkey FE, Fogh J: Int J Cancer 24:733, 1979.
74. Morrissey LW, Sidky YA, Auerbach R: Cancer Res 40:2197, 1980.,
75. Auerbach R, Auerbach W: Science 215:127, 1982.
76. Auerbach R, Morrissey LW, Sidky YA: Cancer Res 38:1739, 1978.
77. Auerbach R, Morrissey LW, Sidky YA: Nature 274:697, 1978.
78. Kyriazis AA, Kyriazis AP: Cancer Res 40:4509, 1980.
79. DeVore DP, Houches DP, Overjera AA, Dill GS, Hutson TB: Exp Cell Biol 48:367, 1980.
80. Tahashi S, Konishi Y, Nakatoni K, Inui S, Kojima K, Shiratori T: JNCI 60:925, 1978.
81. Witte PL, Ber R: JNCI 70:575, 1983.
82. Fidler IJ: JNCI 45:773, 1970.
83. Reid LCM, Sato G: J Cell Biol 70:287, 1976.
84. Reid LCM: Proc Natl Acad Sci USA 78:1171, 1981.
85. Giavazzi IR, Campbell DE, Jessup JM, Cleary K, Fidler IJ: Cancer Res 46:1928, 1986.
86. Naito S, Von Eschenbach AC, Giavazzi IR, Fidler IJ: Cancer Res 46:4109, 1986.
87. Korsaro CM, Pearson ML: Somatic Cell Mol Genet 7:603, 1981.
88. Kozlowski JM, Grayhack JT: In Gillenwater JY, Grayhack JT, Howards SS, Duckett JW (eds): "Adult and Pediatric Urology." Chicago: Year Book Medical Publishers, Inc., 1987, pp 1126–1219.
89. Catalona WJ: "Prostate Cancer." pp 145–171.
90. Byar DP: Bull NY Acad Med 48:751, 1972.
91. Doe RP, Blackard CE: Cancer 26:249, 1940.
92. Rudiger HW, Haenisch S, Metzler M, Oesch S, Glatt HR: Nature 281:392, 1979.
93. Buenaventura SK, Jacobson-Kram D, Dearfield KL, Williams JR: Cancer Res 44:3851, 1984.
94. Mehnert K, Speit G, Vogel W: Cancer Res 45:3626, 1985.
95. Rao PN, Engelberg J: Exp Cell Res 48:71, 1967.

96. Sawada M, Ishidate M Jr: Mutat Res 57:175, 1978.
97. Haukaas SA, Kalland T: The Prostate 3:149, 1982.
98. Luster MI, Boorman GA, Dean JH, Luebke RW, Lawson LD: J Reticuloendothelial Soc 28:561, 1980.
99. Ablin RJ, Bruns GR, Guinan P, Bush IM: J Immunol 113:705, 1974.
100. Haukaas SA, Kalland T: J Urol 128:862, 1982.
101. Boorman GA, Luster MI, Dean JH, Wilson RE: J Reticulo (endothelial Soc 28:547, 1980.
102. Dean JH, Luster MI, Boorman GA, Luebke RW, Lauer LD: J Reticulo (endothelial Soc 28:571, 1980.
103. Kalland T: In Herberman RB (ed): "NK Cells and Other Natural Effector Cells." New York: Academic Press, Inc., 1982, pp 1437–1444.
104. Haukaas S, Kalland T: In Herberman RB (ed): (ed): "NK Cells and Other Natural Effector Cells." New York: Academic Press, Inc., 1982, pp 1317–1321.
105. Kozlowski JM, Fidler IJ, Campbell D, Xu Z, Kaighn ME, Hart IR: Cancer Res 44:3522, 1984.
106. Grayhack JT, Kozlowski JM: Urol Clin North Am 7:639, 1980.
107. Kiessling RE, Klein E, Wigtzell H: Eur J Immunol 5:112, 1975.
108. Shiku H, Bean MA, Old LG, Oettegen HG: JNCI 54:415, 1975.
109. Hanna N, Schneider M: J Immunol 130:974, 1983.
110. Chaproniere DM, McKeehan WL: Cancer Res 46:819, 1986.
111. Grayhack JT, Kozlowski JM: In Gillenwater JY, Grayhack JT, Howards SS, Duckett JW (eds): "Adult and Pediatric Urology." Chicago: Year Book Medical Publishers, Inc., 1987, pp 1062–1125.
112. Cunha GR: In Kimball SA, Buhl AE, Carter DB (ed): "New Approaches to the Study of Benign Prostatic Hyperplasia." New York: Alan R Liss, Inc., 1984, pp 81–102.
113. Cooke DB, Litton GK: The Prostate 7:209, 1985.
114. Kaighn ME: In Fischer G, Wieser RJ (ed): "Hormonally Defined Media: A Tool in Cell Biology." Heidelberg: Springer-Verlag, 1983, pp 418–429.
115. McKeehan WL, Adams PS, Rosser MP: Cancer Res 44:1998, 1984.
116. Chaproniere DM, McKeehan WL: Cancer Res 46:819, 1986.
117. Peehl DM, Stamey TA: In Vitro 20:981, 1984.
118. Liotta LA: In Devita VT Jr, Hellman S, Rosenberg SA (eds): "Important Advances in Oncology 1985." Philadephia: J.B. Lippincott Co., pp 28–41.
119. Liotta LA: Cancer Res 46:1, 1986.
120. Liotta LA, Rao CN, Barsky SH: Lab Invest 49:636, 1983.
121. Nakajima M, Irimura T, Diferrante N, Nicolson GL: J Biol Chem 259:2283, 1984.
122. Liotta LA, Mandler R, Murano G, Katz DA, Gordon RK, Chiang PK, Schiffmann E: Proc Natl Acad Sci USA 83:3302, 1986.
123. Anderson NG, Anderson NL: Anal Biochem 85:331, 1978.
124. Anderson NL, Anderson NG: Anal Biochem 85:341, 1978.
125. O'Farrell PH: J Biol Chem 250:4007, 1975.
126. Tollaksen SL, Anderson NL, Anderson NG: In "Operation of the ISO-DALT SYSTEM," 7th Ed. Argonne, IL: Argonne National Laboratory, Publication #ANL-BIM-84-1, 1984.
127. Bradford M: Anal Biochem 72:248, 1976.
128. Guevara J Jr, Johnston DA, Ramagali LS, Martin BA, Capetillo S, Rodriguez LV: Electrophoresis 3:197, 1982.
129. Harrison HH: Clin Chem 29:1566, 1983.
130. Harrison HH: Clin Chem 30:1981, 1984.
131. Poste G, Fidler IJ: Nature 283:139, 1980.
132. Fidler IJ: Cancer Res 38:2651, 1978.
133. Fidler IJ: Nature 242:148, 1973.
134. Fidler IJ, Hart IR: Science 217:998, 1982.
135. Nicolson GL: Cancer Metastasis Rev 3:25, 1984.
136. Kleinman HK: In Liotta LA, Hart IR (eds): "Tumor Invasion and Metastasis." Boston: Martinus Nijhoff Publishers, 1982, pp 291–308.
137. Kleinman HK, Klebe RJ, Martin GR: J Cell Biol 88:473, 1981.
138. Liotta LA, Thorgeirsson UP, Garbis AS: Cancer Metastasis Rev 1:277, 1982.

139. Murray JC, Liotta LA, Terranova VP: In Liotta LA, Hart IR (eds): "Tumor Invasion and Metastasis." Boston: Martinus Nijohoff Publishers, 1982, pp 310–318.
140. Liotta LA: Cancer Res 46:1, 1986.
141. Liotta LA, Mandler R, Murano G, Katz DA, Gordon RK, Ching PK, Schiffmann E: Proc Natl Acad Sci USA 83:3302, 1986.
142. Terranova VP, Liotta LA, Russo RG, Martin GR: Cancer Res 42:2265, 1982.
143. Varani J, Lovett EJ, McCoy JP, Shibata AS, Maddox D, Goldstein I, Wicha M: Am J Pathol 111:27, 1983.
144. Turpeenniemi-Huganen T, Thorgeirsson UP, Hart IR, Grant SS, Liotta LA: JNCI 74:99, 1985.
145. Liotta LA, Rao CN, Barsky SH: Lab Invest 49:636, 1983.
146. Rao CN, Barsky SH, Terranova VP, Liotta LA: Biochem Biophys Res Commun 111:804, 1983.
147. Terranova VP, Rao CN, Kalebic T, Margulies IMK, Liotta LA: Proc Natl Acad Sci USA 80:444, 1983.
148. Liotta LA, Horan Hand P, Rao CN, Bryant G, Barsky SH, Schlom J: Exp Cell Res 156:117, 1985.
149. Terranova VP, Hujanen ES, Loeb DM, Martin GR, Valentin T, Thornburg L, Glushkov J: Proc Natl Acad Sci USA 83:465, 1985.
150. Albini A, Iwamoto Y, Kleinman HK, Martin GR, Aaronson SA, Kozlowski JM, McEwan RN: Cancer Res 47:3239, 1987.
151. Kleinman HK, McGarvey ML, Liotta LA, Robey PG, Tryggvason K, Martin GR: Biochemistry 21:6188, 1982.
152. Hadley MA, Byers SW, Suarez-Quian CA, Kleinman HK, Dym M: J Cell Biol 101:1511, 1985.
153. Turksen K, Kleinman HK, Kalnins VI: J Cell Biol 101:260a, 1985.

Lymphatic Metastasis

Ian Carr and Norman Pettigrew

Department of Pathology, University of Manitoba (I.C., N.P.) and St. Boniface General Hospital (I.C.), Winnipeg, Manitoba, Canada

This essay discusses some aspects of lymphatic metastasis with a morbid anatomic bias. "The knowledge of morbid structure does not certainly lead to the knowledge of morbid actions, although the one is the effect of the other; yet surely it lays the most solid foundations for prosecuting such inquiries with success." So said Matthew Baillie in 1793 [1]. We touch upon three areas: 1) the lymph node metastasis in human cancer; we emphasize accepted lore, which may be disproved but not ignored; 2) experiments by one author (I.C.) over the years 1971–85 on experimental lymphatic metastasis; 3) our recent investigation into invasion and lymphatic penetration in human colorectal cancer.

Key words: lymphatic metastasis, metastasis, invasion, colorectal cancer

1. The process of lymphatic metastasis results in metastatic deposits in lymph nodes. These may be rather complex. For instance, single cells may permeate sinuses, and then emigrate, or clusters of cells may proliferate and destroy the sinusoid wall. There may be characteristic reactions; these may be angiogenic or fibrogenic, or may involve the gamut of the immune response, whether stimulation of B cell or T cell, or depletion thereof. There may be an inflammatory, histiocytic, or granulomatous response. The reactions may be trivial or massive. The stromal end result often resembles that in the primary. The normal lymphaticovenous connections in the node may open up when lymphatics are blocked by metastasis. The whole process is much more than an accumulation of neoplastic cells in the lymph node. In the human, the nodal metastasis may be a signal, rather than an important part of the process; the nature of any reaction may be of prognostic significance.

2. Over the past 15 years we have constructed models of lymphatic metastasis [2]. Relatively large numbers of tumour cells are injected into the footpad, metastasize consistently to the popliteal lymph node, produce a palpable deposit in 5–7 days, and then spread further to the paraaortic nodes and lungs. The process is reproducible, and the sequential appearance of metastasis indicates that it is mechanism not just signal. This model can be used for studies on immunotherapy and on lymphangiochemotherapy—and might lead to selective regional treatment [3].

In such models tumour cells may enter peripheral lymphatics and leave the lymph

Received April 30, 1987.

© 1988 Alan R. Liss, Inc.

node sinusoids by a variety of mechanisms including active crawling, or diapedesis, the movement of clusters of cells, and the induction of necrosis of the lymphatic endothelium. The latter seemed to be rather artificial because the system used was allogeneic.

An extension of the investigation to the popliteal lymph node in such models shows that if tumour cells adhere readily to a surface in vitro, they move actively through the endothelium in vivo; tumour cells which do not so adhere mature in the sinusoid into large spheroids and penetrate the endothelium by inducing massive destruction [4]. These differences are comparative rather than absolute. In summary—in experimental models tumour cells penetrate lymphatic vessels in at least two ways—diapedesis and destruction.

3. The proper study of mankind is not necessarily the mouse. There are not many choices of human model in which to study lymphatic metastasis; the prerequisite is to have sufficient specimens in which primary and secondary can be examined. Carcinoma of the colon is a useful model and is indeed a classical example of lymphatic metastasis. We have now examined an unselected series of 46 cases of human colorectal cancer, looking for evidence as to the mechanism of invasion and penetration of the lymphatic vessels and of selection in metastasis.

In these cases, we have selected the areas of invasion for careful comparative light and electron examination. The mature carcinoma cells on the luminal aspect of the tumour are differentiated, but at the edge of the tumour undifferentiated cells show reversal of polarity; microvilli of the type usually found on the luminal surface may directly contact such evidently stromal structures as collagen. Reversed polarity of cells infers topographically abnormal synthesis of skeletal and other problems. There may be a relation between the presence of lysosomal dense granules and the presence of degenerative changes in muscle cells. Some of these cells show large cytoplasmic flaps such as are seen in locomoting cells; examination of casual serial sections suggested that these might be single cells.

In tissue culture, small numbers of tumour cells survived, and moved. Distinct single cell movement was apparent, and it seemed clear that these were surviving neoplastic cells [5].

The careful examination of serially and meticulously sectioned large plastic sections of five tumours, cut in such a manner that all the sections were mounted one way up, singly on a slide, found very few examples where it was certain that single cells were detached, if detachment is defined as separation by over 10 μ. There were occasional clusters detached from the main glands. But the vast majority of the apparently detached cells or clusters were in fact parts of long tubules. This is akin to the demonstration of group (or cluster) movement in vitro, and suggests that the tips of neoplastic glands burrow.

A careful search was made in many thick sections for areas where cancer cells were penetrating lymphatics. Penetration of a vessel by single cells after the pattern described in an animal model was not identified. In many specimens large lymphatics were identified surrounded by inflammatory cells, and with disruption of the wall. Clumps of ten or more tumour cells were identified in the gap or within the lumen. Considered in three dimensions such clumps must contain dozens or hundreds of cells. Similar clumps were to be seen in the lymphatic trunks away from, i.e., proximal to the lesion. The disruption of the lymphatic wall was often extensive.

So the evidence for single cell migration is dubious. The lymphatic vessels at the edge of these tumours showed no single cell migration—no diapedesis, but did show a repetition of the finding in the allogeneic Walker rat carcinoma—segmental necrosis of the endothelium of the lymphatic vessels in areas of massive perilymphangitis. It is difficult to see why colorectal cancer cells need to destroy basement membrane—the lymphatics are disrupted and open—and there is little basement membrane anyway. It seems that tumor cells are exported in bulk, and almost by accident, in inflamed areas.

It is clear that there is selection in metastasis, but this is not evident from EM examination. Two further techniques were therefore used. Morphometric examination of electron micrographs of carefully localized, reprocessed, paraffin-embedded material did not show a consistent difference between primary and secondary. But in some instances a morphometrically distinct population was identified at the invasive edge, in transit, and in early nodal metastasis.

DNA flow cytometry analysis was carried out on 11 cases; the material was obtained from paraffin blocks. When tumour was sampled at the invasive edge and at the centre there was no difference in ploidy. In all but one case a lymph node metastasis was also examined. Four of the 11 tumours showed evidence of DNA aneuploidy. Where regional samples were available no difference was noted between the superficial and invasive edges of the tumour. In this small series there was no evidence of DNA aneuploidy in the lymph node deposits.

It may, in fact, be true that there is no difference in DNA ploidy between the superficial and invasive edges of colonic adenocarcinoma. However, it may be that the technique used, i.e., flow cytometry, was too insensitive to detect a small population of cells showing ploidy variation. Image video densitometry or a single nucleus spectrophotometer analysis may be required to detect such a difference. However, the lack of DNA aneuploidy in the lymph node metastases would suggest that certainly no permanent deviation in ploidy is required to accomplish successful metastasis. A significant deviation in DNA ploidy might militate against successful metastasis.

Colorectal cancer is composed of cells that live in clusters, evoke florid inflammatory reactions, and penetrate at least the lymphatics, if not the veins, by mechanisms that involve destruction of the vascular wall. It is appropriate to consider whether cancer is different from any other form of pathologic reaction or is likely to follow the general principles of pathology. The parallel to consider is regeneration, which probably occurs in colonic mucosa, by centrifugal migration of columnar crypt cells without detachment from the sheet.

How then do neoplastic cells invade and penetrate lymphatic vessels in human colorectal carcinoma? A present hypothesis might include the following points: 1) in human colon cancer long columns of cells invade; their morphology suggests active motility at the tip; 2) the process of invasion involves inflammation and fibrosis; 3) invasion of lymphatics involves destruction of lymphatic walls and invasion by clusters of cells. In such a scenario selection is likely to occur not at the rather random level of the necrotic area of lymphatic endothelium but proximally in the lymph node.

SUMMARY

This essay has reviewed the traditional information on metastasis in the human lymph node, and emphasized its complexity. It has reviewed the penetration of lymphatic vessels and lymph node sinusoids in experimental models and suggested twin mechanisms of diapedesis and destruction. And it has suggested the significance of movements of aggregates of cells in invasion in human colorectal cancer, and of segmental endothelial necrosis in metastasis. It is likely that invasion in many other human cancers occurs in a manner different in detail, but similar in principle.

ACKNOWLEDGMENTS

This work has been supported by the National Cancer Institute of Canada, St. Boniface General Hospital Research Foundation, and the Thorlakson Foundation. We acknowledge extensive collaboration with Drs. E. Rector and P. Watson.

REFERENCES

1. Baillie M: "The Morbid Anatomy of Some of the Most Important Parts of the Human Body. London: Johnson & Nicol, 1793.
2. Carr I: Cancer Metastasis Rev 1:307–317, 1983.
3. Carr J, Dreher B, Carr I: Clin Exp Metastasis 1:29–38, 1983.
4. Carr I, Levy M, Orr K, Bruni J: Clin Exp Metastasis 3:125–139, 1985.
5. Carr I, Levy M, Watson P: Clin Exp Metastasis 4:129–139, 1986.

Tumor Cell Surface Lectins and Metastasis

Avraham Raz and Reuben Lotan

Department of Cell Biology, The Weizmann Institute of Science, Rehovot 76100, Israel (A.R.) and Department of Tumor Biology, University of Texas M.D. Anderson Hospital and Tumor Institute, Houston, Texas 77030 (R.L.)

A wide variety of adhesive molecules located on the surface of metastasizing cells have been identified, including laminin, collagens, fibronectin, glycosaminoglycans, and the complementary receptors for them. These adhesive molecules have been shown to influence the spread of various metastatic cells (16) but it is beyond the scope of this article to review them all. Here we summarize progress in the functional and molecular identification of a unique class of cell surface molecules that bind specific carbohydrate sequences (lectins) and are involved in the cognitive interactions among tumor cells and between tumor and host cells.

Key words: endogenous lectins, metastasis

THE METASTATIC CASCADE

Metastasis is defined as the transfer of a neoplastic disease from one organ or part to another, not directly connected with it. Indeed, this ability to invade and metastasize is the only characteristic that is unique to malignant neoplasms and absent in benign tumors. Metastasis is common after surgical removal of the primary tumor and it is the main cause of cancer patient death. Understanding the process of metastasis is of the utmost importance, as it may lead to the development of effective treatment.

Although metastasis is poorly understood, results from experimental animal models and clinical studies indicate that it involves linked, sequential steps which are determined by unique properties of metastatic progenitor cells as well as by host-tumor cell interactions. The process is initiated by the detachment of tumor cells from the primary growth and is followed by their invasion of surrounding tissues and blood vessels. Once in the blood circulation, the tumor cells can disseminate to distant organs where they can arrest, extravasate, and proliferate to form new tumor colonies [for reviews see 7–9]. Because successful metastasis requires that the cells survive many destructive events, and because different properties may be essential at different steps of the process, the question arises whether all the cells within a primary tumor have an equal chance of forming metastases, or whether only specialized cells are capable of forming new tumor foci.

Received April 21, 1987.

© 1988 Alan R. Liss, Inc.

The possibility that cells having different metastatic potential populate the primary tumor was first demonstrated by Koch [10], who selected a highly metastatic subline from an Ehrlich carcinoma. More direct evidence that malignant neoplasms contain cell variants with differing metastatic capabilities was obtained by Fidler and Kripke [11], who performed cell cloning and fluctuation tests with a B16 melanoma parent line and numerous clones derived from it. The metastatic potential of the clones, as seen from the development of pulmonary colonies after inoculation into syngeneic mice, differed from that of the parent line. Furthermore, there was a considerable variation among the clones in the number and site of metastases. A similar heterogeneity in the metastatic potential of cells in the primary tumor has since been demonstrated with a large array of cell types [12,13].

It is generally accepted that the metastatic ability of tumor cells is determined by unique cell properties such as growth rate, cell cycle, cell size, cell surface glycoconjugates, antigenicity, cell surface enzymes, deformability, motility, and the ability to produce angiogenesis factors [1–14]. The relative contribution of each of the above properties is not clear.

The detachment of tumor cells from the primary growth site is a necessary preliminary step for metastasis. This release from the primary tumor mass has been attributed, at least in part, to reduced cell cohesiveness [15–17]. The ability of certain tumors to release hydrolytic enzymes has promoted the idea that the cell surface may be modified, through the action of the secreted enzymes, in a way that facilitates detachment and invasion [18–21].

The penetration of single cells, or small cell clumps, into the circulation may lead to their transport to distant sites. The arrest of some of the cells in organs is influenced greatly by the formation of tumor emboli resulting from interaction of the cells with other tumor cells (homotypic aggregation), and with circulating host cells (heterotypic aggregation) such as platelets and lymphocytes [22–25]. The circulating tumor emboli may be eliminated by host defenses. However, those which survive may be nonspecifically arrested in capillaries, nonspecifically, due to entrapment of large or poorly deformable cell emboli, or they may pass the first capillary bed encountered and arrest specifically [26–28]. The notion of specific arrest evolved from clinical observations in man and in a variety of animal tumor systems which displayed a nonrandom pattern of metastasis [28–31], and from the discovery of tumor cell variants exhibiting preferential implantation in specific organs [1–13]. Once in the capillary bed of the target organ, the metastasizing tumor cells face the endothelial basement membranes, which are resilient structures that present a mechanical barrier to their extravasation. Moreover, it is generally accepted that the extravasation process is similar to cell invasion in the circulation.

THE METASTATIC PHENOTYPE AND CELLULAR INTERACTIONS

Very few, if any, in vitro properties of tumor cells can be correlated with their in vivo metastatic behavior. Elucidation of the tumor properties which are relevant to metastasis was contingent on the development of animal model systems of tumor cells which exhibit high-, low-, or no metastatic potential [1–13,32,33]. Such systems were developed by selection in vivo in syngeneic hosts for enhanced metastasis to a particular organ after intravenous injection of suspended single tumor cells. The most well-characterized system, that of the B16 melanoma, was established by Fidler [32] and has been employed in numerous laboratories. The results of these studies have indicated that intercellular interactions play a considerable role in metastasis. Thus, it was shown that B16 melanoma cell clumps produce more lung metastases after i.v. injection than single cells [34]. Further studies using B16 melanoma variants exhibiting different metastatic potential demonstrated a correlation between the tendency of cells to undergo homotypic and heterotypic aggregation in vitro and their metastatic potential in vivo [32,34–39]. Indirect indications on the role of cell surface components in metastasis have come from studies that have shown that selection for plant lectin resistance [40–42] or isolation of detachment variants [43] of metastatic cells resulted in cells with altered metastatic properties. A more direct demonstration of the importance of cell surface components on B16 melanoma cells in metastasis was achieved by fusing membrane vesicles shed by highly metastatic lung colonizing cells (B16-F10) into less metastatic cells (B16-F1). The modified B16-F1 cells exhibited higher metastatic potential than the unmodified controls after i.v. injection [44]. The nature of the cell membrane molecules which mediate the cell-cell interactions described above is beginning to be elucidated, primarily through the use of antibodies that recognize specific cell surface antigens and affect cellular adhesion and metastasis [45–50].

The involvement of carbohydrate residues in mediation of adhesion between cells was also indicated in reports on the ability of simple sugars, glycopeptides, and glycoproteins to inhibit the aggregation of certain types of cells [51–55]. One possible explanation for these findings is that sugar-binding proteins are present on the surface of the vertebrate cells and that they bind to multivalent glycoproteins which serve as "bridges" between adjacent cells. This idea was supported by an increasing number of reports on the presence of lectins, sugar-binding proteins, on various vertebrate cells and tissues [for reviews see 56–60].

Since intercellular interactions play a key role in various steps of the metastatic process and considering the possibility that endogenous lectins may participate in such interactions, we investigated the presence of lectins on a variety of neoplastic cells.

CHARACTERIZATION OF ENDOGENOUS TUMOR CELL LECTINS

The first indication of tumor cell surface lectin involvement in cell-cell interaction came from the observation that fetuin and its desialylated derivatives bind to the surface of tumor cells and mediate their homotypic aggregation in vitro [61,62]. Fetuin consists of a single polypeptide chain, to which three complex heteropolysaccharide side chains made up of sialic acid, galactose, N-acetyl-D-glucosamine and mannose are attached through asparagine residues, and as well as 3 O-glycosidically linked units composed of sialic acid, galactose, and N-acetyl-D-galactosamine [63,64]. It is conceivable that cell surface lectins recognize and bind galactosyl residues on different side chains of the same fetuin molecule. Thus, the glycoprotein could serve as a cross-linking bridge between adjacent cells and, subsequently, lead to formation of multicell aggregates. The binding of fluorescent derivatives of the above glycoproteins was greatly reduced by lactose (4-0-β-D-galactopyranosyl-D-glucose) [61].

These results suggested the presence of lactose-binding cell surface components on the tumor cells. Indeed, crude extracts of the various malignant cells exhibited lectinlike activities expressed as the ability to agglutinate trypsinized, glutaraldehyde-fixed rabbit erythrocytes. This activity was abolished by treatment with proteolytic enzymes, indicating that the agglutinins are proteins. Of the various sugars tested for their ability to inhibit hemagglutination by tumor cell extracts, lactose was found to be the most potent inhibitor. D-Galactose, D-galactosamine were poor inhibitors, whereas D-mannose, N-acetyl-D-glucosamine and L-fucose were inactive. Our results thus demonstrated the presence of galactoside-specific lectins in tumor cells of different origin and histopathologic type [61,62], supporting the previous demonstration of the presence of β-galactoside specific lectin in mouse neuroblastoma [65]. In the past several years, endogenous tumor cells were found in a wide variety of epithelial and mesenchymal tumors of rodent and human origin: melanomas [61,66], sarcomas [61, 67–70], carcinomas [61, 68–72], testicular and ovarian teratomas [68,70,73,74], T and B lymphoblastoid cells [75,76], Hodgkin's disease cells [77], leukemias [76,78], and hepatomas [70,79]. The sugar specificities varied to include galactoside sequences, mannose, mannan, fucose, fucoidin, heparin, and heparan-sulfate. Various experimental approaches were utilized to identify the tumor cell lectin; tests included hemagglutinating activity, affinity chromatography purification on immobilized sugar ligands or glycoproteins, binding of fluoresceinated neoglycoproteins, and immunological techniques using antilectin antibodies. The molecular weights of the lectins extracted from the various tumors were also variable and ranged between Mr 13,000 and Mr 140,000, and in many cases a tumor cell type was found to express more than one lectin species.

ON THE ROLE OF TUMOR CELL SURFACE LECTINS IN METASTASIS

In the first part of this review we summarized the data showing that intercellular recognition and adhesion among circulating tumor cells and host cells, including platelets, lymphocytes, and endothelial cells, is one of the major driving forces in the formation of tumor emboli. From experimental systems it has become evident that the presence of tumor emboli in the circulation is casually related with metastasis [34,39,80,81]. Pathological observations in humans have revealed that tumor emboli reaching the lungs in the systemic venous blood may have diameters of up to 200 μu and may consist of hundreds of cells [27]. And it was concluded that "almost all metastatic growths in the lungs arise from malignant emboli carried in the circulation" [27]. Having previously found gal-specific lectins in extracts of various tumor cells, we proposed that lectin-mediated intercellular adhesion is responsible for homotypic and heterotypic cell aggregation and embolization [39,61,62]. If indeed gal-specific tumor cell lectins functioned as recognition and adhesion molecules, they had to be cell-surface constituents exposed to the extracellular milieu. The first identification of tumor cell surface carbohydrate-binding proteins came from studies demonstrating binding of FITC-labeled fetuin and asialofetuin to B16-F1 melanoma cells [61]. Subsequently, it was shown that Lewis lung carcinoma and L1210 cells bind to and internalize neoglycoproteins [71,78,82]. Further to that, we produced monoclonal antibodies (mAb) directed against galactose-specific lectins extracted from B16-F1 melanoma cells [83]. The 5D7-mAb antilectin antibody cross-reacted with the Mr 14,000 and Mr 34,000 affinity purified gal-specific tumor lectins [84] and was used for cellular localization and distribution of the lectins in tumor cells.

These endogenous lectins were localized, by indirect immunofluorescence staining, on the surface of different viable cultured tumor cells (murine melanoma and fibrosarcoma, and human melanoma, carcinoma, and neuroblastoma) and, after fixation and permeabilization, in the cytoplasm [83]. The surface distribution was in the form of microclusters, suggesting that the membrane-associated lectin molecules were laterally mobile and subject to rearrangement by exogenous ligands (mAb or glycoproteins). Recently, a similar lectin localization in two cellular compartments (membrane and intracellular) was found in 3T3 fibroblasts, by utilizing the Mr 35,000 antilectin antibodies [85]. The presence of both the Mr 14,500 and Mr 34,000 lectins on the surface of various tumor and transformed cells was demonstrated also by labeling the proteins exposed on the surface of viable cells with iodine-125 by lactoperoxidase-catalyzed iodination, followed by cell soulobolization and immunoprecipitation with polyclonal antilectin antibodies prepared in rabbits against affinity purified lectins [86]. The presence of other sugar-binding proteins at the cell surface of tumor cells was also demonstrated by other techniques, e.g., rosetting with red blood cells [73,87], binding of ^{125}I-asialoglycoprotein [79], binding of glycoprotein-containing micelles [75], and affinity purification of lectins extracted from isolated membranes of human malignant melanoma [66].

These results and the availability of specific antilectin antibodies and of cell lines and clones from experimental mouse tumor systems which exhibit different metastatic potentials (B16 and K-1735 melanomas and UV-2237 fibrosarcoma) enabled us to directly probe the question of the possible relation between lectin cell surface expression and the metastatic capacity. The membrane expression of the cell surface endogenous galactoside-specific lectin was identified and quantitated by indirect immunofluorescent staining of viable cells with 5D7 antilectin mAb, followed by analysis in a fluorescence-activated cell sorter [84]. It was found that among related tumor cells of these three tumor systems, cells exhibiting a higher lung-colonizing potential were more intensely labeled and there was a higher percentage of positively labeled cells in the samples than in their corresponding, less metastatic cell counterparts [84]. These results were further verified when we analyzed a recently developed BALB/c mouse angiosarcoma system consisting of cells at four different stages of tumor progression: untransformed immortalized, anchorage-independent nontumorigenic, transformed tumorigenic, and metastatic [33]. We studied the relationship between endogenous lectin expression and the acquisition of a metastatic phenotype in these stages and found a gradual increase in the total cellular and cell surface lectins with increasing malignancy. Lectin expression on the cell surface increased most considerably, however, when the tumorigenic cells acquired metastatic properties.

A different approach to studying the involvement of tumor cell lectins in metastasis was to analyze the effect of the 5D7 antilectin mAb on cell adhesiveness in vitro and on organ colonization in vivo. It was found that both the asialofetuin-induced aggregation and the spontaneous adhesion of B16 melanoma and UV-2237 fibrosarcoma cells to the substratum could be inhibited by asialofetuin glycopeptides and that these cellular interactions were also inhibited by the 5D7 antilectin mAb [88]. This strongly supported the hypothesis that cell surface lectins mediate at least part of the cell-to-cell and cell-to-substratum adhesion by binding with galactose-containing glycoconjugates. That endogenous lectins might be involved in cellular adhesion was already proposed several years before [89]. Endogenous hepatic lectin was found to mediate the adhesion of hepatocytes to tissue culture dishes coated with desialylated ceruloplasmin [90] or collagen [91]. The promotion of attachment of HeLa-S3 carcinoma cells to glass by fetuin [92] may also be explained by the presence of endogenous lectin molecules on the HeLa cell surface [61,83]. The adhesion of metastatic rat hepatocarcinoma to endothelial cells was also carbohydrate mediated, as it was inhibited by methyl-α-D-mannopyranoside and N-acetyl-D-galactosamine [93]. A good correlation between adhesion of tumor cells in vitro to tissue culture dishes and lung colonization potential has been established in experiments that produced mAb to B16 melanoma cells and screened for hybridomas secreting mAbs capable of inhibiting adhesion of the cells to the substratum [45,46]. Some mAbs were found that not only decreased cell-substratum adhesion but also suppressed lung colonization when preabsorbed on the melanoma cells [46]. Polyclonal antibodies against fetal rat liver cells that block liver cell-cell aggregation were found to bind to RAW117 rat lymphosarcoma sublines in relation to their metastatic potential, to decrease adhesion of the lymphosarcoma cells to embryonic murine liver cells in vitro, and to inhibit experimental blood-borne metastasis [47,48]. The antigens recognized by such antibodies have been identified, but their function in cell adhesion and metastasis is not known. When the effect of the 5D7 antilectin mAb on metastatic ability of B16 melanoma and UV-2237 fibrosarcoma cells was explored, a decrease of up to 90% in the appearance of tumor lung colonies was noted [88], implying that the reduced lung-colonizing ability is associated with the reduced cell adhesiveness, as manifested by the antilectin mAb effects.

The process of metastasis is very complex and its outcome is influenced by various properties of the tumor cells and of different host cells. It is also probable that factors controlling tumor dissemination vary among different tumor cells and even among different target organs in the same host. Despite such variability, common denominator processes for metastasis must exist. We have focused here on a novel class of tumor cell surface molecules that bind specific carbohydrates and can contribute to cognitive interactions between metastasizing cells and host cells. Such molecules could be candidates for a common functional constituent which contributes to the overall metastatic phenotype of malignant cells.

ACKNOWLEDGMENTS

We thank Ms. Malvine Baer for excellent assistance in manuscript preparation. The work described here was supported by PHS grant CA-31330 awarded by the National Cancer Institute, NIH (to R.L. and A.R.), by M.D. Anderson Annual Campaign Funds (to R.L.), and by the Minerva Foundation, Federal German Republic (to A.R.). A.R. is the incumbent of the Sophi M.T. and Richard S. Richards Career Development Chair in Cancer Research in perpetuity.

REFERENCES

1. Nicolson GL: Biochim Biophys Acta 495:113–176, 1982.
2. Roos E: Biochim Biophys Acta 738:263–284, 1984.
3. Ruoslahti E: Cancer Metastasis Rev 3:43–52, 1984.
4. McCarthy JB, Basara ML, Palm SL, Furch LT: Cancer Metastasis Rev 4:125–152, 1985.
5. Geiger B, Volk T, Raz A: Exp Biol Med 10:39–53, 1985.
6. Raz A, Ben-Ze-ev A: Cancer Metastasis Rev, 1987 (in press).
7. Fidler IJ, Gersten DM, Hart IR: Adv Cancer Res 38:149–250, 1978.
8. Nicolson GL: Exp Cell Res 150:3–22, 1984.
9. Schirrmacher V: Adv Cancer Res 43:1–73, 1985.
10. Koch FE: Z Krebsforsch 48:495, 1939.
11. Fidler IJ, Kripke ML: Science 192:893–895, 1983.
12. Poste G: Cancer Metastasis Rev 1:141–199, 1982.

13. Heppner GH, Miller BE: Cancer Metastasis Rev 2:5–23, 1983.
14. Folkman J, Klagsbrun M: Science 235:442–447, 1987.
15. Coman DR: Cancer Res 13:397–404, 1953.
16. Weiss L, Ward PM: Cancer Metastasis Rev 2:111–127, 1983.
17. Gabbert H: Cancer Metastasis Rev 4:293–309, 1985.
18. Liotta LA, Rao CN: Lab Invest 49:636–649, 1983.
19. Sloane BF, Honn KV: Cancer Metastasis Rev 3:249–263, 1984.
20. Mignatti P, Robbins E, Rifkin DB: Cell 47:487–498, 1986.
21. Bernacki RJ, Niedbala MJ, Korytnk W: Cancer Metastasis Rev 4:81–101, 1985.
22. Gasic GJ: Cancer Metastasis Rev 3:99–116, 1984.
23. Honn KV, Menter DG, Onoda JM, Taylor JD, Sloane BF: In Nicolson GL, Milas L (eds): "Cancer Invasion and Metastasis: Biological and Therapeutic Aspects." New York: Raven Press, 1984, pp 361–368.
24. Warren BA: BrJ Exp Pathol 53:301–313, 1972.
25. Fidler IJ, Bucana C: Cancer Res 37:3945–3956, 1977.
26. Zeidman I: Cancer Res 17:157–162, 1957.
27. Willis RA: "The Spread of Tumors in the Human Body." London: Butterworth, 1973.
28. Hart IR: Cancer Metastasis Rev 1:5–16, 1982.
29. Paget S: Lancet 1:571–574, 1889.
30. Kinsey DL: Cancer 13:674–676, 1960.
31. Fidler IJ, Nicolson GL: J Natl Cancer Inst 58:1867–1872, 1977.
32. Fidler IJ: Nature (New Biol) 242:148–149, 1973.
33. Zvibel I, Raz A: Int J Cancer 36:261–272, 1985.
34. Fidler IJ: Eur J Cancer 9:223–227, 1973.
35. Winkelhake JL, Nicolson GL: J Natl Cancer Inst 56:285–298, 1976.
36. Nicolson GL, Winkelhake JL: Nature 255:230–232, 1975.
37. Raz A, Bucana C, McLellan W, Fidler IJ: Nature 284:363–364, 1980.
38. Fidler IJ, Nicolson GL: Cancer Biol Rev 2:1–53, 1981.
39. Lotan R, Raz A: Cancer Res 43:2088–2093, 1983.
40. Dennis JW, Donaghue TP, Kerbel RS: J Natl Cancer Inst 66:129–139, 1981.
41. Finne J, Tao TW, Burger MM: Cancer Res 40:2580–2587, 1980.
42. Reading CL, Belloni PN, Nicolson GL: J Natl Cancer Inst 64:1241–1249, 1980.
43. Briles EB, Kornfeld S: J Natl Cancer Inst 60:1217–1222, 1978.
44. Poste G, Nicolson GL: Proc Natl Acad Sci USA 77:399–403, 1980.
45. Vollmers HP, Birchmeier W: Trends Biochem Sci 8:452–455, 1983.
46. Vollmers HP, Birchmeier W: Proc Natl Acad Sci USA 80:3729–3733, 1983.
47. Nicolson GL, Mascali JJ, McGuire EJ: Oncodev Biol Med 4:149–159, 1982.
48. McGuire EJ, Mascali JJ, Grady SR, Nicolson GL: Clin Exp Med 2:213–222, 1984.
49. Steinemann C, Fenner M, Parish RW, Binz H: Int J Cancer 34:407–414, 1984.
50. Middelkoop OP, Roos E, Van De Pavert IV: J Cell Sci 56:461–470, 1982.
51. Asao MI, Oppenheimer SB: Exp Cell Res 120:101–110, 1979.
52. Vicker MG: J Cell Sci 21:161–173, 1976
53. Costello M, Fiedel BA, Gewurz H: Nature 286:677–678, 1979.
54. Rauvala H, Carter WG, Hakomori SI: J Cell Biol 88:127–137, 1981.
55. Huang RT: Nature 276:624–626, 1978.
56. Simpson DL, Thorne DR, Loh HH: Life Sci 22:727–748, 1978.
57. Monsigny M, Kieda C, Roche AC: Biol Cell 47:95–110, 1983.
58. Barondes SH: Science 23:1259–1264, 1984.
59. Sharon N, Lis H: Annu Rev Biochem 55:35–67, 1986.
60. Raz A, Lotan R: Cancer Metastasis Rev, 1987 (in press).
61. Raz A, Lotan: Cancer Res 41:3642–3647, 1981.
62. Raz A, Lotan R: In Galeotti T, Cittadini A, Neri G, Papa S (eds): "Membranes in Tumor Growth." Amsterdam: Elsevier Biomedical, 1982, pp 213–221.
63. Baenziger KI, Fiete D: J Biol Chem 254:789–795, 1979.
64. Spiro RG, Bhoyroo VD: J Biol Chem 249:5704–5717, 1974.
65. Teichberg VI, Silman I, Beitsch DD, Resheff G: Proc Natl Acad Sci USA 72:1383–1387, 1975.
66. Gabius HJ, Vehmeyer K: Naturwissenschaften 74:S37, 1987.

67. Jiang PH, Chang-Fournier F, Fobert-Galliot B, Sarragne M, Chang C: J Biol Chem 258:12361–12367, 1983.
68. Gabius HJ, Engelhardt R, Rehm S, Carmer F: J Natl Cancer Inst 73:1348–1357, 1984.
69. Gabius HJ, Engelhardt R, Sartoris DJ, Carmer F: Cancer Lett 31:139–145, 1986.
70. Gabius HJ, Engelhardt R, Rehm S, Barondes SH, Cramer F: Cancer J 1:19–21, 1986.
71. Roche AC, Barzilay M, Midoux P, Jungqua S, Sharon N, Monsigny M: J Cell Biochem 22:131–140, 1983.
72. Gabius HJ, Engelhardt R, Cramer F, Batge R, Nagel GA: Cancer Res 45:253–257, 1985.
73. Grabel LB, Glabe CR, Singer MS, Martin GR, Rosen SD: Biochem Biophys Res Comm 102:1165–1171, 1981.
74. Carrol SB, Ippolito LM, Bewolf WC: Biochem Biophys Res Comm 109:1353–1359, 1982.
75. Apgar JR, Cresswell P: Eur J Immunol 12:570–576, 1982.
76. Carding SR, Thrope SJ, Thrope R, Feizi T: Biochem Biophys Res Comm 127:680–686, 1985.
77. Paietta E, Stockert RJ, Morell AG, Diehl V, Wiernik PH: Proc Natl Acad Sci USA 83:3451–3455, 1986.
78. Monsigny M, Roche AC, Midoux P: Biol Cell 51:187–196, 1984.
79. Schwartz AL, Fridovich SE, Knowles BB, Lodish HF: J Biol Chem 258:11249–11255, 1983.
80. Liotta LA, Kleinerman J, Saidel GM: Cancer Res 36:889–894, 1976.
81. Glaves D: Br J Cancer 48:655–673, 1983.
82. Kieda C, Monsigny M: Invasion Metastasis 6:347–366, 1986.
83. Raz A, Meromsky L, Carmi P, Karkash R, Lotan D, Lotan R: EMBO J 3:2979–2983, 1983.
84. Raz A, Meromsky L, Lotan R: Cancer Res 46:3667–3672, 1986.
85. Moutsatsos IK, Davis JM, Wang JL: J Cell Biol 102:477–483, 1983.
86. Raz A, Meromsky L, Zvibel I, Lotan R: Int J Cancer, 1987 (in press).
87. Roos E, Tulp A, Middlekoop OP, Van De Apavert IV: J Natl Cancer Inst 72:1173–1180, 1984.
88. Meromsky L, Lotan R, Raz A: Cancer Res 46:5270–5275, 1986.
89. Harrison FL, Chesterton CJ: FEBS Lett 122:157–165, 1980.
90. Hook M, Rubin K, Oldberg A, Orbrink B, Vaheri A: Biochem Biophys Res Comm 79:726–733 1977.
91. Rubin K, Oldberg A, Hook M, Obrink B: Exp Cell Res 117:165–177, 1978.
92. Fisher HW, Puck TT, Sato G: Proc Natl Acad Sci USA 44:4–10, 1958.
93. Stanford DR, Starkey J, Magnuson JA: Int J Cancer 37:435–444, 1986.

Expression of Cell Adhesion Molecules During Embryogenesis and Malignancy

Robert Brackenbury and Gerald M. Edelman

The Rockefeller University, Laboratory of Developmental and Molecular Biology, New York, New York 10021

It has been believed for over 40 years that changes in cell–cell interactions may be one key determinant of metastatic potential. Recent advances in the identification and characterization of molecules involved in these interactions (cell adhesion molecules [CAMs]) have made it possible to describe changes in the expression and activity of specific CAMs that occur during cell transformation. Initial studies revealed that transformation of neuroepithelial cells by Rous sarcoma virus results in decreased expression of a well-characterized neural cell adhesion molecule, N-CAM. Cloned cDNA sequences of N-CAM are being used to investigate the mechanism of transformation-induced changes in N-CAM expression and to evaluate the role these changes play in the malignant behavior of tumor cells.

Key words: tumor cell detachment, cell motility, invasiveness, cell adhesion, neural cell adhesion molecule, N-CAM

Although most tumors originate from a single transformed cell, the cells in a growing tumor rapidly become heterogeneous in many properties, including such clinically critical factors as growth rate, drug resistance, and metastatic capacity [for reviews, see 1–3]. Some cells may acquire the ability to detach from the tumor mass and locally invade the surrounding tissue, a critical step in the progression from a benign to a malignant tumor. Tumor cell detachment undoubtedly involves many cellular processes (see Fig. 1), but it is reasonable to assume that changes in cell–cell adhesion are important. Our approach to understanding how such changes might be involved in malignancy has been to identify and characterize CAMs expressed by normal cells, to describe the means by which their expression or activity is regulated, and to evaluate how their expression changes during transformation [4–6].

The first vertebrate CAM to be identified [7,8], and the best characterized, is N-CAM [9], a large and abundant cell-surface glycoprotein [10] that mediates the calcium-independent adhesion of nerve cells [11]. About one-third of the mass of N-CAM is carbohydrate, including an exceptionally large amount of sialic acid [10], which is attached as long, unbranched polymeric chains [12]. N-CAM is highly conserved during evolution and is present in all vertebrates [13]. Although several different po-

Received August 14, 1987.

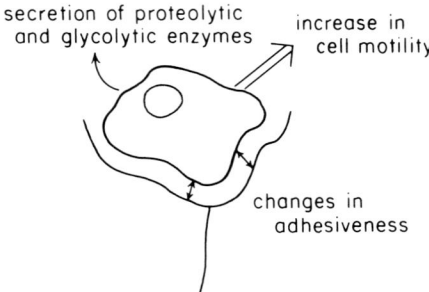

Fig. 1. Factors affecting tumor cell detachment. Cell transformation is frequently accompanied by changes in cell adhesiveness or motility, and secretion of proteolytic and glycolytic enzymes. It is not yet known whether changes in any one of these factors is sufficient to cause detachment of tumor cells, or whether specific combinations or temporal patterns of changes are required.

lypeptide forms have been identified, N-CAM is encoded by a single gene [14], which has been mapped to chromosome 9 in mice [15] and chromosome 11 in humans [16].

Alternative splicing of the N-CAM transcript gives rise to three major polypeptides in neural tissue (see Fig. 2) [17–19]. When fully deglycosylated, these polypeptides migrate on sodium dodecyl sulfate (SDS) gels with apparent molecular weights of 160,000, 130,000, and 110,000 [20–22]. Analysis of the isolated polypeptides [20] and of cDNA clones derived from the different mRNAs [19,23–25] indicates that the three polypeptides are identical from their amino termini up to the region where they associate with the plasma membrane. The amino-terminal portion of this extracellular region contains the N-CAM binding site [20]. The polysialic acid is attached outside of the binding region. Both the Mr 160,000 and Mr 130,000 polypeptides span the membrane, but their cytoplasmic domains differ [19,20,26]. The largest chain (ld polypeptide) contains a 30,000-dalton cytoplasmic segment, encoded by a single large exon, that is absent from the 130,000 (sd) and 110,000 (ssd) chains [17,18]. The ssd chain does not contain the membrane spanning domain, but instead contains a different hydrophobic-rich segment that is attached to the membrane by a phosphotidylinositol linkage [24,27].

The most striking feature of the amino acid sequence of N-CAM, as deduced from the sequence of cDNA clones, is the presence of five segments that are homologous to each other and to members of the immunoglobulin gene superfamily [19,23,25] (see Fig. 2). This amino-terminal portion of the molecule, which is common to all three chains, contains the binding region of N-CAM [19,20]. Because N-CAM binding is homophilic (N-CAM on one cell binds to another N-CAM on an apposed cell), interactions among immunoglobulin-like domains play a role in N-CAM binding. However, in contrast to the immunoglobulin genes, there is no evidence for any heterogeneity in sequence that might allow for variations in binding specificity.

Factors that modulate N-CAM binding have been revealed by assays that use purified N-CAM reconstituted into synthetic vesicles [28]. These studies have revealed that the polysialic acid is not necessary for N-CAM binding, but does modulate the level of binding: the A-form, or low-sialic acid form, of N-CAM mediates binding at four times the rate of the E-, or high-sialic acid, form of N-CAM. These studies also showed a high-order dependence of binding on the concentration of N-CAM.

The distribution of N-CAM during embryogenesis suggests some of its roles during

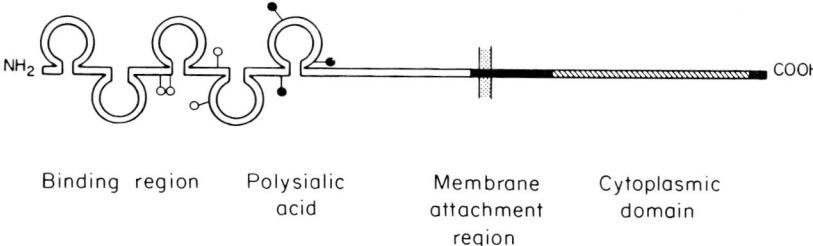

Fig. 2. Regional specialization of the N-CAM polypeptides. All three N-CAM polypeptides contain five immunoglobulin-like domains (loops), which extend away from the cell surface. This common extracellular portion contains the binding region and carbohydrate. Potential attachment sites for asparagine-linked oligosaccharides are shown as attached circles; the filled circles represent attachment sites for polysialic acid. Both the Mr 180,000 (ld) and Mr 140,000 (sd) polypeptides contain identical hydrophobic segments that span the cell membrane (stippled vertical bar). These two polypeptides differ in the extent of their cytoplasmic domains: the ld chain, which is found only in neural tissue, contains a unique region (crosshatched) coded by a single large exon that is included via a tissue-specific splicing event. Unlike the larger chains, the Mr 120,000 (ssd) chain does not span the membrane, but instead is synthesized with a different hydrophobic-rich segment and attaches to the membrane via a phosphatidylinositol linkage.

development [9]. The molecule is found on all neurons and is concentrated at the neuromuscular junction in striated muscle, implying a role in neuromuscular junction formation. N-CAM is also present on early pregastrula cells, and appears transiently during embryogenesis on somites, placodes, kidney, and some other cells. These results suggest that adhesion mediated by N-CAM is a fundamental process that is used repeatedly in various developmental contexts.

A particularly striking example is the program of N-CAM expression during the development of neural crest cells [29]. These cells express substantial amounts of N-CAM when they are clustered at the dorsal surface of the neural tube. N-CAM is not detectable on crest cells during the period when they are migrating but is re-expressed when crest cells coalesce to form spinal ganglia. Although direct evidence is lacking, these observations suggest that changes in the expression of N-CAM are causally involved in the crest cell migration/aggregation sequence.

The coordination of N-CAM expression and cell motility during neural crest cell migration is important when considered in light of its possible significance for tumor cell detachment and invasion. Both increases in cell motility and decreases in cell–cell adhesiveness have been suggested to play important roles in tumor cell mobilization [30,31]. The availability of specific probes for N-CAM made it possible to test whether transformation by oncogenic viruses caused changes in its expression or activity.

We carried out two parallel sets of studies to test whether transformation by Rous sarcoma virus (RSV) affected N-CAM expression. In the first study [32], we used cell lines derived from rat cerebellum that were established by transformation with a temperature-sensitive mutant of RSV. When these cells were grown at the nonpermissive temperature (conditions that inactivate the *src* gene product) they expressed large amounts of N-CAM and adhered effectively. However, when grown at the permissive temperature, the cells became morphologically transformed, lost N-CAM, and adhered poorly.

RSV transformation also decreased N-CAM expression in primary chick neuroepithelial cells [33] (Fig. 3). In these experiments, retinal neuroepithelial cells were obtained from embryos and placed into culture before most of the cells became postmitotic. When cultured with RSV, up to 70% of these cells became morphologically transformed within 3–5 days. Cells in the control cultures collected into tight clusters, but the transformed cells remained more evenly dispersed over the surface of the dish. Immunofluorescent staining, immunoblotting, and immunoprecipitation analyses showed that the transformed cell cultures expressed about one-tenth the normal level of N-CAM, with a corresponding reduction in cell–cell adhesiveness.

How does RSV reduce the level of N-CAM? In preliminary experiments we have found that RSV-transformed cells have substantially lower levels of N-CAM mRNAs. This result implies that pp60^{src} primarily affects the transcription or processing of N-CAM mRNAs, although direct effects on the stability of N-CAM protein have not been excluded. Although many transformation-induced changes occur within hours, the change in N-CAM expression occurs slowly [32], suggesting that it is an indirect or secondary consequence of transformation.

In addition to the changes in cell–cell adhesiveness, time-lapse cinematographic observations [33] showed that the transformed cells had become highly motile, migrating rapidly over the culture dish and under or through aggregates of cells. The

Fig. 3. RSV transformation causes a reduction in N-CAM. Primary cultures of chick neuroepithelial cells were incubated with the Schmidt-Ruppin strain A of RSV (SR-RSV-A), a transformation-defective strain (td 107), or without virus. To reveal the amounts and forms of N-CAM present, extracts of these cultures were fractionated by SDS polyacrylamide gel electrophoresis, transferred to nitrocellulose, incubated with antibodies to N-CAM followed by ^{125}I-labeled protein A, and autoradiographed. The control cultures (Normal) contained high levels of the Mr 180,000 and Mr 140,000 forms of N-CAM, whereas the RSV-transformed cells (SR-RSV-A) contained only about one-tenth the amount of these forms. Cells infected with the transformation-defective (td 107) strain, retained normal levels of N-CAM, indicating that transformation, and not simply viral replication or production, is necessary to induce the change in N-CAM expression.

changes in motility and cell–cell adhesiveness seem likely to be important in the invasive behavior of RSV-transformed neuroepithelial cells.

It is important to note that decreases in N-CAM have not been observed in cells transformed by agents other than RSV; for example, several chemically transformed cell lines express normal levels of N-CAM [32,34]. The invasiveness of these various cells has not been examined, but these observations are consistent with the view that enhanced invasiveness may result from changes in different cellular processes in different tumors or even in different cells from the same tumor.

A major aim of our current research is to determine how the changes in cell–cell adhesiveness that we have observed affect the behavior of tumor cells. This has been difficult in the past because of the variety of changes that are induced during transformation and the inability to isolate and analyze individual changes. A significant advantage of the RSV system is that it offers the opportunity to analyze the effect of changes in adhesiveness that are occurring throughout the population of transformed cells. Our current strategy is to compare the invasiveness of fully transformed cells (that have lost N-CAM) with "partially transformed" cells in which N-CAM has been re-expressed by transfection with full-length cDNA clones. Differences in the behavior of these cells should be directly due to the difference in their N-CAM-mediated adhesiveness.

REFERENCES

1. Fidler IJ, Gersten DM, Hart, IR: Adv Cancer Res 28:149–250, 1978.
2. Poste G, Fidler, IJ: Nature 283:139–146, 1980.
3. Nicolson G: Biochim Biophys Acta 695:113–176, 1982.
4. Edelman GM: Science 219:450–457, 1983.
5. Edelman GM: Annu Rev Biochem 54:135–169, 1985.
6. Brackenbury R: Cancer Metastasis Rev 4:41–58, 1985.
7. Brackenbury R, Thiery J-P, Rutishauser U, Edelman GM: J Biol Chem 252:6835–6840, 1977.
8. Thiery J-P, Brackenbury R, Rutishauser U, Edelman GM: J Biol Chem 252:6841–6845, 1977.
9. Edelman GM: Annu Rev Cell Biol 2:81–116, 1985.
10. Hoffman S, Sorkin BC, White PC, Brackenbury R, Mailhammer R, Rutishauser U, Cunningham BA, Edelman, GM: J Biol Chem 257:7720–7729, 1982.
11. Brackenbury R, Rutishauser U, Edelman, GM: Proc Natl Acad Sci USA 78:387–391, 1981.
12. Finne J, Finne V, Deagostini-Bazin H, Goridis C: Biochem Biophys Res Commun 112:482–487, 1983.
13. Hoffman S, Chuong C-M, Edelman GM: Proc Natl Acad Sci USA 81:6881–6885, 1984.
14. Owens GC, Edelman GM, Cunningham BA: Proc Natl Acad Sci USA 84:294–298, 1987.
15. D'Eustachio P, Owens GC, Edelman GM, Cunningham BA: Proc Natl Acad Sci USA 82:7631–7635, 1985.
16. Nguyen C, Mattei M-G, Mattei J-F, Santoni M-J, Goridis C, Jordan BR: J Cell Biol 102:711–715, 1986.
17. Murray BA, Hemperly JJ, Prediger EA, Edelman GM, Cunningham, BA: J Cell Biol 102:189–193, 1986.
18. Murray BA, Owens G, Crossin KL, Edelman GM, Cunningham BA: J Cell Biol 103:1431–1439, 1986.
19. Cunningham BA, Hemperly JJ, Murray BA, Prediger EA, Brackenbury R, Edelman GM: Science 236:799–806, 1987.
20. Cunningham BA, Hoffman S, Rutishauser U, Hemperly JJ, Edelman GM: Proc Natl Acad Sci USA 80:3116–3120, 1983.
21. Rougon G, Deagostini-Bazin H, Hirn M, Goridis C: EMBO J 1:1239–1244, 1982.
22. Rothbard JB, Brackenbury RW, Cunningham BA, Edelman GM: J Biol Chem 257:7720–7729, 1982.

23. Hemperly JJ, Murray BA, Edelman GM, Cunningham BA: Proc Natl Acad Sci USA 83:3037–3041, 1986.
24. Hemperly JJ, Edelman GM, Cunningham BA: Proc Natl Acad Sci USA 83:9822–9826, 1986.
25. Barthels D, Santoni M-J, Wille W, Ruppert C, Chaix J-C, Hirsch M-R, Fontecilla-Camps JC, Goridis C: EMBO J 6:907–914, 1987.
26. Gennarini G, Rougon G, Deagostini-Bazin H, Hirn M, Goridis C: Eur J Biochem 142:57–64, 1984.
27. He H-T, Barbet J, Chaix J-C, Goridis C: EMBO J 5:2489–2494, 1986.
28. Hoffman S, Edelman GM: Proc Natl Acad Sci USA 80:5762–5766, 1983.
29. Thiery J-P, Duband J-L, Rutishauser U, Edelman GM: Proc Natl Acad Sci USA 79:6737–6741, 1982.
30. Strauli P, Weiss L: Eur J Cancer 13:1–22, 1977.
31. Coman D: Cancer Res 4:625–629, 1944.
32. Greenberg ME, Brackenbury R, Edelman GM: Proc Natl Acad Sci USA 81:969–973, 1984.
33. Brackenbury R, Greenberg ME, Edelman GM: J Cell Biol 99:1944–1954, 1984.
34. Friedlander DR, Grumet M, Edelman GM: J Cell Biol 102:413–419, 1986.

Interactions of Human Carcinoma Cells With Extracellular Matrix

R.J. Bernacki, K. Pavelic, C.L. Sullivan, G. Leto, M.A. Bulbul, Y.M. Rustum, M.J. Niedbala, and K. Crickard

Department of Experimental Therapeutics, Grace Cancer Drug Center, Roswell Park Memorial Institute (R.J.B., K.P., C.L.S., G.L., M.A.B., Y.M.R., M.J.N.) and Department of Gynecology and Obstetrics, Buffalo General Hospital (K.C.), Buffalo, New York 14263

> Our experience with culture dishes coated with extracellular matrix (ECM), produced by bovine corneal endothelial cells, has shown that ECM can serve as a biochemically complex, biologically relevant substrate that supports primary epithelial (ovarian and urological) human tumor cell growth in vitro. Growth success for different ovarian and urological carcinomas (prostatic, bladder, kidney, and testicular) following enzymatic digestion was compared after seeding fresh surgical explants onto ECM and plastic culture flasks. Tumor cells demonstrated rapid attachment to ECM with subsequent proliferation of tumor cell colonies. A high percentage of fresh surgical samples grew cell colonies on ECM. Ovarian, renal, and prostatic tumors had excellent success rates, with bladder and testicular tumors being more difficult to culture. Poorly differentiated, metastatic renal, prostatic, or ovarian carcinomas generally caused visual degradation of ECM. There appeared to be a correlation between the release of certain tumor hydrolases, such as β-N-acetylglucosaminidase, cellular degradation of ECM, and invasive potential. This ECM-tumor model system has been found to be useful for establishing human tumor colonies in vitro and for investigating mechanisms of tumor cell attachment, invasion, and drug sensitivity.

Key words: cellular attachment, tissue degradation, hexosaminidase, human urological and ovarian tumors

Many elements affect tumor cell growth, differentiation, and metastasis including various growth and differentiation factors and their receptors, oncogene expression, and cell-to-cell and cell-to-substratum interactions. This report will be focused mainly on the latter topic, cell-to-substratum interactions (Fig. 1).

Cells interact with exogenous substrates in numerous ways. They attach to specific substrates and once adherent spread, migrate, and proliferate. In some cases tumor cells also have the ability to degrade and penetrate tissue matrix. This act constitutes an important step in tumor cell invasion, and one which facilitates tumor metastasis [1,2].

In order to study certain aspects of tumor metastasis in more detail extracellular

Received October 19, 1987.

© 1988 Alan R. Liss, Inc.

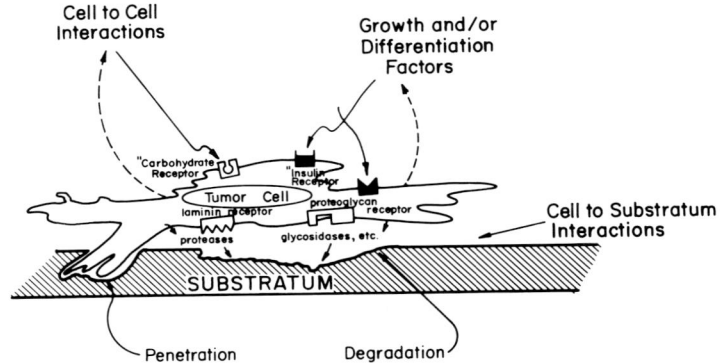

Fig. 1. Factors influencing tumor cell growth, differentiation, and metastasis.

matrix (ECM), produced by bovine corneal endothelial cells (BCEC), was utilized as a model substrate for studying human tumor cell attachment, proliferation and degradative potential in vitro [3]. Fresh human tumor explants, or cell lines recently isolated from these tissues [4,5], were evaluated for their growth success and their ability to attach and degrade ECM. The results of these studies suggest that the use of ECM improves the growth success for fresh human tumors in vitro by providing a substrate to which tumor cells avidly attach and in some cases subsequently degrade [6–8]. In these instances there appeared to be an association between tumor cell-mediated degradation of ECM and tumor cell secretory β-N-acetylglucosaminidase activity. A search for inhibitors of these cellular enzymes and processes is described herein with the expectation that such agents may have therapeutic potential.

MATERIALS AND METHODS
Materials

Falcon plastic culture dishes (6 and 10 cm in diameter) and 2-cm 24-well plates were obtained from Becton Dickinson (Oxnard, CA). N-2-Hydroxyethyl-piperazine-N-2-ethanesulfonic acid, spermidine, and dextran were purchased from Sigma Chemical Co. (St. Louis). Trypsin-ethylenediamine tetraceutic acid (EDTA), heat-inactivated fetal calf serum (HIFCS), calf serum, RPMI 1640 medium, glutamine, fungizone, and gentamicin were purchased from Grand Island Biological Co. Laboratories (Grand Island, NY); and methyl-[^{3}H]thymidine (specific activity, 20 Ci/mmol), [5,6-^{3}H]uridine (specific activity, 38.9 Ci/mmol), and [4,5-^{3}H(N)]leucine (specific activity, 50 Ci/mmol) were from New England Nuclear (Boston). Testosterone was obtained from Upjohn Company (Kalamazoo, MI), platelet-derived growth factor, insulin-like growth factor II, and epidermal growth factor were from Collaborative Research, Inc. (Lexington, MA); endothelial cell growth factor and fibroblast growth factor were from Seragen (Boston); insulin was from Novo (Copenhagen); and human growth hormone was from Hoechst (San Diego). Collagenase II and DNAse were obtained from Worthington Biochemicals (Freehold, NJ). Calcium channel blockers—verapamil (Searle Research and Development Division, G.D. Searle and Co., Stokie, IL), nimodipine (Miles Laboratories Inc., New Haven, CT), nifedipine (Pfizer Laboratories Division, New York, NY)—the calmodulin antagonist W-13, N-(4-aminobutyl)-5-chloro-2-naphthalene sulfonamide hydrochloride (Seikagaku America Inc., St. Petersburg, FL), tunicamycin, isolated from *Streptomcyes lysosuperficius* (from the National Cancer Institute), and leupeptin (Sigma Chemical Co., St. Louis) were tested as inhibitors of tumor cell attachment and growth.

Tumor Specimens

Fresh surgical specimens from human bladder, renal, prostatic, and testicular carcinoma were washed with RPMI 1640 medium containing 10% HIFCS and defatted, and their malignant nature was confirmed by frozen section pathological and cytological examination prior to processing. Specimens were disaggregated into cell suspensions enzymatically as described by Slocum et al. [9]. Briefly, tumor tissue slices, 0.5 mm in thickness, were incubated with a mixture of 0.8% collagenase II and 0.002% DNAse. Disaggregated cells were characterized by trypan blue exclusion (viability), cytological examination, and flow cytometric DNA ploidy determination. Following these procedures cell suspensions were seeded and cultured on different substrates in vitro.

Similarly, human ovarian tumor cells were derived from primary tumor tissue (A-121 ovary), ascitic effusions (A-1, A-69 and A-121 ascites), and a distant inguinal node metastasis (A-90). The isolation procedures and characterization of these tumor cells and resultant lines have been described previously [18]. These tumor cell lines were established on ECM and have been maintained continually in vitro as short-term cultures (P_{10}–P_{30}) for less than 1 year. Normal cell lines included human mesothelial cells and human ovarian fibroblasts and were utilized between passage numbers 1 and 4 [4,10].

All cells were maintained in the presence of Roswell Park Memorial Institute (RPMI)-1640 medium supplemented with 20% heat-inactivated fetal calf serum (HIFCS), 25 mM 4-(2-hydroxyethyl)-1-piperazine ethane-sulfonic acid (HEPES), 2 mM glutamine, gentamycin (50 μg/ml), and fungizone (2.5 μg/ml) as previously described [4].

Preparation of Plates Coated with Extracellular Matrix

Primary cultures of bovine corneal endothelial cells that synthesize ECM were established from steer eyes [11]. BCEC cells were plated at an initial density of 1×10^4 cells/ml per well in Dulbecco's modified Eagle's medium supplemented with 5% fetal calf serum, 5% calf serum, 5% Dextran T-40, fungizone (1%), and gentamycin (2%) in a 24-well tissue culture plate. Epidermal growth factor (1 ng/ml) was added every other day. Once the cultures reached confluency (ordinarily within 6 days) the media were renewed, and the cultures were incubated for another 6 days Following these procedures the cultures were washed with phosphate-buffered saline and exposed for 5 min to 0.02 M NH_4OH in distilled water to remove the BCEC cells. Once the underlying ECM became visible, the culture plates were washed 3 times with phosphate-buffered saline to prepare stock plates with ECM.

Cell Attachment Assay

Cell attachment assays were performed using ECM coated and uncoated plastic culture dishes. Tumor cell suspensions were prelabeled for 24 hr at 37°C using [^{3}H]thymidine (0.5 μCi/ml) in medium supplemented with HIFCS. Subsequently, all labeled cells were removed from ECM-coated plates using trypsin-EDTA (0.2 g EDTA/1.5 min at 37°C) and washed several times in RPMI 1640 containing 20% HIFCS. Radiolabeled cells were then added to the various culture vessels. Following incubations at 37°C for 30, 60, and 180 min unattached cells were removed, and each well was rinsed several times with phosphate-buffered saline (0.2 g KCl, 0.2 g KH_2PO_4, 8 g NaCl, and 1 g Na_2HPO_4 per liter, pH 7.2). Attached cells were harvested on filter paper using an automated cell harvester. Radioactivity of incorporated cellular [^{3}H]-thymidine was measured by use of scintillation counting methods [7].

Growth Inhibition Studies

Human carcinoma cells (10^5/ml) were preplated in each well of 24-well plates 1 day prior to the addition of drugs. Cells were incubated for 3–5 days at 37°C, 5% CO_2. Drug effect was determined by measuring cell number or protein content [12] and comparing it with control cultures.

β-N-Acetylglucosaminidase (β-NAG) Assay

Intracellular β-NAG activity for the various cell types grown in vitro was determined following dissociation of the cells in 4 volumes of 0.1% of Triton X-100 with 30 strokes in a Dounce homogenizer at 4°C. This cellular homogenate was used as a crude enzyme source. Extracellular β-NAG activity associated with cell-free conditioned medium was also determined in the presence of twice heat inactivated (56°C for 30 min) fetal calf serum for the various cell types. The amount of respective glycosidase activity present in cellular homogenates or cell-free conditioned medium was determined at pH 4.3 using commercially available p-nitrophenyl-βNAG (Sigma Chemical Co., St. Louis) as described previously [13].

RESULTS
Cellular Growth and Degradation of ECM

Following solubilization of the bovine corneal endothelial cell layer with 0.02 N NH_4OH, the underlying extracellular matrix (ECM) was exposed and made ready for use as a substrate for subsequent attachment and growth studies of human carcinoma cells in vitro. Human ovarian A-1 tumor cells, recently derived from human ovarian ascites tumor, demonstrated rapid attachment to ECM versus plastic and the subsequent formation of numerous colonies of proliferating tumor cells with a structurally intact ECM (Fig. 2A). Human ovarian A-90 tumor cells, derived from a lymph node metastases, however, demonstrated digestion of ECM following 3 days in culture (Fig. 2B). Similarly, an A-121(p) ovarian tumor cell line obtained from a human primary tumor and a line of cells derived from that patient's ascites A-121(a) both demonstrated visual evidence, by phase microscopy, of ECM invasion and degradation (micrographs not shown).

Other studies with primary human urological tumor cells, derived from enzymatically digested surgical tumor samples, demonstrated rapid attachment of tumor cells to ECM with subsequent proliferation of tumor cell colonies followed in some cases by degradation of ECM components. Thirty-eight out of 48 surgical tumor samples (80%) grew cell colonies on ECM. Renal (16/17) and prostatic tumors (8/9) had excellent success rates, with bladder (12/19) and testicular tumors (2/3) being more difficult to culture. Twelve high-grade and metastatic tumors caused visual degradation of ECM. Human prostate tumor demonstrated degradation of ECM after 5 days in culture (Fig. 2C).

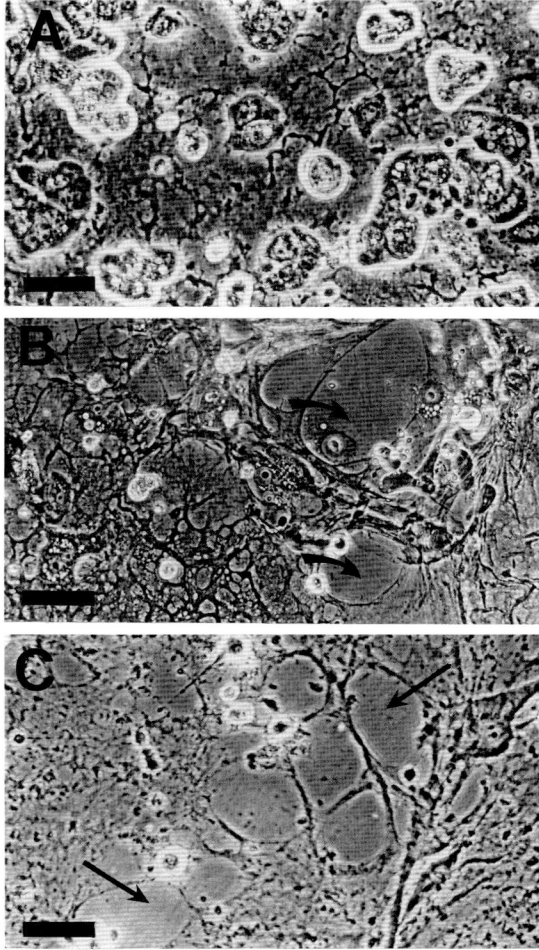

Fig. 2. Human tumor cell attachment, growth, and degradation of extracellular matrix (ECM) in vitro. **A:** Human ovarian adenocarcinoma A-1 cell clusters proliferating on ECM. Bar = 20 μm. **B:** Human ovarian adenocarcinoma cells derived from a distant lymph metastasis demonstrating digestion (arrows) of ECM after 3 days in culture. Bar = 10 μm. **C:** Degradation of ECM (arrows) by clinically invasive prostate carcinoma, day 15. Bar = 10 μm.

Biological Aspects of Degradation

The degradative potential of various cell types grown on ECM was quantitated by use of metabolically prelabeled ECM-coated 16-mm culture dishes. These plates were prepared by incubating bovine corneal endothelial cells with tritium-labeled precursors ([^{3}H]-fucose, -galactose, -glucosamine, or -proline), which were subsequently incorporated into ECM macromolecular components. Degradation potential was assayed by measuring release of radioactivity into the cellular medium, 40 hr after seeding of radiolabeled ECM with cells. Metastatic ovarian A-90 and A-121 and endometrial HEC-1 cells released high amounts of radioactive components into the medium, while the noninvasive human ovarian tumor A-1 and normal human mesothelial (HMC-70)

TABLE I. Degradative Potential of Various Cell Types Grown on ECM*

Cell type	Percentage of [^{3}H]-isotope released			
	Fucose	Galactose	Glucosamine	Proline
Invasive tumor cells				
Ovarian A-90 lymph node metastasis	8.6	0.6	8.1	2.7
Ovarian A-121 primary	8.0	2.8	9.1	5.0
Ovarian A-121 ascites	9.4	.1	11.6	6.6
Ovarian A-69 ascites	4.8	0.9	0.1	0.1
Endometrial HEC-1	14.2	6.6	2.8	21.6
Noninvasive cells				
Ovarian A-1 tumor	0	0.2	0.4	1.3
Mesothelial HMC-70	0	2.1	0.1	0.5
Fibroblast HOF-1	0.2	0	0	1.0

*Bovine corneal endothelial cell monolayers were pulse-labeled with 20 µCi/ml of various [^{3}H]-metabolic precursors for 72 hr just prior to cellular confluency. At 6 days postconfluency endothelial cells were removed and the radiolabeled ECM washed three times prior to seeding with the cell-types indicated (5×10^4 cells/ml/well). Degradative potential was assayed after 40 hr incubation by determining the amount of radiolabel released into the culture medium. Values are expressed as the percentage of radioactivity released from radiolabeled ECM following subtraction of spontaneous release, which was less than 15%. Assays were performed in triplicate, and standard deviations among replicate samples were less than 10%.

and fibroblast (HOF-1) cells did not release significant amounts of radiolabeled components (Table I). The percentages of [^{3}H]-isotope released varied for the different cell lines, with the A-90 line releasing fucose and glucosamine, the A-121 line releasing these two sugars and proline, the A-69 line releasing fucose, and the HEC-1 line releasing fucose, galactose, and proline. These results indicate a heterogeneity in the mechanisms responsible for tumor invasion. The noninvasive ovarian tumor A-1 and normal mesothelial and fibroblast cell lines released little radioactivity from the ECM.

Secretion of various hydrolytic enzymes may account for the degradation of ECM components. A systematic search for various glycosidase activities was performed on cells and media from the various cell lines. α and β-galactose, α and β-glucosidase, α and β-fucosidase, α-mannosidase, β-B-acetylgalactosaminidase, β-N-acetylglucosaminidase, and acid phosphatase activities were quantitated using p-nitrophenyl-substrates for both intra- and extracellular enzyme activity. Several glycosidases were elevated in the media of cultures containing tumor cells capable of degrading ECM as compared with normal cells [8]. β-N-Acetylglucosaminidase activity, measured with p-nitrophenol-β-N-acetylglucosaminide substrate, secreted into the tissue culture media correlated with ECM degradation. HEC-1A, A-90, A-69, and A-121 tumor cells (primary or ascites-derived) released high amounts of this enzyme activity into the culture medium. In contrast, noninvasive A-1 ovarian tumor cells and the normal human mesothelial and fibroblast cells secreted low amounts of this enzyme (Fig. 3). Evidence from other work has shown that purified tumor hexosaminidase is capable of releasing radioactivity from [^{3}H]-glucosamine-labeled ECM [6].

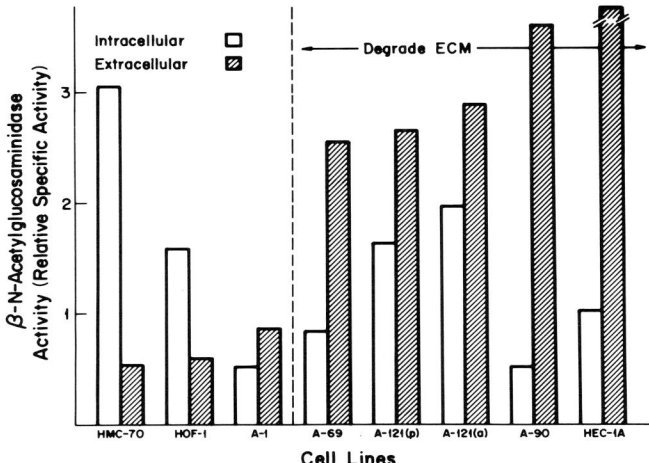

Fig. 3. β-N-acetylglucosaminidase activity associated with various human cell lines. HMC-70, human mesothelial cells, HOF-1, human ovarian fibroblasts, and A-1 human ovarian tumor cells demonstrated lower secretory enzyme activity as compared with the ovarian tumor lines A-69, A-121(p) primary or (a) ascites, A-90, or HEC-1A human endometrial carcinoma cells in vitro, which all degrade extracellular matrix (ECM).

Attachment Assays

Initial studies measuring A-121(a) human ovarian tumor cell attachment confirmed earlier work, which demonstrated a rapid and selective attachment of tumor cells to extracellular matrix (ECM) as compared to plastic substrate (Fig. 4). Within 15 min, greater than 50% of the cells attached to ECM. On plastic more than 1 hr was needed for 50% of cell attachment to occur. At a concentration of tunicamycin (1×10^{-6} M), which decreases glycoprotein biosynthesis and alters membrane agglutination within 24 hr [14], a significant decrease in the rate of attachment of tumor cells to either plastic or ECM was noted (Fig. 4). Tunicamycin exposure used in these experiments was not growth inhibitory for A-121 tumor cells. In comparison, at non-growth-inhibitory concentrations for several calcium channel blockers—verapamil (5×10^{-6} M), nifedipine (1.25×10^{-4} M), and nimodipine (5.0×10^{-6} M)—no effect on cellular attachment to plastic or ECM was noted (data not shown). On the other hand, W-13, a calmodulin antagonist (1×10^{-5} M) significantly decreased ovarian A-121 cell attachment to plastic and to extracellular matrix, also at a non-growth-inhibitory concentration (Fig. 5). Maximal significant inhibition of cellular attachment to plastic (35%) occurred after 180 min of drug exposure. A more immediate decrease in cellular attachment to ECM (22%) was noted 30 min after drug exposure, with maximal effectiveness (30% inhibition) occurring at 180 min, in a time-dependent fashion.

DISCUSSION

The majority of cancer patients fail therapy as a result of disseminated disease or drug resistance. Ovarian and urological cancers generally metastasize in early stages of tumor growth, often before clinical detection. The inability to prevent primary tumors

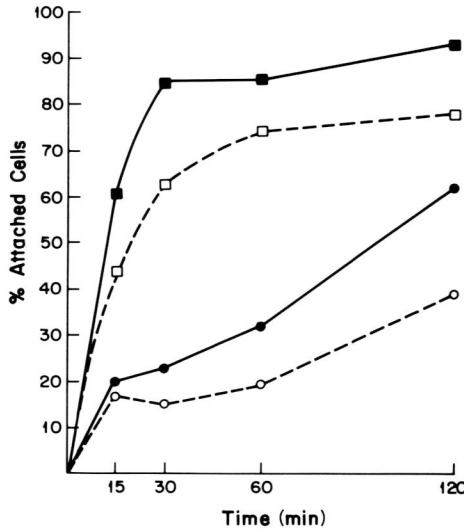

Fig. 4. Attachment kinetics of human A-121 ovarian tumor cells. A-121 cells (1 × 10⁴ cells/ml) were allowed to attach to ECM (■,□) or plastic (●,○) following a 24-hr incubation in the absence (■,●) or presence (□,○) of 1 × 10⁻⁶M tunicamycin. At the indicated times cell attachment was measured by counting attached cells. All points are the mean of triplicate determinations performed on three separate occasions.

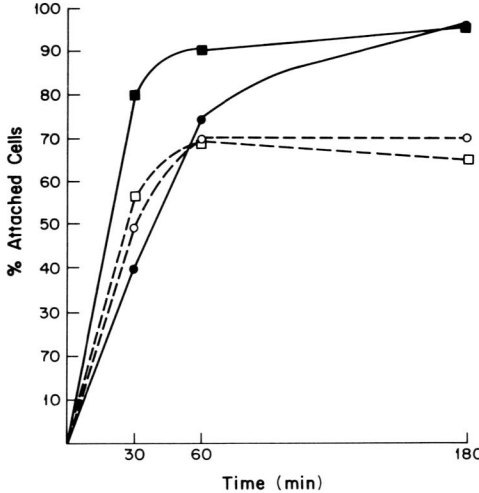

Fig. 5. Attachment kinetics of A-121 human ovarian tumor cells. A-121 cells were allowed to attach to ECM (■,□) or plastic (●,○) in the absence (■,●) or presence (□,○) of 1 × 10⁻⁵M calmodulin antagonist, W13. Attachment was measured as described in Figure 4. Results are the mean of triplicate determinations performed on more than two separate occasions.

from spreading to surrounding tissue and distant sites remains a significant obstacle to cancer treatment. Research studies are now aimed at characterizing events in tumor cell invasion and metastasis in hopes of defining new targets for therapeutic exploitation.

Our studies have focused on growing fresh human tumors in vitro using a naturally produced extracellular matrix (ECM) to support epithelial tumor cell attachment and proliferation. Initial studies by Vlodavsky et al. [15] and Crickard et al. [5] have demonstrated the utility of this model system for growing fresh human tumor explants in vitro. Using similar methodology we have obtained a high degree of success for growing fresh human urological tumors in vitro and have observed that clinically aggressive tumors often have the ability to degrade ECM [7]. Using a series of tumor and normal cell lines, some of which were recently established by us on ECM [4], a correlation was observed between cellular degradation of ECM and the release of β-N-acetylglucosaminidase activity (Fig. 3). Additionally, using radiolabeled ECM metabolically prelabeled by bovine corneal endothelial cells with either [^{3}H]-fucose or [^{3}H]-proline, evidence was obtained implying that other enzymes, including collagenases, may be involved in matrix degradation. That series of experiments (Table I) suggested that each invasive tumor cell line may degrade matrix differently; however, it was noted that all the tumor cell lines demonstrating ECM degradation released substantial amounts of one or more hydrolytic enzyme, in particular, β-N-acetylglucosaminidase activity. These findings complement a number of other studies that have implicated proteases, collagenases, and endoglycosidases in tumor cell invasion and metastasis [1,2,16]. However, it should be noted that metastasis is a highly inefficient process involving many different steps prior to the establishment of secondary tumor foci and that it is very difficult to establish clearly a primary cause and effect relationship for metastasis. In the initial stages of tumor cell detachment from the primary tumor and local tissue invasion the involvement of hydrolytic enzymes would aid tumor metastases; however, at a subsequent stage of tumor cell arrest such enzymes may be deleterious. Therefore, one must be cautious with the interpretation of the present findings, which correlate higher β-N-acetylglucosaminidase (β-NAG) activity with ECM degradation and invasion.

Subsequent to tumor cell extravasation and hematogenous migration to a distant site is tumor cell arrest and reattachment to subendothelial basement membrane. In many respects cellular attachment to ECM in culture is similar. The extracellular matrix (ECM) in these in vitro studies is produced and secreted basally by bovine corneal endothelial cells and is composed of interstitial collagen types I–III and basement membrane collagen types IV + V as well as elastin, fibronectin, and basement membrane-specific laminin [17]. Laminin and fibronectin are the major components involved in the cell-attachment mechanisms. Tumor cells have cell surface receptors for these basement membrane components. Interference between these cell surface receptors and their ligands should result in inhibition of cellular attachment. Membrane modifiers such as calcium channel blockers and calmodulin antagonists and tunicamycin, an inhibitor of N-linked glycosylation, were selected to be candidates for interfering with these processes.

In an effort to select for attachment inhibition, only relatively non-growth-inhibitory concentrations of these drugs were investigated. No effect on blocking attachment was observed with the calcium channel blockers at the concentrations tested. W-13, a calmodulin antagonist, however, did reveal an inhibitory effect upon ovarian A-121 tumor cell attachment at a non-growth-inhibitory concentration of 1×10^{-5} M. Cells were exposed to the drug immediately upon plating to allow for attachment interference.

The results obtained with tunicamycin demonstrated that this antibiotic is able to decrease the rate of A-121 tumor attachment to both plastic and ECM provided that the cells were preincubated with this drug for 24 hr. Since tunicamycin is known to inhibit the first step in the synthesis of glycoproteins containing asparagine-linked oligosaccharides, it is reasonable to suggest that membrane glycoproteins are involved in the process of cell attachment.

In conclusion, studies with culture dishes coated with ECM, produced by bovine corneal endothelial cells, have shown that ECM can serve as a biochemically relevant substrate, which supports primary epithelial human tumor cell growth in vitro and may be used to determine the invasive potential of these tumors. A correlation was observed between the ability of a variety of cell types to invade ECM as determined by light microscopy and their ability to solubilize metabolically prelabeled ECM. The degree of solubilization and the specificity of radiolabeled ECM components degraded by invasive tumor cells varied in each case. Some cell types were observed to degrade proline-enriched ECM components avidly; others specifically hydrolyzed carbohydrate-rich ECM moieties, while others hydrolyzed both. There appears to be a correlation between the release of certain tumor cell hydrolases, such as β-N-acetylglucosaminidase, their degradation of ECM, and their invasive potential.

This extracellular matrix model system may be useful for investigating mechanisms of tumor cell attachment and invasion and also may lead to the development of new chemotherapeutic agents and modalities designed to limit tumor cell growth and metastasis.

ACKNOWLEDGMENTS

These studies were supported by NCI grants CA-42898 and CA-13038. The excellent technical and secretarial assistance of Jean Veith and Sandra Trafalski is greatly appreciated.

REFERENCES

1. Liotta LA, Tryggvason K, Garbisa S, Hart I, Foltz CM, Schafie S: Nature 284:67, 1980.
2. Bernacki RJ, Niedbala MJ, Korytnyk W: Cancer Metastasis Rev 4:81, 1985.
3. Niedbala MJ, Crickard K, Bernacki RJ: Exp Cell Res 160:499, 1985.
4. Crickard K, Niedbala MJ, Crickard U, Yoonessi M, Sandberg AA, Okuyama K, Bernacki RJ, Stachidand SK: Gynecol Oncol 1988 (in press).
5. Crickard K, Crickard U, Yoonessi M: Cancer Res 43:2762, 1983.
6. Niedbala MJ, Crickard K, Bernacki RJ: Clin Exp Metastasis 5:181, 1987.
7. Pavelic K, Bulbul M, Slocum HK, Pavelic ZP, Rustum YM, Niedbala MJ, Bernacki RJ: Cancer Res 46:3653, 1986.
8. Niedbala MJ, Madiyalakan R, Matta K, Crickard K, Sharma M, Bernacki RJ: Cancer Res 47:4634, 1987.
9. Slocum HK, Pavelic ZP, Rustum YM, Creaven PJ, Karakousis C, Takita H, Greco WR: Cancer Res 41:1428, 1981.
10. Niedbala MJ, Crickard K, Bernacki RJ: J Cell Sci 85:133, 1986.
11. Gospodarowicz D, Mescher AL, Birdwell CR: Exp Eye Res 25:75, 1977.
12. Lowry OH, Rosebrough NJ, Farr AL, Randall RJ: J Biol Chem 193:265, 1951.
13. Dobrossy L, Pavelic ZP, Vaughan M, Porter N, Bernacki RJ: Cancer Res 40:3281, 1980.
14. Morin MJ, Bernacki RJ: Cancer Res 43:1669, 1983.
15. Vlodavsky I, Liu GM, Gospodarowicz D: Cell 19:607, 1980.
16. Nakajima M, Irimura T, DiFerrante DT, DiFerrante N, Nicolson GL: Science 220:611, 1983.
17. Tseng SCG, Savion N, Gospodarowicz D, Stern R: J Biol Chem 256:336, 1981.

Basement Membranes, Reconstituted to Assess the Invasiveness of Tumor Cells

Adriana Albini, Sharon L. Aukerman, Antonella Melchiori, Erik W. Thompson, Reuven Reich, Thomas B. Shima, George R. Martin, and Yukihide Iwamoto

LDBA, NIDR (E.W.T., R.R., T.B.S., G.R.M., Y.I.), and NEI (A.A.), NIH, Bethesda, Maryland 20892; Department of Cell Biology, M.D. Anderson Hospital, Houston, Texas 77030 (S.L.A.); Istituto Scientifico Tumori, 16132 Genova, Italy (A.M.)

Current concepts suggest that malignant cancer cells possess specific activities that allow the tumor cells to penetrate through biological barriers and form satellite lesions [1,2]. Such barriers are created both by cells and their extracellular matrices. A variety of in vitro models have been developed for studying the invasiveness of tumor cells utilizing organs as well as tissues such as the lens, bladder wall, amnion, and chorioallantoic membrane, fragments of tissues such as heart and muscle, and cultures of epithelial cells and hepatocytes [for review, see ref.2]. Typically, amnion, lens, or chorioallantoic membranes can be freed of cells, flattened, and placed as a barrier between the two chambers of a modified Boyden chamber device. Invasive cells added to the upper chamber will traverse the tissue and can be quantitated [3,4].

Observations on malignant tumors both in vivo and in vitro suggest that basement membranes represent critical barriers to the passage of tumor cells [1,2]. The dissolution of basement membranes by the tumor cells and the invasion of tumor cells into adjacent tissue is a necessary step in the progression of the tumor to malignant status [5–7]. Therefore, one should expect correlations between invasion in "in vitro" systems and malignant potential.

Basement membranes are composed mostly of laminin, collagen IV, heparan sulphate proteoglycan, and entactin/nidogen. [8,9]. It is generally believed that in the basement membrane, a network of collagen IV molecules linked end to end forms the principle structural element. Laminin binds to the collagen IV network, to itself, to entactin, and to heparan sulfate proteoglycan, forming different structures in the basement membrane depending on the number and type of its associations with these matrix components [9,10]. Laminin has diverse biological activities, which include binding to cells and influencing their morphology, differentiation, and function [11]. The heparan sulfate proteoglycan is known to create a filtration barrier in capillaries and in the glomerulus and thus restricts the passage of proteins [12]. Additionally, it seems to inhibit the passage of cells through basement membrane [13].

Received June 30, 1987.

© 1988 Alan R. Liss, Inc.

We have tested purified basement membrane components as barriers to cellular invasion in vitro. In one system, collagen IV and laminin were pressed into flattened discs, which were placed between the compartments of a modified Boyden chamber device [14]. Such barriers were found to prevent the passage of normal cells, while metastatic tumor cells were able to cross them over a 48-hr period. It was also noted that chemoattractants greatly increased the passage of the malignant cells through the barrier [14,15].

A RECONSTITUTED BASEMENT MEMBRANE GEL AS AN INVASION BARRIER

Recent studies indicate that the components of basement membranes will bind to one another and can be reconstituted into a firm gel under physiological conditions [16]. Such basement membrane gels contain laminin, collagen IV, heparan sulfate proteoglycan, and entactin, as well as other proteins [16]. Analysis of the reconstituted basement membrane (matrigel) shows that the extract is relatively deficient in collagen IV and heparan sulfate proteoglycan compared to authentic basement membranes. Supplementing the extract with these two factors induces the formation of a much stronger gel (Fig. 1).

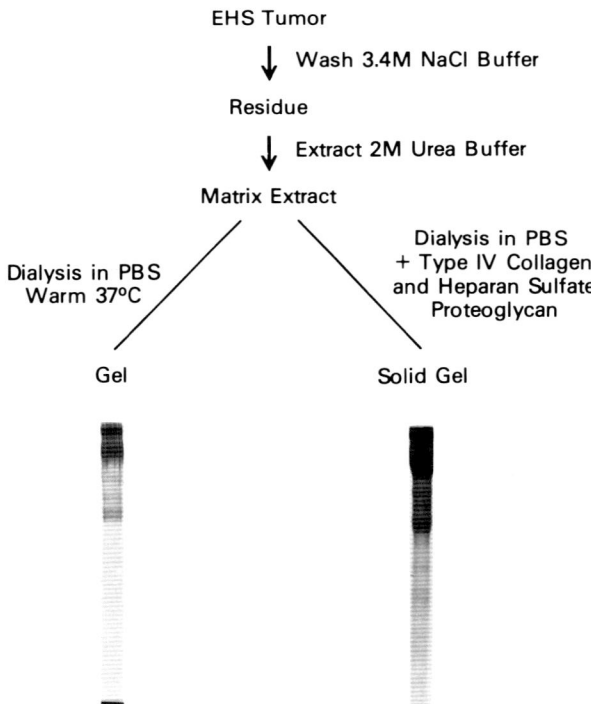

Fig. 1. Method used for preparing matrigel or supplemented matrigel and analysis of its components by electrophoresis. PBS, phosphate-buffered saline.

Matrigel itself is biologically active and can induce the differentiation of a variety of epithelial cells, nerves, and endothelial cells [16–18]. This material offers the opportunity to fabricate three-dimensional substrates for biological tests both in vivo and in vitro. When plated on matrigel, nonmetastatic cells remain isolated on the surface in clumps while metastatic tumor cells disperse and penetrate into the gel leaving tunnels behind them [19].

We have developed a rapid in vitro invasion assay employing a layer of reconstituted matrigel as the barrier in a Boyden chamber device. The matrigel is supported on a porous polycellulose filter (Nucleopore). Figure 2a shows a cross-section of a Nucleopore filter that has been coated with matrigel. The matrigel was applied at 4°C as a thin even coat over the filter and then allowed to reconstitute into a gel-like layer at 37°C. For use in the invasion assay [20], the filters are first coated with matrigel and then placed in the Boyden chamber. The appearance of the surfaces of a typical assay filter several hours after adding cells to the upper chamber is shown in Figure 2b. Highly invasive

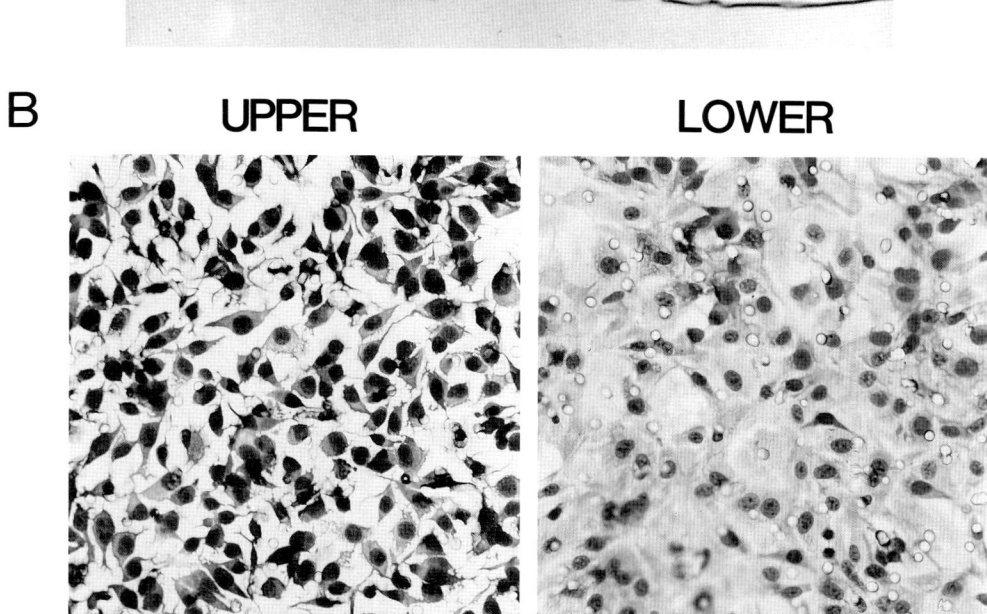

Fig. 2. The matrigel invasion assay. **A:** A cross-section of a polycarbonate filter coated with matrigel is shown. Note the homogenous gel covering the surface of the filter and preventing access to the pores. **B:** Attachment of highly invasive MDA-MB 231 breast cancer cells to the matrigel coating on the upper filter surface and their ability to penetrate the matrigel and be retained on the lower surface of the filter.

MDA-MB 231 breast cancer cells adhere well to the matrigel and coat the upper surface of the filter. They also have crossed the filter in large numbers. Noninvasive cells also bind to the matrigel but are unable to cross it. Additionally it was found that increased amounts of matrigel caused a proportional increase in the time required to cross the filter [20] as did supplementation of the matrigel with collagen IV (unpublished).

In order to invade the reconstituted matrix, cells must 1) adhere, 2) degrade the matrix, and 3) migrate. Murine melanoma and human fibrosarcoma cells were found to produce proteases in the assay chamber, particularly collagenase IV and plasminogen activator. These act in concert to degrade the basement membrane barrier (unpublished). In particular, collagenase IV appears to be a key enzyme in degrading the basement membrane, and the production of this enzyme shows some correlation with malignant potential [6,21].

CORRELATION BETWEEN INVASIVE ACTIVITY AND METASTATIC POTENTIAL

A number of murine and human tumor cells of known malignant activity have been assessed for invasive activity [20,22]. In general, highly malignant cells such as rhabdomyosarcoma and prostatic carcinoma demonstrate a high degree of invasiveness [20], while fibroblasts, smooth muscle cells, and endothelial cells exhibit little ability to penetrate through the basement membrane barrier (Fig. 3). Additionally, cells derived from Kaposi's sarcoma exhibit invasiveness comparable to that of malignant cells [22]. A direct comparison of invasive activity in vitro and metastatic activity in vivo is shown in three tumor lines cloned from the K1735 murine melanoma [23] (Table I). In this case, the metastatic cell lines are approximately 10 times more invasive in vitro and

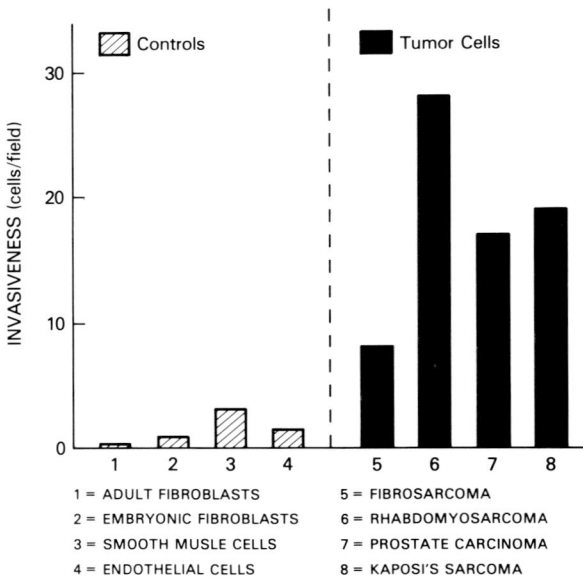

Fig. 3. The relative invasive activity of normal cells, benign tumor cells, and tumor cells of known malignant origin.

TABLE I. Comparison of In Vitro Invasion of Matrigel and In Vivo Metastatic Activity of Tumor Cells

Cell line	Invasive cells/field	Animals with metastasis (IV injection)
K-1735 Cl 10	4 ± 1	0/10
K-1735 M2	44 ± 2	10/10
K-1735 M4	53 ± 6	10/10

form pulmonary metastases in all animals when injected intravenously. The nonmetastatic line is poorly invasive in vitro and only rarely metastatic.

ISOLATION OF INVASIVE CELLS

It is possible to isolate the cells that have penetrated through the matrigel-filter barrier to the bottom of the filter (Albini, unpublished) (Fig. 4). After removal of the media (0.1% bovine serum albumin [BSA] in Dulbecco's modified Eagle's medium

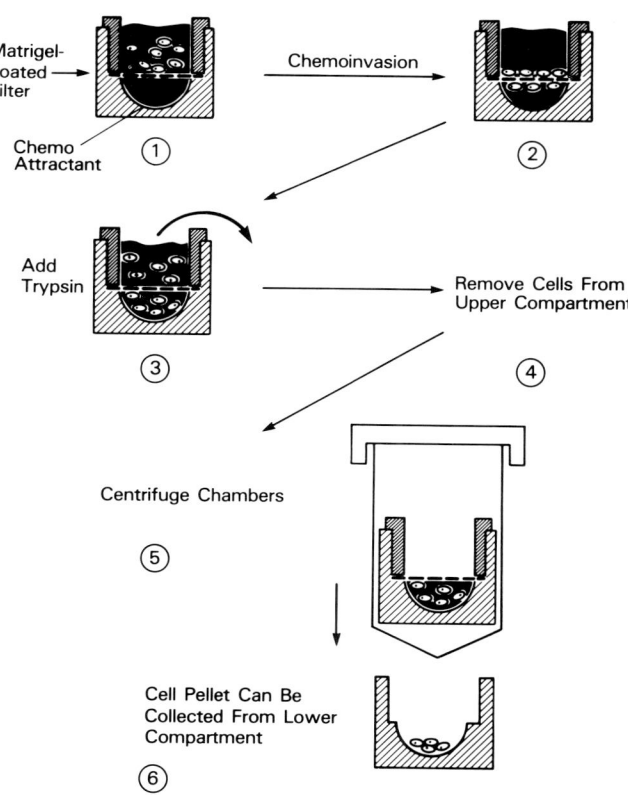

Fig. 4. The technique used to isolate the invasive population of cells by releasing them with trypsin from the lower surface of the filter and collecting them by centrifuging the Boyden chamber.

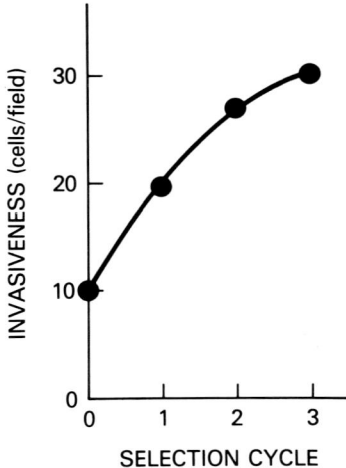

Fig. 5. Selection of invasive cells. Cells penetrating through matrigel were grown and cycled through the chamber again. Increases in their ability to invade were noted consistent with the isolation of an invasive subpopulation of tumor cells.

[DMEM]), trypsin (0.05%) is added to the upper chamber to release the cells on each side of the filter [24]. The entire chamber is centrifuged, and the cells that have penetrated through the filter are collected as a pellet in the lower chamber. The invasive cells are transferred into culture for further study. An example of the behavior of cells selected in this fashion is shown in Figure 5. In this case, human teratocarcinoma-derived PA-1 cells [25], which showed an intermediate degree of penetration through the matrigel barrier, were isolated after invasion, expanded in culture, and retested for invasiveness. Three such selection cycles produced a cell line that showed an approximate threefold increase in invasive activity.

We have found that a variety of metastatic cells when tested in the in vitro assay are invasive [20]. However, tumor cells may be invasive but not metastatic as shown in Table II. In this study, the invasive and metastatic activity of cells transfected with certain oncogenes is reported. Human breast cancer cells transfected with v-ras are highly invasive in vitro and in vivo [26,27]. Similarly, murine cells transfected with v-ras are highly invasive and metastatic [28–30]. In contrast, transfection of a line of murine

TABLE II. Effect of Oncogene Transfection on Matrigel Invasion

Cell type	Transfection	Invasiveness in vitro	Malignancy in vivo
MCF-7	None	Low	No
breast cancer	Eco-gpt	Low	No
cell	v-ras^H + gpt	High	Yes
NIH-3T3	None	None	No
fibroblastic cell	c-ras^H	High	Yes
K1735 C110	None	Low	Low
melanoma cell	Neo	Low	Low
	v-myc + neo	High	Low

melanoma cells with v-myc induced invasive capacity in vitro but not malignant activity in vivo. Such behavior is undoubtably due to the multifactorial nature of the metastatic process in which the tumor cells must complete all aspects of the process to form lesions [31].

USE OF IN VITRO ASSAYS TO SCREEN FOR ANTIMETASTATIC SUBSTANCES

Current concepts suggest that the invasion of basement membrane by tumor cells proceeds in discrete steps [1,2]. These include the attachment of the cells to the basement membrane [2] and the production of collagenase IV [21] and heparinases [32,33], which destroy the basement membrane barrier and allow the movement of the cells into normal tissues. Each of these steps represents a specific potential target for unique drugs that could block the formation of metastases.

Metastatic cells have a high affinity for laminin and attach preferentially to this molecule [11,34]. Since laminin is found exclusively in basement membranes, this interaction may ensure the initial attachment to the target organ. Metastatic cells have a high number of cell surface receptors (M_r = 67,000) for laminin [35–37]. The binding of the metastatic cells to laminin stimulates the production of enzymes required for degrading basement membrane [38] and induces invasion [39].

Recently, an amino acid sequence on laminin, tyrosine-isoleucine-glycine-serine-arginine (YIGSR), has been found to have receptor binding activity [40]. That is, it appears to be a cell attachment site in laminin. Cells can attach to YIGSR when the peptide is coated onto substrates, and the peptide in solution can inhibit competitively the attachment of cells to laminin. This peptide has been tested in vitro in invasion assays and in vivo in experimental metastases tests and has been found to inhibit the invasive and metastatic activity of melanoma cells [41]. This may be due to its ability to compete with laminin for binding to tumor cells, although this has not yet been shown directly.

The formation of active collagenase has been found to involve a proteolytic cascade [7]. Collagenase IV is produced as an inactive proenzyme, and the generation of active enzyme is accomplished via plasminogen activator and plasminogen (Reich, unpublished). Inhibitors of serine protease and antibodies to plasminogen activator were found to prevent the activation of collagenase IV and to inhibit the ability of tumor cells to invade through the basement membrane barrier in vitro (Reich, unpublished). A newly developed collagenase IV inhibitor was also tested (A gift from Dr. G. Fuller, Searle Co., Skokie, IL). This compound mimics the profile of the collagen helix and is bound to the active site of collagenases via a hydroxamic acid group, which chelates to zinc. This compound was found to inhibit tumor cell invasion in vitro and the formation of lung lesions in mice injected with malignant melanoma cells (Reich, unpublished). Its ability to inhibit metastases indicates the essential role of collagenase in metastasis and raises the possibility of developing therapeutic regimens against this step. Heparitanase is involved in the degradation of basement membrane proteoglycan, and inhibitors of this enzyme reduce tumor cell invasion through the amnion in vitro and reduce experimental metastases [13].

Finally, it has been suggested that interferon may increase the metastatic activity of tumor cells [42]. Since interferon has diverse actions on the normal cells of the host [43], it was of interest to test its actions on the invasive behavior of tumor cells. Cells transformed by two distinct oncogenes were studied (Fig. 6). Interferon was found to

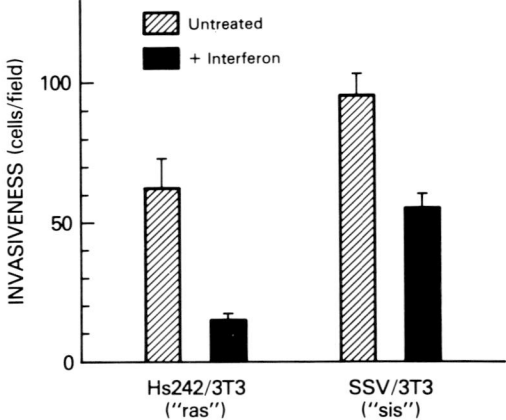

Fig. 6. Inhibition of basement membrane invasion following treatment of metastatic cells with interferon.

reduce the invasiveness of both ras- and sis-transformed cells [44]. These data suggest that interferon treatment does not necessarily directly increase the metastatic activity of tumor cells. Rather, it would appear that metastatic activity is subject to regulation and that metastasis can be suppressed when these pathways are identified.

SUMMARY

We describe the use of a reconstituted basement membrane formed as a barrier over a porous filter to assess the invasiveness of tumor cells. Examination of a number of human and animal tumor cell lines of known metastatic activity showed that the malignant tumor cells, but not benign cells are able to invade through the barrier. However, certain cells that become invasive following transformation with the myc oncogene do not exhibit metastatic activity in vivo. This system was also found to be useful in screening for compounds that block invasiveness. In some cases, anti-invasive drugs were also found to inhibit experimental metastases.

ACKNOWLEDGMENTS

Portions of this work and one of the authors (E.W.T.) were supported by the Breast Cancer Study Group, Medical Breast Cancer Section, Medicine Branch, NCI, NIH.

REFERENCES

1. Liotta LA: Am J Pathol 117:339, 1984.
2. Terranova VP, Hujanen ES, Martin GR JNCI 77:311, 1986.
3. Liotta LA, Lee WC, Morakis DJ: Cancer Lett 11:141, 1980.
4. Hendrix MJC, Gehlsen KR, Wagner HN, Rodney SR, Misiorowski, RL, Meyskens, FL: Clin Exp Metastasis 3:221, 1985.
5. Jones PA, DeClerck YA: Cancer Res 40:3222, 1980.
6. Nakajima M, Welch DR, Irimura T, Nicolson GL: In Welch DR, Bhuyan BK, Liotta LA (eds):

"Cancer Metastasis: Experimental and Clinical Strategies." (eds) New York: Alan R. Liss, Inc., 1986 pp 113–122.
7. Mignatti P, Robbins E, Rifkin DB: Cell 47:487, 1986.
8. Laurie GW, Leblond CP, Martin, GR: J Cell Biol 95:340, 1982.
9. Timpl R, Fujiwara S, Dziadek M, Aumailley M, Weber S, Engel J: In Porter R, Whelan J (eds): "Basement Membranes and Cell Movement." London: Pitman, 1984, pp 25–74.
10. Martin GR, Timpl R: Annu Rev Cell Biol 3:57–85, 1987.
11. Kleinman HK, Cannon FB, Laurie GW, Hassell JR, Aumailley M, Terranova VP, Martin GR, Dubois-Dalcq M: J Cell Biochem 27:317, 1985.
12. Hassell JR, Kimura JH, Hascall, VC: Annu Rev Biochem 55:539, 1986.
13. Irimura T, Nakajima M, Nicolson GL: Biochemistry 25:5322, 1986.
14. Terranova VP, Hujanen ES, Loeb DM, Martin GR, Thornburg L, Glushko V: Proc Natl Acad Sci USA 83:465, 1986.
15. Hujanen ES, Terranova VP: Cancer Res 45:3517, 1985.
16. Kleinman HK, McGarvey ML, Hassell JR, Star VL, Cannon FB, Laurie GW, Martin GR: Biochemistry 25:312, 1986.
17. Bissell MJ: Proc Natl Acad Sci USA 84:136, 1987.
18. Kleinman HK, Graf J, Iwamoto Y, Kitten GT, Ogle RC, Sasaki M, Yamada Y, Martin GR, Luckenbill-Edds L: Ann NY Acad Sci (in press).
19. Kramer RH, Bensch KK, Wong J: Cancer Res 40:1980, 1986.
20. Albini A, Iwamoto Y, Kleinman HK, Martin GR, Aaronson SA, Kozlowski JM, McEwan RN: Cancer Res 47:3239–3245, 1987.
21. Liotta LA, Thorgeirsson UP, Garbisa S: Cancer Metastasis Rev 1:277, 1982.
22. Albini A, Mitchell CD, Thompson EW, Seeman R, Martin GR, Wittek AE, Quinnan GV: J Cell Biochem (in press).
23. Aukerman SL, Price JE, Fidler IJ: JNCI 77:915, 1986.
24. Albini A, Muller PK, Parodi S: Biosci Rep 4:311, 1984.
25. Zeuthen J, Norgaard JOR, Avner P, Fellous M, Wartiovaara J, Vaheri A, Rosen A, Giovannella BC: Int J Cancer 25:19, 1980.
26. Albini A, Graf J, Kitten GT, Kleinman HK, Martin GR, Veillette A, Lippman ME: Proc Natl Acad Sci USA 83:8182, 1986.
27. Kasid A, Lippman ME, Papageorge AG, Lowy DR, Gelmann EP: Science 238:725, 1985.
28. Thorgeirsson UP, Turpeenniemi-Hujanen T, Williams JE, Westin EJ, Heilman CA, Talmadge JE, Liotta LA: Mol Cell Biol 5:259, 1985.
29. Greig RG, Koestler TP, Trainer L, Corwin SP, Milen U, Kline T, Sweet R, Yokayama S, Poste G: Proc Natl Acad Sci USA 82:3698, 1985.
30. Bondy GP, Wilson S, Chambers AF: Cancer Res 45:6005, 1985.
31. Fidler IJ: Cancer Res 38:2651, 1978.
32. Nakajima M, Irimura T, DiFerrante N, Nicolson GL: J Biol Chem 25:2283, 1984.
33. Vlodovsky I, Fuks Z, Bar-Ner M, Ariav Y, Schirrmacher V: Cancer Res 43:2704, 1983.
34. Terranova VP, Liotta LA, Russo RG, Martin GR: Cancer Res 42:2265, 1982.
35. Rao CN, Barsky SH, Terranova VP, Liotta LA: Biochem Biophys Res Commun 111:804, 1983.
36. Wewer UM, Liotta LA, Jaye M, Ricca GA, Drohan WN, Claysmith AP, Rao CN, Wirth P, Coligan JE, Albrechtsen R, Mudryj M, Sobel ME: Proc Natl Acad Sci USA 83:7137, 1986.
37. Terranova VP, Rao CN, Kalebic T, Margulies IM, Liotta LA: Proc Natl Acad Sci USA 80:444, 1983.
38. Turpeenniemi-Hujanen T, Thorgeirsson UP, Rao CN, Liotta LA: J Biol Chem 261:1883, 1986.
39. Terranova VP, Williams JE, Liotta LA, Martin GR: Science 226:982, 1984.
40. Graf J, Iwamoto Y, Sasaki M, Martin GR, Kleinman HK, Robey FA, Yamada Y: Cell 48:989, 1987.
41. Iwamoto Y, Robey FA, Graf J, Sasaki M, Kleinman HK, Yamada Y, Martin GR: Science 238:1132–1134, 1987.
42. Seigal GP, Thorgeirsson, VP, Russo RG, Wallace DM, Liotta LA, Berger SL: PNAS 79:4064, 1982.
43. Gressner I, Tovey MG: Biochim Biophys Acta 516:231, 1987.
44. Melchiori A, Allavena G, Bohm J, Remy W, Schmidt J, Parodi S, Santi L, Albini A: Anticancer Res (in press).

Interactions Between Tumor Cells and Liver Cells During Liver Metastasis Formation

Ed Roos, John G. Collard, Folkert F. Roossien, and Geertje La Rivière

Division of Cell Biology, Antoni van Leeuwenhoek Huis, The Netherlands Cancer Institute, 1066 CX Amsterdam, The Netherlands

Tumor cells colonizing the liver have to adhere to, and invade between, sinusoidal endothelial cells and hepatocytes. Adhesion is mediated by several different adhesion molecules, specific for tumor type and possibly also for liver. On lymphoma cells one of these molecules is LFA-1. For lymphoid tumor cells, invasion depends on signals transduced by a pertussis-toxin-sensitive G-protein. Experiments with T-cell hybridoma cells suggest that the invasion mechanism of at least some malignant lymphoma cells is similar to that of normal activated T-lymphocytes. Both invasiveness and metastatic potential can be induced in benign lymphoma cells by transfection of the ras-oncogene. In human lymphoma cells genes essential for invasiveness are located on human chromosome 7.

Key words: invasion, lymphoma, T-cell hybridoma, pertussis toxin, LFA-1

The liver is a major target organ for metastasis, especially for abdominal carcinomas, and a preferred metastatic site for lymphomas [1]. Invasion of blood-borne tumor cells occurs in the capillaries [5,11], which are unique in that no basement membrane is present under the endothelial cells. Therefore, tumor cells do not have to adhere to and pass through a basement membrane as, e.g., in the lungs. They only have to interact with endothelial cells and with hepatocytes. We have used short-term cultures of isolated rat liver cells to investigate the mechanisms underlying these interactions.

ENDOTHELIAL CELLS

Sinusoidal endothelial cells were isolated from collagenase-dispersed livers and purified by gradient sedimentation at 1g [16] or centrifugal elutriation. Tumor cells were added a few hours after isolation. Highly metastatic lymphoma cells adhered to the endothelial cells, but low- or nonmetastatic lymphoma cells and also metastatic [12] TA3 mammary carcinoma cells did not [16]. Adhesion to liver endothelial cells is therefore apparently not necessary for arrest in the liver, which is 100% efficient for all

Received April 12, 1987.

© 1988 Alan R. Liss, Inc.

of these tumor cells. Furthermore, this adhesion does not seem to be a prerequisite for liver metastasis formation by the TA3 cells. However, it may be important for lymphoma metastasis. Lymphoma cell adhesion was inhibited by the same polyclonal antisera that inhibited adhesion to hepatocytes (see below), indicating that the same adhesion molecules might be involved. We have therefore mainly used hepatocyte cultures in our attempts to identify these molecules.

HEPATOCYTES

Isolated hepatocytes were cultured overnight before addition of tumor cells. TA3 carcinoma cells and certain lymphoma cells attached to the upper surface of the hepatocyte monolayer [19]. A small fraction of the TA3 carcinoma cells invaded very slowly, but some lymphoma cells infiltrated very rapidly. Invasiveness of lymphoma cells correlated with their in vivo behaviour: MB6A [5,11] and ESb [22] cells, which diffusely infiltrated the liver, rapidly invaded in vitro, whereas GRSL leukemia cells, which formed a limited number of nodular metastases [16], and BW5147 cells, which were not metastatic [4], did not invade. Furthermore, among a panel of T-cell hybridomas (see below), invasion correlated with metastatic capacity [13].

T-CELL HYBRIDOMA CELLS

Activated T-lymphocytes share properties with metastatic tumor cells, e.g., the ability to degrade extracellular material and to invade endothelial cell monolayers [21]. We found that activated T-cells also invade hepatocyte cultures [17]. In vivo fusion of noninvasive BW5147 T-lymphoma cells with host T-cells has been observed, and the resulting hybridomas acquired both invasive and metastatic potential [4]. This suggested that invasiveness, and as a consequence metastatic capacity, was derived from the normal T-cell. We have confirmed this notion using T-cell hybridomas generated in vitro from nonmetastatic BW5147 cells and activated T-lymphocytes [13]. These hybridomas were highly invasive and metastasized readily, predominantly to the liver, but also to kidneys, ovaries, and lymphoid tissue.

After segregation of chromosomes carrying relevant genes, the hybrids lost invasiveness. By selection and cloning we could therefore generate a large panel of invasive and noninvasive hybridomas, which differed in several properties not correlated with invasive capacity [13,32]. The properties of part of this panel are shown in Table I. Comparison of these cell lines should enable us to focus on the relevant properties.

INVASION INTO FIBROBLAST MONOLAYERS

Activated T-cells tend to move under fibroblasts in culture, in contrast to nonstimulated T-cells [2]. Verschueren et al. [29] have shown that metastatic T-cell hybridoma cells behave similarly. We have found that fibroblast cultures are quite suitable for the selection of invasive subpopulations, because cells usually attach less strongly to the upper surface of fibroblasts than of hepatocytes; therefore, adherent cells that have not invaded can be relatively easily removed by mechanical agitation. Selection was very efficient: invasive T-cell hybridoma cells could be selected from a 1:500,000 mixture with noninvasive BW5147 cells [33].

Remarkably, MB6A lymphoma cells, which metastasized only to the liver and the

TABLE I. Invasiveness, Metastasis, and DNA Content of T-Cell Hybridomas

Cell line[a]	Invasive[b]	Infiltration index[c]	% DNA[d]	Additional chromosomes[e]	Metastases Day[f]	Mice
BW5147	No	0.0	100	0	32	0/10
TAM202	Yes	1.0	205	46	40	14/14
TAM8A6	Yes	1.1	150	22	18	5/5
TCM6B2	Yes	0.5	134	15	40	10/11
TAM11I1	Yes	0.8	109	4	n.d.[g]	
TAM11B1	Yes	0.4	107	3	n.d.	
TAS9B5	No	0.02	108	4	63	0/5
TAS5.C4.1.2	No	0.05	115	7	59	0/5
TAS9A2	No	0.06	115	7	50	0/5
TAS5C6	No	0.01	115	7	62	0/7

[a]Representative examples of a larger series are shown.
[b]Infiltration index > 0.1; for discussion see [13].
[c]For explanation see [13,18].
[d]Assessed with impulse cytophotometry.
[e]Estimated from % DNA.
[f]Autopsy, days after i.v. injection of 10^6 cells.
[g]n.d., not determined.

spleen [5] and which were highly invasive in hepatocyte cultures, hardly invaded fibroblast monolayers [32], in contrast to the T-cell hybridoma cells, which also formed kidney, ovary, and lymph node metastases [13]. This indicates that the mechanisms of invasion into the two types of cultures are different. It is conceivable that MB6A cells do not form kidney and ovary metastases, because they are unable to invade into these tissues.

ras-TRANSFECTED BW5147 CELLS

Transfection of the mutated *ras*-oncogene has been reported to induce or increase metastatic capacity in fibroblasts [28] and carcinoma cells [30]. We found that similarly transfected BW5147 cells simultaneously acquired invasive and metastatic capacity, albeit at lower levels than the T-cell hybridomas [3]. Thus, it seems that the mutated *ras*-protein mimics to a certain extent the activity of (a) normal protein(s) produced by activated T-cells as part of the invasive machinery. Strikingly, the pattern of dissemination was similar to that of T-cell hybridomas. For instance, in contrast to the transfected fibroblasts and carcinoma cells, no lung metastases were formed. Thus, although *ras* is a general inducer of metastatic capacity, the mechanisms affected are apparently cell-type-specific.

GENES ON HUMAN CHROMOSOME 7 INVOLVED IN INVASIVE CAPACITY

Human activated T-cells and certain human lymphoma cells invaded the rat hepatocyte monolayers similarly as comparable murine cells. Thus, it was feasible to study (human × mouse) T-cell hybrids generated by fusion of these human cells with mouse BW5147 cells, and some were found to be quite invasive. (Human × mouse) hybrids quickly segregate human chromosomes, and therefore invasiveness was rapidly lost, except when invasive cells were continuously selected on fibroblast monolayers. Among a series of hybrids containing a few human chromosomes, invasiveness was 100% correlated with the presence of human chromosome 7, and finally invasive hybrids were selected that contained only this chromosome [33]. Therefore, a gene or genes located on chromosome 7 appear(s) to be indispensable for invasiveness and metastatic capacity of at least some human lymphoid malignancies.

INHIBITION OF INVASION BY PERTUSSIS TOXIN

Pertussis toxin inhibits particular signal transduction pathways because it irreversibly inactivates certain G-proteins [27], e.g., the one inhibiting adenylate cyclase [7]. The pathways affected are not yet fully elucidated, but are likely to differ between cell types. The toxin is known to cause accumulation of lymphocytes in the blood, because of inhibition of recirculation through lymph nodes and invasion into tissues such as the skin [24,25]. We found that the toxin strongly inhibits invasion into hepatocyte ([34], see Fig. 1) and fibroblast [32] monolayers. This result and the effects of *ras*, which has been shown to encode a signal-transducing protein [31], suggest that the invasion-relevant genes, activated in T-cell hybridomas and certain lymphomas, encode components of signal transduction pathways.

Pertussis toxin is an ideal reagent for *in vivo* studies, because invasiveness remained suppressed for at least 5 days after a preincubation for 4 hr with 1 μg/ml and because it did not affect proliferation. Liver metastasis formation of toxin-pretreated T-cell hybridoma cells, measured as liver weight increase after a fixed time period, was reduced to approximately 20% of controls [34], once again indicating that invasiveness is an important aspect of the metastatic phenotype, and showing that the toxin-affected mechanisms are relevant *in vivo*. Extrahepatic metastasis was less easy to quantitate, and toxin effects were either not observed or were less evident. However, the results obtained were not sufficiently clear to conclude that the toxin has no effect.

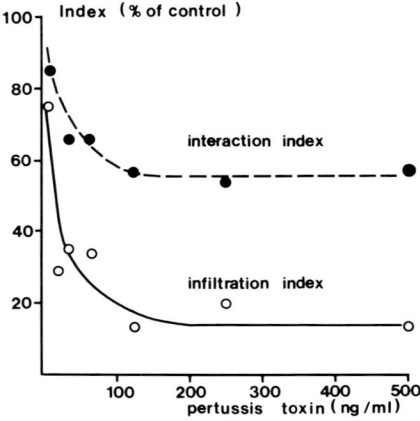

Fig. 1. Effect of pertussis toxin on interaction, and on invasion, of MB6A cells in hepatocyte cultures, as measured by counting cells in sections using light microscopy. **Solid circles,** Interaction index; **open circles,** Infiltration index, as percentage of control values (for explanation see [13] and [18]). From [34].

ADHESION MOLECULES

Adhesion to the upper surface of hepatocytes is an essential first step in the invasion process, and inhibition of this step leads to a corresponding reduction of invasion [9,18]. Antisera obtained from different rabbits immunized with liver plasma membranes differentially inhibited adhesion of lymphoma and carcinoma cells [9,14], suggesting that the two tumor cell types interact with different hepatocyte adhesion molecules. This notion was confirmed when we generated a monoclonal antibody against rat hepatocytes, designated OPAR-1, which inhibited adhesion of various carcinoma, but not melanoma or lymphoma cells to hepatocytes [10].

On Western blots the OPAR antibody reacted with different bands in the 110 to 140-kDa region. In the liver, the antigen was abundantly present on the sinusoidal hepatocyte surface but was absent from endothelial cells, in line with the lack of adhesion of carcinoma cells to these endothelial cells (see above). Outside the liver, the antigen was only detected in the skin, but not in any major metastatic site, suggesting that the OPAR adhesion molecule is specific for liver. However, the possibility that the OPAR antibody reacts with a liver-specific carbohydrate epitope, which may be present on different proteins including a more generally important adhesion molecule, has not yet been excluded.

LEUCOCYTE FUNCTION-ASSOCIATED ANTIGEN-1 (LFA-1)

We recently found that a monoclonal antibody to LFA-1 inhibited adhesion of MB6A lymphoma and TAM2D2 T-cell hybridoma cells (Fig. 2) to hepatocytes, in contrast to isotype-matched control antibodies, of similar affinity and binding levels, directed against Thy.1 and T200 [15]. LFA-1 is thus likely to be involved in lymphoma liver metastasis formation. LFA-1 is an adhesion molecule, first detected to be important

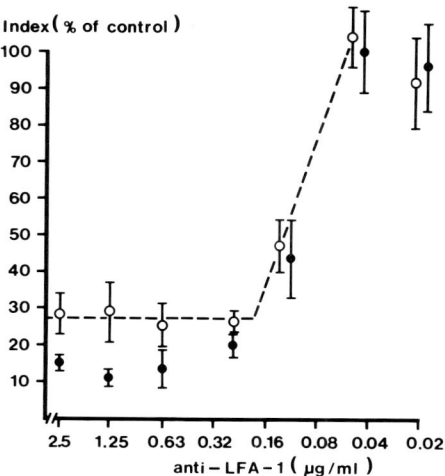

Fig. 2. Inhibition by a monoclonal anti-LFA-1 antibody of adhesion and invasion of TAM2D2 cells in hepatocyte cultures 4 hr after addition of the cells, as determined by counting cells in sections of embedded cultures. **Open circles,** the *interaction index*; and **closed circles:** the *infiltration index* (for explanation see [13] and [18]), as percentage of control values (from [15]).

for the interaction between cytotoxic T-cells and their target cells, but now known to be generally involved in adhesion between leucocytes and also between leucocytes and endothelial cells [8,26].

Our results were surprising in that adhesion of cytotoxic lymphocytes to epithelial target cells had been shown to be LFA-1 independent [23] and in that a putative counterstructure of LFA-1, ICAM-1, had been reported to be absent from human hepatocytes [6]. However, our results show that T-cells and lymphoma cells can use LFA-1 to mediate adhesion to an epithelial cell, the hepatocyte, and suggest that an LFA-1 counterstructure different from ICAM-1 is present on the latter cell. Remarkably, the maximal percentage inhibition by the anti-LFA-1 antibody was the same for MB6A and TAM2D2 cells, despite the fact that LFA-1 density on the former cells was tenfold lower than on the latter. Apparently, LFA-1-dependent adhesion does not correlate with LFA-1 surface density.

OTHER LYMPHOMA ADHESION MOLECULES

Previously, we had found that Fab fragments prepared from a rabbit antiserum against MB6A lymphoma cells inhibited their adhesion to hepatocytes. We have investigated whether the antigen involved was LFA-1 (Roossien, F.F. et al., unpublished results). The antiserum did precipitate LFA-1 α- and β-chain and also a band with a molecular weight similar to Mac-1 [20] from a detergent extract of ^{125}I-labeled MB6A cells, indicating that at least part of the anti-LFA-1 antibodies was directed against the common β-chain of LFA-1 and Mac-1. The Mac-1 band was not precipitated from T-cell hybridoma cells (Fig. 3).

The anti-LFA-1 Fab fragments were absorbed from the antiserum by repeated exposure to Sepharose-coupled LFA-1, purified from TAM2D2 T-cell hybridoma cells. Absorption did not reduce their inhibitory capacity. Furthermore, we have recently prepared Fab fragments from a different rabbit anti-MB6A serum, which strongly inhibited adhesion of MB6A, but not of TAM2D2 cells (Fig. 4), and this antiserum did not precipitate LFA-1. Thus, in addition to LFA-1, other adhesion molecules appear to participate in lymphoma-hepatocyte adhesion, and these molecules appear to be different, or to contain different epitopes, on MB6A cells and T-cell hybridoma cells.

We have recently generated a monoclonal antibody against MB6A cells, provisionally designated Moab 520, which reduced adhesion of MB6A cells to hepatocytes to approximately 65% of control values but had no effect on adhesion of T-cell hybrids (F.F. Roossien et al., unpublished results) and may therefore be directed against the additional MB6A adhesion molecule discussed above. Moab 520 further reduced adhesion of cells maximally inhibited by saturating concentrations of anti-LFA-1 antibody. On Western blots Moab 520 appears to react with a band of approximately 35 kDa. Further characterization of the antigen is in progress.

CONCLUSIONS

We have shown for a set of lymphoid malignancies that invasiveness in hepatocyte cultures is associated with the ability to metastasize to the liver. This suggests that invasion into liver tissue is an essential step in liver metastasis formation. Invasive T-cell hybridomas, which have derived their invasiveness from the normal T-cell fusion partner, were shown to have acquired metastatic capacity. This suggests that at least

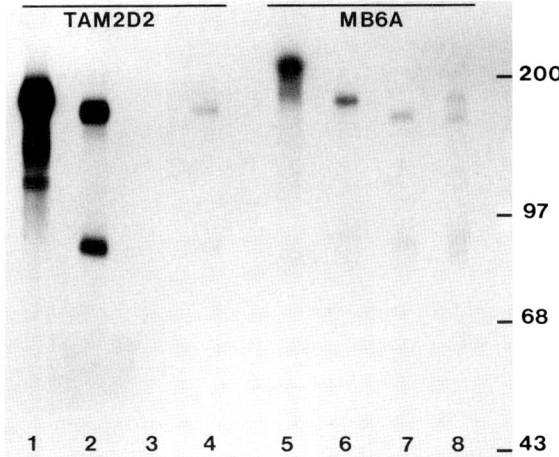

Fig. 3. Immune precipitation from detergent extracts of MB6A lymphoma and TAM2D2 cells. The same number of both types of cells was iodinated under the same conditions, and an equivalent amount of extract of both cell types was used. **Lanes 1–4:** TAM2D2 cells. **Lanes 5–8:** MB6A cells. The primary antibodies were monoclonal anti-T200 (lanes 1, 5), monoclonal anti-LFA-1 (lanes 2, 6), monoclonal anti-Mac-1 (lanes 3, 7), and polyclonal Fab fragments absorbed from polyclonal anti-MB6A Fab fragments on Sepharose-coupled purified LFA-1 (lanes 4, 8).

some lymphomas may become metastatic by activation of their inherent lymphoid invasive machinery. This notion is supported by the effect of pertussis toxin on invasion and metastasis formation, which was similar for the regular MB6A lymphoma and the TAM2D2 T-cell hybridoma. The pertussis toxin effects and the induction of invasion by the mutated *ras*-oncogene indicate that particular signal transmission pathways play an essential role. It is thus conceivable that in other lymphomas invasiveness is due to the unregulated autonomous activity of oncogenes that form part of these pathways.

The invasion process in the liver would appear relatively simple as compared to

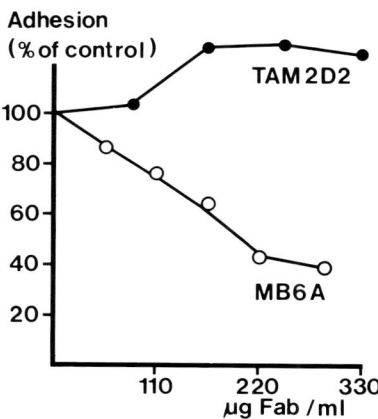

Fig. 4. Effect of Fab fragments prepared from a rabbit anti-MB6A antiserum, which did not precipate LFA-1, on adhesion of ^{51}Cr-labeled MB6A and TAM2D2 cells to hepatocyte cultures. **Solid symbols,** TAM2D2; **open circles,** MB6A. Values given are percentages of controls.

other organs, because it involves a limited number of only intercellular interactions. Our results show, however, that the process is quite complex and involves several different cellular constituents the activity of which may be highly specific for tumor cell type and also for the liver. The initial adhesion to liver cells is mediated by adhesion molecules, which are distinct for carcinoma and lymphoma cells, but also among lymphoma cells, which share molecules such as LFA-1, additional adhesion mediators appear to be different. Furthermore, since there is no correlation between invasiveness in hepatocyte and fibroblast cultures, invasion mechanisms are at least in part specific for the tissues to be invaded. We anticipate that a further elucidation of the molecular details of these processes will enable us to explain differences in metastatic behaviour between tumor cell types.

REFERENCES

1. Bross ID, Viadana E, Pickren JW: Virchows Arch [A] 365:91–101, 1975.
2. Chang TW, Celis E, Eisen HN, Solomon F: Proc Natl Acad Sci USA 76:2917–2921, 1979.
3. Collard JG., Schijven JF, Roos E: Cancer Res 47:754–759, 1987.
4. De Baetselier P, Roos E, Brys L, Remels L, Feldman M: Int J Cancer 34:731–738, 1984.
5. Dingemans KP: JNCI 51:1883–1895, 1973.
6. Dustin ML, Rothlein R, Bhan AK, Dinarello CA, Springer TA J Immunol 137:245–255, 1986.
7. Katada T, Ui M: Proc Natl Acad Sci USA 79:3129–3133, 1982.
8. Martz E: Hum Immunol 18:3–37, 1987.
9. Middelkoop OP, Roos E, Van de Pavert IV: J Cell Sci 56:461–470, 1982.
10. Middelkoop OP, Van Bavel P, Calafat J, Roos E: Cancer Res 45:3825–3835, 1985.
11. Roos E, Dingemans KP, Van de Pavert IV, Van den Bergh-Weerman MA: JNCI 58:399–407, 1977.
12. Roos E, Dingemans KP, Van de Pavert IV, Van den Bergh-Weerman MA: Br J Cancer 38:88–99, 1978.
13. Roos E, La Rivière G, Collard JG, Stukart MJ, De Baetselier P: Cancer Res 45:6238–6243, 1985.
14. Roos E, Middelkoop OP, Van de Pavert IV: JNCI 73:963–969, 1984.
15. Roos E, Roossien FF: J Cell Biol, 105:553–559, 1987.
16. Roos E, Tulp A, Middelkoop OP, Van de Pavert IV: JNCI 72:1173–1180, 1984.
17. Roos E, Van de Pavert IV: Clin Exp Metastasis 1:173–180, 1983.
18. Roos E, Van de Pavert IV: J Cell Sci 55:233–245, 1982.
19. Roos E, Van de Pavert IV, Middelkoop OP: J Cell Sci 47:385–397, 1981.
20. Sanchez-Madrid F, Nagy JA, Robbins E, Simon P, Springer TA: J Exp Med 158:1785–1803, 1983.
21. Savion N, Vlodavsky I, Fuks Z: J Cell Physiol 118:169–178, 1984.
22. Schirrmacher V, Shantz G, Clauer K, Komitowski D, Zimmermann HP, Lohmann-Mathes ML: Int J Cancer 23:233–244, 1979.
23. Shimonkevitz R, Cerottini JC, MacDonald HR: J Immunol 135:1555–1557, 1985.
24. Spangrude GJ, Araneo BA, Daynes RA: J Immunol 134:2900–2906, 1985.
25. Spangrude GJ, Braten BC, Daynes RA: J Immunol 132:354–362, 1984.
26. Springer TA, Davignon D, Ho MK, Kürzinger K, Martz E, Sanchez-Madrid F: Immunol Rev 68:171–195, 1982
27. Stryer L, Bourne HR: Annu Rev Cell Biol 2:391–419, 1986.
28. Thorgeirsson UP, Turpeenniemi-Hujanen T, Williams JE, Westin EH, Heilman CA, Talmadge JE, Liotta LA: Mol Cell Biol 5:259–262, 1985.
29. Verschueren H, Dekegel D, De Baetselier P: Invasion Metastasis 7:1–15, 1987.
30. Vousden KH, Eccles SA, Purvies J, Marshall CJ: Int J Cancer 37:425–433, 1986.
31. Wakelam MJO, Davies SA, Houslay MD, McKay I, Marshall CJ, Hall A: Nature 323:173–176, 1986.
32. La Rivière G, Schipper C, Collard JG, Roos E: Cancer Res, (in press).
33. Collard JG, Van de Poll M, Scheffer A, Roos E, Hopman AHM, Geurts Van Kessel AHM, Van Dongen JJM: Cancer Res 47:6666–6670, 1987.
34. Roos E, Van de Pavert IV: Cancer Res 47:5439–5444, 1987.

Use of the Nude Mouse Model to Investigate Human Colorectal Cancer Metastases

Raffaella Giavazzi

Mario Negri Institute for Pharmacological Research, 24100 Bergamo, Italy

The malignant potential of human colorectal carcinomas can be investigated in athymic nude mice. The metastatic potential of tumor cells varies with the site of initial implantation. Thus, both tumor cells and host properties need to be taken into account in designing an experimental model for investigating the biology and therapy of cancer metastases. Since the most common site of colorectal carcinoma metastasis is the liver, we investigated the capacity of human colorectal-derived tumor cells to produce metastases in the liver of nude mice. Human colorectal carcinomas, originating from primary neoplasms and/or hepatic metastases of different patients, were enzymatically dissociated, and single-cell suspensions were injected into different sites of nude mice. Tumor cells transplanted into the subcutis or muscularis of nude mice produced only local tumors without macroscopic visceral metastases. However, the same tumor cells given intrasplenically gave rise to liver tumors. The capacity to proliferate in the liver of nude mice was a distinct characteristic of each cell line and marked tumor cells with different malignant potential. Human colorectal tumors were established as continuous cell lines in the nude mouse, and their metastatic potential was maintained at different passages.

Key words: colorectal carcinoma, nude mouse, intrasplenic injection, liver metastases

Colorectal carcinoma is one of the most devastating malignant neoplasms. Patients frequently already have clinical evidence of tumor dissemination at diagnosis; many more show local or distant recurrent disease shortly after surgical excision of the primary tumor [1]. There is an urgent need to identify an active therapy for colorectal cancer metastases, and the design of such therapeutic modalities, to be effective, must be based on considerations of the biology of malignancy.

Animal models have proved invaluable in cancer research. In the recent years the use of the nude mouse mutant, T-lymphocyte deficient [2] as a recipient of xenotransplanted tumors, has progressively increased. However, this model's utility in relation to cancer metastasis has been limited by the fact that human tumors transplanted into nude mice rarely produce metastases [3–6]. Nevertheless, it was recently shown that under

Received May 18, 1987.

© 1988 Alan R. Liss, Inc.

appropriate experimental conditions human tumors grafted into nude mice can metastasize in a consistent fashion [3–6]. In this context we review studies of human colorectal carcinoma (HCC) transplanted into nude mice and discuss our experience in establishing an experimental model for investigating the biology and therapy of colorectal cancer metastases.

METASTATIC BEHAVIOUR OF HUMAN COLORECTAL NEOPLASM TRANSPLANTED INTO NUDE MOUSE

The metastatic process comprises a sequence of linked events that tumor cells have to complete [7]. To form metastases, tumor cells that leave the primary tumor have to possess all the characteristics necessary to invade, survive in the circulation, arrest in a distant capillary bed, extravasate, and finally grow in a secondary organ, all this in a continuous interaction between host and tumor cells.

It is now commonly accepted that neoplasms are biologically heterogeneous [8–10] and continuous emergence of clonal populations with different biological phenotypes, including metastatic potential, has been proposed during tumor progression [11]. Such biological heterogeneity has been observed not only within primary tumors and between primary tumor and metastases and among metastases, but also within an individual metastasis. For instance, for human colon cancer, subpopulations of cells with different tumorigenicity and malignant potential have been described [10,12,13] in nude mice. Biological differences were also described for xenografted tumors originating from two distinct metastases of a patient with a colon carcinoma [13]. This complexity in the pathogenesis of metastasis may explain why the process is inefficient and why only a few of the tumor cells that leave the primary tumor are indeed able to form metastases. It also shows that the study of tumor biology and therapy cannot be confined to the primary tumor.

Much work has been published on the metastatic behaviour of rodent tumors, whereas studies on the metastasis of human tumors in experimental models, of immunosuppressed or genetically athymic animals, are fewer [3–6]. Since the first report by Giovanella with a human melanoma cell line that formed metastases to the lung and lymph nodes [14], reports on human tumor metastasis in the nude mouse have gradually accumulated. Human colon cancer lines that produce micro- and/or macroscopic metastases in the nude mouse lung and lymph nodes have also been described [6,10,15–20].

The majority of studies on human tumor metastases in nude mice deals with cultured cell lines. In our laboratory we began to investigate the malignant behaviour in nude mice of freshly isolated HCC. Tumor cells derived from primary HCC or liver metastases were injected at different sites in nude mice (16). Subsequent to transplantation into the subcutis or the muscularis, the formation of macroscopic metastases was rare, even in mice that survive up to 6 months after surgical removal of the tumor graft.

In the metastatic process the first step that tumor cells have to complete is to detach themselves from the primary tumor, to invade and enter the circulation, then grow in a defined environment. With this in mind, the tumor implantation site may influence not only the growth of the primary tumor but also the formation of distant metastases. It is becoming increasingly evident that production of metastases in nude mice is in fact modulated by the site of tumor cell implantation. For instance, tumor cells implanted subcutaneously (s.c.) in the cranial aspect of the nude mouse's flank produced more metastases than tumor cells implanted in the posterior aspect [19].

Several investigators have shown that human tumors that were not invasive when growing s.c. as solid tumors produced ascites with local infiltration and distant metastases when injected intraperitonealy (i.p.) [6,18,21,22]. This is the case of a colon line, which, when injected s.c., grew locally completely encapsulated in dense connective tissue and metastases were associated with extensive invasion of the capsula, but were limited to regional lymph nodes. The same tumor cells injected i.p. disseminated in the abdominal organs and formed metastases to mediastinal lymph nodes and lungs [18]. Furthermore, a poorly differentiated colon carcinoma produced ascitic carcinoma and distant metastases after i.p. injection, while three better-differentiated colon carcinomas grew in the peritoneum of the mice as solid tumors with no evidence of distant metastases [6]. It is important to consider that in most of the studies referred to, human tumor cells were grafted into a site that does not correspond to their anatomical origin. Orthotopic transplantation in nude mice, associated with metastasis formation, has been described for s.c. injected human melanomas [23], a human pancreatic tumor cell line injected into the duodenal lobe of the pancreas [24], and a hormone-responsive human mammary carcinoma injected into the mammary fat pad [25]. For colon tumors, orthotopic transplantation into the intestine of syngeneic mice and liver metastasis formation has been described for a chemically induced murine adenocarcinoma. The same tumor transplanted s.c. or injected directly intraportally was not followed by liver metastasis, suggesting that growth at the primary site promoted hepatic metastasis formation [26].

More recently, in nude mice, the injection of two human colon carcinomas in the dissecting part of the large bowel was reported as being followed by infiltration of the colonic wall and mesenteric lymph nodes. This is in contrast to two human melanomas that were not invasive in the same experimental conditions. However, no hepatic metastases were reported in that study [6,20].

EXPERIMENTAL NUDE MOUSE MODEL TO INVESTIGATE HUMAN COLORECTAL CARCINOMA HEPATIC METASTASES

Metastasis can be considered the major problem in treating patients with colorectal carcinoma. More than 50% of patients already have micro- or macrolymphatic and hematogenous (mainly liver) tumor cell dissemination at diagnosis [1]. To date treatment of recurrent colon carcinoma metastases has given poor results. In order to develop new, efficacious therapies we need appropriate experimental models to investigate their biology and therapy. The response of tumors to therapy can be influenced by the interaction between tumor cell properties and host environment such as anatomical location, defense mechanisms, or growth factors.

As shown above, human tumors, including colorectal carcinoma, have usually been transplanted in the subcutis of nude mice, a site rarely metastasizing, and certainly not to the liver. To bypass local tumor growth at the injection site and study tumor production in the liver, murine and human tumor cells have been injected in the spleen (intrasplenically [i.s.]) of recipient animals [16,17,27–29]. From here they gain access easily to the bloodstream, reach the liver, and eventually grow as secondary tumors. We have shown in fact that [^{125}I]-IdUrd-labeled human colon cancer cells arrest in the nude mouse liver shortly after injection into the spleen [30]. We found that intrasplenic injection of HCC cells was followed by the tumor growth in the spleen and tumor foci in the liver of nude mice. The malignant potential of the HCC lines was determined from the liver tumor burden at autopsy [16].

We have investigated HCC derived from primary neoplasms or from metastases of different patients [16,30]. The incidence of mice with liver tumors and the number of liver tumor foci differed between the HCC lines. In fact, i.s. injection of HCC cells followed by tumor growth in the liver distinguished HCC with different malignant potential. The most dramatic expression of malignant potential in the liver was observed for two HCC derived from patient's hepatic metastasis [16]. The growth of a "primary" tumor in the spleen of nude mice did not significantly influence the formation of tumor cells in the spleen as we found in experiments in which splenectomy was done after tumor cell injection in the spleen [30]. That liver tumor formation was not associated with tumor growth in the spleen was shown by the finding that all the HCC examined grew in the spleen, but their growth was not correlated to liver tumor formation [16].

These data taken together suggest that the final outgrowth of liver metastases depends on the ability of tumor cells to proliferate in the liver. Kozlowki and coworkers investigated the metastatic behaviour of human cell lines of different histological origin injected i.s. in nude mice; the mice developed metastases depending on the site of injection and ultimately depending on the nature of the tumor cells [17]. More recently we reported that variants of an early established human renal carcinoma were highly metastatic to the lung when grown s.c. or in the kidney of nude mice but rarely produced tumors in the liver when injected in the spleen [31].

HCC were maintained as continuous tumor lines in nude mice. Single cell suspensions were obtained by enzymatic digestion of the s.c. growing tumors and injected i.s. into nude mice [30]. Tables I–III show the different malignant potential of three HCC derived from a primary tumor, a liver metastasis, and a lymph node metastasis. Cells from the hepatic metastasis-derived line produced extensive liver tumors in all mice by 30 days after injection. Cells from the primary tumor-derived and from the lymph node metastasis-derived lines produced fewer liver tumor foci and took longer. The three HCC lines maintained their characteristic malignant behaviour after passages in nude mice. Their capacity to proliferate in the liver of the nude mouse slightly increased with passages, but their relative malignant potential appeared stable. This increased metastatic ability was more evident for the primary-derived tumor cells, suggesting a possible progressive selection of malignant cell populations within a tumor. The histological characteristics of the original neoplasm were maintained in the liver tumors in the nude mouse [16,30], and the human nature of these tumors was ascertained by isoenzyme analysis. Liver foci from nude mice consisted of cells with human karyotype.

TABLE I. Production of Liver Tumors in Nude Mouse by a Primary Tumor-Derived HCC*

Passage No.[a]	Autopsy day	Mice with spleen tumors[b]	Mice with liver tumors	Median liver tumor foci (range)
3	90	5/5	2/6	0 (0–1)
5	50	5/5	4/5	9 (0–11)
6	90	6/6	5/6	11 (0–>100)

*From Giavazzi et al. [30].
[a]Passage after the implantation of surgical specimen into nude mice.
[b]$1-2 \times 10^6$ cells were injected i.s. into nude mice.

TABLE II. Production of Liver Tumors in Nude Mouse by a Lymph Node Metastasis-Derived HCC*

Passage No.[a]	Autopsy day	Mice with spleen tumors[b]	Mice with liver tumors	Median liver tumor foci (range)
4	90	5/5	1/5	0 (0–2)
7	30	5/5	2/5	0 (0–4)
8	40	6/6	4/6	5 (0–20)

*From Giavazzi et al. [30].
[a]Passage after the implantation of surgical specimen into nude mice.
[b]Nude mice were given $1-2 \times 10^6$ tumor cells in the spleen.

TABLE III. Production of Liver Tumors in Nude Mouse by a Hepatic Metastasis-Derived HCC*

Passage No.[a]	Autopsy day	Mice with spleen tumors[b]	Mice with liver tumors	Median liver tumor foci (range)
6	33	8/8	8/8	All >300
7	29	5/5	5/5	300 (10–>300)
9	26	5/6	5/6	101 (0–>300)
12	28	5/5	5/5	300 (14–>300)

*From Giavazzi et al. [30].
[a]Passage after the implantation of surgical specimen into nude mice.
[b]$1-2 \times 10^6$ tumor cells injected i.s. into nude mice.

The basic characteristics of the original karyotype were maintained with only slight modifications [32].

CONCLUSIONS

These data collectively show that HCC can metastasize in the nude mouse, but it depends on the experimental conditions. The site of tumor cell implantation influences tumor growth and metastasis formation, but the final tumor outgrowth depends on the tumor cells' intrinsic characteristics. Injection of HCC in the spleen of the nude mouse led to liver tumor formation. The ability to proliferate in the liver parenchyma marks tumor cell populations with different malignant potential, and it appears to be a distinct characteristic of each tumor cell population. The HCC-liver tumor model in the nude mouse offers an experimental system for investigating liver-tumor cell interactions in the metastatic process and for assessing antimetastatic therapy.

REFERENCES

1. August DA, Ottow RT, Sugarbaker PH: Cancer Metastasis Rev 3:303–324, 1984.
2. Rygaard J, Povlsen CO: Acta Pathol Microbiol Immunol Scand 77:758–760, 1969.
3. Fidler IJ: Cancer Metastasis Rev 5:29–52, 1986.
4. Giovanella BC, Fogh J: Adv Cancer Res 44:70–120, 1985.
5. Sharkey FE, Fogh J: Cancer Metastasis Rev 3:341–360, 1984.

6. Sordat BCM, Ueyama Y, Fogh J: In Fogh J, Giovanella BC (eds): "The Nude Mouse in Experimental and Clinical Research." New York: Academic Press, 1982, pp 95–147.
7. Poste G, Fidler IJ: Nature 283:139–146, 1980.
8. Fidler IJ, Hart IR: Science 217:998–1003, 1982.
9. Heppner GH: Cancer Res 44:2259–2265, 1984.
10. Spremulli EN, Dexter DL: J Clin Oncol 1:496–509, 1983.
11. Nowell PC: Science 194:23–28, 1976.
12. Brattain MG, Levine AE, Chakrabarty S, Yeoman LC, Willson JKV, Long B: Cancer Metastasis Rev 3:177–191, 1984.
13. Spremulli EN, Scott C, Campbell DE, Libbey NP, Shochat D, Gold DV, Dexter DL: Cancer Res 43:3828–3835, 1983.
14. Giovanella BC, Yim SO, Morgan AC, Stehlin JS, Williams LJ Jr: JNCI 50:1051–1053, 1973.
15. Fermor B, Umpleby HC, Lever JV, Symes MO, Williamson RCN: JNCI 76:347–349, 1986.
16. Giavazzi R, Campbell DE, Jessup JM, Cleary K, Fidler IJ: Cancer Res 46:1928–1933, 1986.
17. Kozlowski JM, Fidler IJ, Campbell D, Xu Z, Kaighn ME, Hart IR: Cancer Res 44:3522–3529, 1984.
18. Kyriazis AP, DiPersio L, Michael GJ, Pesce AJ, Stinnett JD: Cancer Res 38:3186–3190, 1978.
19. Kyriazis AP, Kyriazis AA, McCombs WB III, Kereiakes JA: Cancer Res 41:3995–4000, 1981.
20. Wang WR, Sordat B, Piguet D, Sordat M: In Sordat B (ed) "4th International Workshop on Immune-Deficient Animals in Experimental Research." Kargel, Basel, 1984, pp 239–245.
21. Lockshin A, Giovanella BC, De Ipolyi PD, Williams JL Jr, Mendoza JT, Yim SO, Stehlin JS Jr: Cancer Res 45:345–350, 1985.
22. Takahashi S, Konishi Y, Nakatani K, Inui S, Kojima K, Shiratori T: JNCI 60:925–927, 1978.
23. Giovanella BC, Stehlin JS, Santamaria C, Yim SO, Morgan AC, Williams CJ Jr, Leibovitz A, Fialkow PJ, Mumford DM: JNCI 56:1131–1142, 1976.
24. Mong HT, Chu TM: Tumor Biol 6:89–98, 1985.
25. Shafie SM, Liotta LA: Cancer Lett 11:81–87, 1980.
26. Tan RH, Holyoke ED, Goldrosen MH: JNCI 59:1537–1544, 1977.
27. Kopper L, van Hanh T, Lapis K: J Cancer Res Clin Oncol 103:31–38, 1982.
28. Lafreniere R, Rosenberg SA: JNCI 76:309–315, 1986.
29. Leduc EH: Cancer Res 19:1091–1095, 1959.
30. Giavazzi R, Jessup J. Milburn, Campbell DE, Walker SM, Fidler IJ: JNCI 77:1303, 1986.
31. Naito S, Von Eschenbach AC, Giavazzi R, Fidler IJ: Cancer Res 46:4109–4115, 1986.
32. Giavazzi R, Jessup JM, Pathak S, Morikawa K, Fidler IJ: In Moyer MP, Poste GH (eds): "Colon Cancer Cells" (in press).

New Approaches to Achieve Systemic Activation of Macrophages for Destruction of Disseminated Cancer Cells

Isaiah J. Fidler

Department of Cell Biology, The University of Texas M. D. Anderson Hospital and Tumor Institute at Houston, Houston, Texas 77030

Tumoricidal macrophages can recognize and destroy neoplastic cells in vitro and in vivo while leaving nonneoplastic cells unharmed. These macrophages can be activated to become tumoricidal by interaction with phospholipid vesicles (liposomes) containing various immunomodulators, such as lymphokines, bacterial products, and synthetic molecules. In the activation process, intravenously administered liposomes are cleared from the circulation by phagocytic cells. The endocytosis of the liposomes containing the immunomodulators generates cytotoxic properties in the macrophages in situ in a process independent of the thymus: it can be achieved in mice without functional T cells such as athymic nude mice or mice immunosuppressed by cyclosporin A. The multiple administration of liposomes containing immunomodulators eradicates cancer metastases in several rodent-tumor systems, but success is limited by the ratio of effector to target cells. Thus, small metastases are destroyed, but once metastases exceed a certain number of cells, therapeutic efficacy is diminished. For this reason, we have been investigating various methods to reduce the overall metastatic burden by modalities such as chemotherapy or radiotherapy before liposomal activation. The results of these investigations suggest that the systemic activation of macrophages provides an effective modality for treatment of metastases.

Key words: macrophages, metastasis, liposomes, therapy

By the time of diagnosis, human neoplasms can contain multiple populations of cells with different biological properties, such as growth rate, antigenic and immunogenic status, response to cytotoxic agents, presence of cell surface receptors and products, invasiveness, and metastatic potential [1–3]. Recent data indicate that metastases can arise from the nonrandom spread of specialized subpopulations of cells that preexist within the primary tumor [4], and that metastases can be clonal in their origin [5–7] and even result from the proliferation of a single cell [8]. Biological heterogeneity of cancer metastases is also due to phenotypic and genotypic instability of some metastatic cells, which can readily become resistant to chemotherapy [9]. Collectively, these data indicate that to be successful, the therapy of metastases must circumvent the problems

Received May 4, 1987.

© 1988 Alan R. Liss, Inc.

of biological diversity and the development of resistance by tumor cells. In this review, I discuss the evidence that appropriately activated macrophages can be used to eradicate metastases and emphasize the approaches undertaken to increase the efficiency of tumor cell destruction by such macrophages.

ACTIVATION OF MACROPHAGES TO THE TUMORICIDAL STATE

Normal macrophages do not lyse tumor cells [1]. Rather, in order to destroy tumor cells, macrophages must first undergo a series of events collectively referred to as "activation." "An activated macrophage" is a working definition and its use in the literature has been extended to describe a large number of macrophage characteristics that may or may not correlate with the capacity of macrophages to recognize and destroy microorganisms, parasites, or cancer cells [1,10]. In this paper, however, the term "activated macrophages" is reserved for those cells capable of lysing tumorigenic, but not normal, cells.

There are two major physiological pathways to achieve activation of macrophages to cytotoxicity against cancer cells. Although macrophages are readily activated by interaction with microorganisms or their products, the in vivo use of microorganisms to activate macrophages has been accompanied by significant toxicity. The notable exception is the water-soluble, low-molecular-weight (M_r 459), synthetic moiety muramyl dipeptide (MDP), which has potent effects on a variety of host defense cells, including macrophages [10–15]. Recently, a lipophilic MDP derivative, muramyl tripeptide phosphatidylethanolamine (MTP-PE), has been synthesized [11,15]. Although muramyl peptides influence several macrophage functions in vitro, comparable effects have not been observed in vivo because these molecules are rapidly cleared after parenteral administration [16,17]. Even when injected at very high doses, MDP fails to induce significant macrophage-mediated antitumor activity [15].

The other category of activating agents with the potential for therapeutic use in vivo are the lymphokines, generally referred to as macrophage-activation factors (MAF) [18], which include gamma-interferon (IFN-γ) [19–21]. In general, attempts to use lymphokines to activate macrophages in situ to enhance host defense against cancer have also been unsuccessful, probably owing to the very short half-life of lymphokines in the circulation [18,24]. Regardless of the method of their activation, tumoricidal macrophages acquire the ability to recognize and destroy neoplastic cells both in vitro and in vivo while leaving nonneoplastic cells unharmed. The mechanism for this is not known but appears to be nonimmunologic in nature and to require intimate cell-to-cell contact [22,23].

THE USE OF LIPOSOMES TO DELIVER SIGNALS TO PHAGOCYTIC CELLS

Phospholipid vesicles (liposomes) provide a unique carrier vehicle for the delivery of biologically active materials to phagocytic cells in vivo. Following intravenous administration, >90% of liposomes are removed by phagocytic cells in the liver, spleen, lymph nodes, and bone marrow and by circulating monocytes [25,26]. This physiological fact allows "targeting" of liposome-encapsulated materials to macrophages in vivo [15,25,26].

In order for liposomes to serve as vehicles for the delivery of compounds to macrophages, they must bind to and be phagocytosed by the cells. We have found that macrophages can recognize certain classes of phospholipids. Specifically, liposomes containing negatively charged phosphatidylserine (PS) are phagocytosed up to 10-fold faster than are liposomes of the same size and configuration that contain positively charged stearylamine or those consisting only of negatively charged phosphatidylcholine (PC) [15,25–27]. The presence of PS in the phospholipid bilayer of small unilamellar liposomes or large uni- or multilamellar liposomes results in their enhanced binding to and phagocytosis by all cells of the reticuloendothelial system, including mouse peritoneal macrophages, mouse Kupffer cells, mouse or rat alveolar macrophages, human alveolar macrophages, and human peripheral blood monocytes [1].

The in vivo distribution and fate of liposomes is influenced by the size, surface charge, and lipid composition of the vesicles [25–27]. We have found that large multitilamellar vesicles (MLV) consisting of PC and PS (7:3 molar ratio) were the most effective vehicle for the delivery of encapsulated compounds to fixed macrophages in organs rich in RES activity and to blood monocytes in the lung. The monocytes then migrated out of the circulation and differentiated into lung macrophages [28].

Regardless of the source of macrophages, development of the activated phenotype requires the phagocytic uptake of liposomes followed by a lag period of several hours before expression of tumoricidal activity [1,15]. Studies on the mechanism of activation by liposome-encapsulated activators indicate that participation of macrophage cell surface receptors is not required and that activation results from the interaction of immunomodulating molecules with intracellular targets [20,21].

SYSTEMIC ACTIVATION OF MACROPHAGES FOLLOWING INJECTION OF LIPOSOMES CONTAINING IMMUNOMODULATORS

The intravenous injection of appropriate MLV containing MDP or MTP-PE immunomodulators produced in situ activation of mouse lung macrophages [15]. This activation did not occur by an indirect action of the immunomodulator on T cells and a consequent release of lymphokines that activate macrophages [29]. This conclusion is based on data from experiments in which alveolar macrophages of mice with impaired T cell function—mice exposed to UV radiation, thymectomized adult mice exposed to x-rays, and athymic nude mice [29], and mice treated with cyclosporin A [30]—were all rendered tumoricidal by the systemic administration of liposome-encapsulated MTP-PE but not by control liposome preparations.

SYSTEMIC ACTIVATION OF MACROPHAGES AND TREATMENT OF METASTASIS FOLLOWING INJECTION OF LIPOSOMES CONTAINING IMMUNOMODULATORS

The B16-BL6 melanoma cell line, which is syngeneic to C57BL/6 mice, was used as the primary model to determine the effectiveness of liposome-encapsulated materials in the treatment of metastases. After implantation in the footpad, this tumor metastasizes to lymph nodes and the lungs in more than 90% of mice [30]. Mice were given injections of the melanoma cells, and 4–5 weeks later, when the tumors had reached a size of 10 to 12 mm, the leg bearing the tumor, including the popliteal lymph node, was amputated. Three days later, the mice was injected i.v. with MLV prepared from chromatographically pure PC and PS and containing immunomodulators or a control preparation, twice weekly for 4 weeks (8 i.v. injections). We used these liposomes because they are arrested efficiently in the lungs as well as in organs of the reticuloendothelial system following i.v. injection [1,15], and they are not toxic at the dose used [31].

Spontaneous metastases in the lungs and lymph nodes were well established at the time treatment with liposomes began. Mice treated with saline, with free lymphokines, with free MDP, or with liposomes containing saline died by day 90 of the experiment, i.e., 60 days after the amputation of the tumor-bearing leg. Significantly, 65–70% of mice injected intravenously with liposome-encapsulated lymphokines or MDP were alive when the experiments were terminated at 200 days. At the time of first liposome treatment, we estimate that the metastases in this tumor system contained at least 10^7 tumor cells. Since the median survival time of mice injected with as few as 10 viable B16 cells (admixed with 10^6 dead cells) is 40 to 50 days, we speculate that the tumor burden in the successfully treated mice (alive on day 200) must have been reduced to less than 10 viable cells [1,15]. Similar data on the treatment of other murine metastatic tumors by the systemic administration of liposomes containing different immunomodulators have been published [32–36].

OPTIMIZATION AND LIMITATIONS OF LIPOSOME-IMMUNOMODULATORS THERAPY

Even under controlled laboratory conditions, 30% of the mice treated with liposomes containing immunomodulators died of extensive disease. These fatal tumor cells, however, were not resistant to macrophage-mediated lysis [37]. Several questions thus remain unanswered: 1) Could manipulation of the schedule of liposome-MTP-PE administration influence the outcome of the treatment? 2) What is the major factor distinguishing "treatment success" from "treatment failure" mice? 3) Were the surviving mice free of dormant metastatic cells in the lung?

In the above studies, liposomes were injected twice per week for 4 weeks. In the present study, we determined whether varying this schedule of administration could influence therapeutic efficacy. Groups of mice whose primary B16-BL6 melanomas were resected 3 days previously received i.v. injections of liposomes containing MTP-PE according to the following schedules: once a week for 8 weeks; twice weekly for 1 week; twice weekly for 2 weeks; twice weekly for 3 weeks; and twice weekly for 4 weeks. Control mice were injected twice weekly for 4 weeks with liposome preparations containing saline. All animals were monitored daily for 250 days. Dead or moribund animals were necropsied to ascertain the presence or absence of melanoma metastases. Animals surviving at least 200 days after the last liposome treatment were considered to be free of disease [38].

The most effective schedule for treatment of lung metastases was the twice weekly injection for 4 weeks: 68% of the mice were alive on day 200 of the experiment ($P<0.001$). Less impressive, but still statistically significant, survival was observed in the groups treated once weekly for 8 weeks (40% survival, $P<0.01$); twice weekly for 2 weeks (44% survival, $P<0.01$) and twice weekly for 3 weeks (45% survival, $P<0.001$).

The tumor burden in the lung and lymph node metastases on day 3 after leg amputation has been estimated to be between 5×10^6 and 1×10^7 cells [1,15]. The volume doubling time of B16-BL6 melanoma lung metastases ranges between 3 and 5 days [1]. For this reason, we wished to determine whether the timing of the first liposome administration was critical to the outcome of the treatment. In the next set of experiments, the first i.v. injection of liposomes was administered to groups of mice either 3 days,

7 days, or 10 days after the amputation of the hind footpad with the primary implanted melanoma. Control groups of mice were injected i.v. with liposomes containing saline solution. All mice were treated twice weekly for 4 weeks and then monitored daily for up to 250 days.

The systemic administration (8 i.v. injections) of liposomes containing saline had no therapeutic benefits regardless of the time of initial treatment. Treatment with liposomes containing MTP-PE had significant therapeutic benefits, but the degree of success depended upon the timing of the first treatment. The most impressive survival was observed in mice receiving the first treatment on day 3 after surgical removal of the primary tumor (65% survival, $P<0.001$). If the first treatment began on day 7, 45% of the mice survived ($P<0.01$), and if the first treatment began on day 10, only 33% of the mice survived ($P=0.2$).

We also investigated whether the lungs of animals surviving to day 200–250 of the study contained dormant melanoma cells. Lung cells of mice were dissociated, and 5×10^6 lung cells were injected s.c. into normal syngeneic recipients. No subcutaneous tumors developed in the mice injected with 5×10^6 cells disassociated from lungs of tumor-free mice. In contrast, 5×10^6 lung cells from normal mice admixed with 100 viable B16 melanoma cells produced subcutaneous tumors in 19 of 20 injected mice [38]. Collectively, these results show that the schedule of administrating liposomes containing MTP-PE that optimally activates tumoricidal properties in macrophages is also optimal for the treatment of systemic metastases.

SYNERGISTIC ACTIVATION OF MACROPHAGES BY LIPOSOMES CONTAINING MULTIPLE IMMUNOMODULATORS

Recent studies from our laboratory and many others have shown that free or liposome-encapsulated lymphokines (MAF, IFN-γ) and bacterial products (LPS, MDP) can act synergistically to activate the tumoricidal properties in macrophages [19–21,39,40]. Because liposomes can deliver more than one compound to macrophages in situ, we investigated whether the combination of MAF and MDP (within the same liposome) could produce synergistic activation of lung macrophages in vivo and enhance destruction of lung melanoma metastases [41].

Synergistic activation of the tumoricidal properties in lung macrophages by unencapsulated MAF and MDP has been previously shown to occur in vitro [19–21,39,40]. Neither the i.v. injection of free MAF nor free MDP, however, led to systemic activation of macrophages in situ. The i.v. administration of MLV containing optimal doses of MAF or MDP generated tumoricidal properties in lung macrophages [41]. On the other hand, i.v. administration of MLV containing a 1/20 dilution of MAF or 1/20 dilution of MDP did not activate the lung macrophages to become tumor cytotoxic. However, when these subthreshold doses of MAF and MDP were combined and encapsulated within the same MLV, significant in situ activation was produced.

Therapeutic experiments were carried out in mice with relatively large metastases. We postponed the start of the treatment until 7 days after the resection of the primary neoplasms to allow examination of the hypothesis that MAF and MDP encapsulated within the same liposme would act synergistically to activate macrophages in situ to destroy a larger number of metastatic tumor cells. At the time of first i.v. treatment, spontaneous pulmonary metastases were well established, with some lung metastases being 1 mm in diameter. Liposomes were injected twice weekly for 4 weeks (8 injections).

Practically all the mice receiving saline alone and MLV containing encapsulated, diluted MAF or diluted MDP died by day 90 of the experiment. Multiple i.v. injections of liposomes containing either optimal MDP or optimal MAF resulted in the long-term survival (>250 days) of 27% of the animals (5 of 18). Mice treated with MLV containing both MAF and MDP at individual subthreshold concentrations resulted in 50% survival at day 250 ($P=0.0007$) [41].

LOCAL THORACIC X-IRRADIATION FOLLOWED BY SYSTEMIC ACTIVATION OF MACROPHAGES

As discussed above, there is a second limiting factor in the treatment of metastases by activated macrophages: the tumor burden in metastases may exceed the destructive capability of the available activated macrophages. For this reason, we designed a study to determine whether the combination of local thoracic x-irradiation (LTI) with activation of blood monocytes would be beneficial for the treatment of large lung tumor colonies. Ionizing radiation has been shown to produce a logarithmic decrease in tumor cell survival [42], which thus reduces metastatic burden. Radiation also induces blood vessel damage and inflammation in irradiated tissues [43]. We reasoned that this might promote the arrest and influx of macrophages into the inflamed, damaged tissue. We combined LTI and systemic activation of macrophages by i.v. administration of liposomes containing MTP-PE to treat experimental lung metastases of a murine fibrosarcoma.

In the first set of experiments, we determined the dose of LTI that would not interfere with systemic activation of macrophages by MLV-MTP-PE. Two days after LTI of 5 or 8 Gy, mice were given i.v. injections of MLV containing saline or MLV containing 20 μg MTP-PE, as were control mice. One day thereafter, lung macrophages were harvested and assayed for cytotoxicity to B16-BL6 tumor cells in vitro. The results demonstrated that both 5- and 8-Gy LTI markedly decreased the number of recoverable lung macrophages. In contrast, the cytotoxicity of lung macrophages from mice treated with MLV containing MTP-PE was not reduced by prior LTI.

We next investigated the kinetics of the decrease in the number of lung macrophages at various intervals after 8-Gy LTI. A 60% decrease in the number of recoverable lung macrophages was found at 3 days after irradiation. Thereafter, the number increased gradually but remained below the control value even at 12 days after irradiation. These data suggested that liposomes containing immunomodulators should be administered at least 5 days after LTI, when recovery in the number of harvested lung macrophages occurs.

In the next set of experiments, mice were given i.v. injections of 1×10^5 fibrosarcoma cells and 5 days later they were exposed to 8-Gy LTI or sham irradiation (anesthetized). After 5 additional days, the mice were given i.v. injections of MLV containing saline or MTP-PE. The data demonstrate that the i.v. administration of MLV-MTP-PE (but not MLV-placebo) activated tumoricidal properties in alveolar macrophages of all groups of mice (normal, untreated, or irradiated mice with lung tumor colonies). Thus, the presence of micrometastases in the lung did not affect the magnitude of macrophage activation in normal or irradiated mice.

In the final experiments, we determined whether LTI, followed by systemic administration of liposomes containing MTP-PE, produced increased destruction of lung metastases. Mice were given i.v. injections of 1×10^5 fibrosarcoma cells. Five days later, treatment with LTI alone, liposomes alone, or combinations of the treatments began. The mice were observed daily for up to 120 days. Moribund or dead mice were autopsied. The experiment was carried out twice with very similar results. Practically all the mice (24 of 25) with lung tumor colonies that received no treatment died. The median survival time of mice with lung tumor colonies was 50 days (range, 20–101). Treatments with liposomes containing saline or MTP-PE did not decrease the median number of lung tumor colonies or significantly increase the overall survival of the mice. Treatment with irradiation alone followed by MLV containing saline prolonged the median survival and led to long-term survival of 8 of 25 mice (32%) ($P<0.01$, χ^2 test). The median number of lung tumor colonies in these treatment groups was reduced to 29 and 23, respectively. The most remarkable therapeutic results were achieved in mice given LTI and twice weekly (4 weeks) i.v. injections of liposomes containing MTP-PE. On day 120 of the experiment in this treatment group, 15 of 25 mice were alive. Even in the treatment failure mice, the median number of lung tumor colonies was significantly reduced, to 9 (range, 1–37) ($P<0.01$). Thus, the combined therapeutic modalities of LTI with liposomes containing MTP-PE produced a highly significant ($P<0.001$, χ^2 test) survival rate of 60%. Mice surviving on day 140 of the study were killed and necropsied. No cancer was found in these mice [44].

CONCLUSIONS

The successful therapy of disseminated metastases must circumvent the problem of neoplastic biological heterogeneity and the development of resistance to therapy by tumor cells. The major limitation in the treatment of disseminated cancer with macrophages activated in situ is not tumor cell resistance per se but rather the inability of macrophages to destroy large numbers of tumor cells. For this reason, it is important to begin studies on the use of combination of different therapies for metastases and to use tumoricidal macrophages for the destruction of tumor cells that resist conventional therapies.

ACKNOWLEDGMENTS

This work was supported by the R.E. "Bob" Smith Chair in Cell Biology.

REFERENCES

1. Fidler IJ: Cancer Res 45:4714–4726, 1985.
2. Fidler IJ, Poste G: Semin Oncol 12:209–222, 1985.
3. Fidler IJ, Balch CM: Curr Probl Surg 24:137–209, 1987.
4. Fidler IJ, Kripke ML: Science 197:893–895, 1977.
5. Talmadge JE, Wolman SR, Fidler IJ: Science 217:361–363, 1982.
6. Hu F, Wang RY, Hsu TC: JNCI 78:153–163, 1987.
7. Talmadge JE, Zbar B: JNCI 78:315–320, 1987.
8. Fidler IJ, Talmadge JE: Cancer Res 46:5167–5171, 1986.
9. Cifone MA, Fidler IJ: Proc Natl Acad Sci USA 78:6949–6952, 1981.
10. Chedid L, Carelli L, Audibert F: J Reticulo Endothel Soc 26:631–641, 1979.
11. Fidler IJ, Fogler WE, Tarcsay L, Schumann G, Braun DG, Schroit AJ: Adv Immunopharmacol 2:235–253, 1983.
12. Fogler WE, Fidler IJ: In Chirigos MA, Fenichel RL (eds): "Immune Modulation Agents and their Mechanisms." New York: Marcel Dekker, 1984, pp 498–512.
13. Gisler RH, Dietrich FM, Baschang G, Brownbill A, Schumann NG, Tarcsay L, Wachsmuth ED,

Dukor P: In Turk JL, Danker D (eds): "Immune Responsiveness." London: Macmillan, 1979, pp 133–160.
14. Lederer E: J Med Chem 23:819–825, 1980.
15. Fidler IJ: In Tomlinson E, Davis SS (eds): "Site Specific Drug Delivery." London: John Wiley & Sons, 1986, pp 111–134.
16. Fogler WE, Wade R, Baundish DE, Fidler IJ: J Immunol 135:1372–1377, 1985.
17. Parent M, Parant F, Chedid L, Yapo A, Petit JF, Lederer E: Int J Immunopharmacol 1:35–41, 1979.
18. Fidler IJ: Lymphokine Res 3:41–54, 1984.
19. Saiki I, Fidler IJ: J Immunol 135(1):684–688, 1985.
20. Saiki I, Sone S, Fogler WE, Kleinerman ES, Lopez-Berestein G, Fidler IJ: Cancer Res 45:6188–6193, 1985.
21. Fidler IJ, Fogler WE, Kleinerman ES, Saiki I: J Immunol 135:4289–4294, 1985.
22. Bucana CD, Hoyer LC, Schroit AJ, Kleinerman E, Fidler IJ: J Pathol 112:101–111, 1983.
23. Hibbs JB Jr: JNCI 53:1487–1492, 1974.
24. Poste G: Am J Pathol 96:595–606, 1979.
25. Schroit AJ, Hart IR, Madsen J, Fidler IJ: J Biol Response Mod 2:97–100, 1983.
26. Poste G, Kirsh R, Bugelski P: In Sunkara PS (ed): "Liposomes as a Drug Delivery System in Cancer Therapy: Novel Approaches to Cancer Chemotherapy." New York: Academic Press, 1984, pp 166–221.
27. Schroit AJ, Fidler IJ: Cancer Res 42:161–167, 1982.
28. Key ME, Talmadge JE, Fogler WE, Bucana C, Fidler IJ: JNCI 69:1189–1198, 1982.
29. Fidler IJ: J Immunol 127:1719–1720, 1981.
30. Fidler IJ: Science 208:1469–1471, 1980.
31. Hart IR, Fogler WE, Poste G, Fidler IJ: Cancer Immunol Immunother 10:157–166, 1981.
32. Deodhar SD, Barna BP, Edinger M, Chiang T: J Biol Response Mod 1:27–34, 1982.
33. Lopez-Berestein G, Mehta K, Mehta R, Juliano RL, Hersh EM: J Immunol 130:1500–1504, 1983.
34. Lopez-Berestein G, Milas L, Hunter N, Mehta K, Eppstein D, VanderPas MA, Mathews TR, Hersh EM: Clin Exp Metastasis 2(2):366–367, 1984.
35. Phillips NC, Mora ML, Chedid L, Lefrancier P, Bernard J: Cancer Res 45:128–135, 1985.
36. Talmadge JE, Lenz BF, Klabansky R, Simon R, Riggs C, Guo S, Oldham RK, Fidler IJ: Cancer Res 46:1160–1164, 1986.
37. Fogler WE, Fidler IJ: Cancer Res 45:14–18, 1985.
38. Fidler IJ: Cancer Immunol Immunother 21:169–173, 1986.
39. Sone S, Fidler IJ: J Immunol 125:2454–2460, 1980.
40. Sone S, Fidler IJ: Cell Immunol 57:42–50, 1981.
41. Fidler IJ, Schroit AJ: J Immunol 133(1):515–518, 1984.
42. Suit HD: In Fletcher GH (ed): "Radiation Biology: A Basis for Radiotherapy." Textbook of Radiotherapy. Philadelphia: Lea and Febiger, pp 65–97, 1966.
43. Poste G, Bucana C, Raz A, Bugelski P, Kirsh R, Fidler IJ: Cancer Res 42:1412–1422, 1982.
44. Saiki I, Milas L, Hunter N, Fidler IJ: Cancer Res 46:4966–4970, 1986.

Use of a Virus-Modified Tumor Cell Vaccine for Postoperative Immunotherapy of Metastases in an Animal Model System

Volker Schirrmacher, Paul von Hoegen, and Rüdiger Heicappell

Institut für Immunologie und Genetik, Deutsches Krebsforschungszentrum, D-6900 Heidelberg, Federal Republic of Germany

Key words: tumor vaccines, immunotherapy of metastases, cytotoxic T lymphocytes

The aim of our study was the postoperative activation of tumor-specific T-cells as a means to achieve immune control of minimal residual disease. In contrast to unspecific immune stimulation, the activation of specific T-cell reactivity can lead to long-lasting antitumor immunity. In several instances, immunization with modified tumor cells led to the induction of tumor immunity against the original nonmodified tumor cells. The rationale of our approach was therefore to develop a modified tumor vaccine that combined a specific component (tumor cells expressing a tumor-associated antigen) with a nonspecific adjuvant component. Our concept of postoperative immunotherapy consisted of 1) reduction of the total tumor burden by surgery, and 2) postoperative immunization with a modified highly immunogenic tumor vaccine. We postulate that tumor-bearing animals or tumor patients might be sensitized at the level of cell-mediated immunity against the corresponding tumor but that the sensitization is not sufficient to activate this cell-mediated immunity. Upon vaccination a cell-mediated immune reaction will be initiated at the site of the vaccine inoculation, thereby recruiting and activating the host's tumor-specific T-cell-mediated immune system. Among the recruited cells we might selectively enrich for the tumor-specific immune cells and thereby achieve a selective activation of these tumor-specific clones. Tumor-specific precursor T-cells might then become activated to tumor-specific effector T-cells, such as cytotoxic T-cells via a second signal mediated through the virus (or another immune-activating component), and these activated cells should recirculate, detect, and destroy micrometastases. This active specific immunization (ASI) procedure might become an adjuvant therapy in combination with surgery in conditions where cell-mediated immune responses against cancer cells play a role and where micrometastases have already been established. In other situations (too-large tumor burden, advanced disease progression, suppression of immune responsiveness) this procedure is not expected to function. In this overview we summarize our

Received May 14, 1987.

© 1988 Alan R. Liss, Inc.

findings that have led to the development of this concept and our experiments concerning the mechanism of action of the virus-modified tumor vaccine.

THE ESb TUMOR MODEL SYSTEM

The mouse tumor line ESb is a spontaneous, highly metastatic variant of the methylcholanthrene-induced T-cell lymphoma L5178YE (Eb) [1,2]. The etiology of this variant, which most likely arose by fusion with a host macrophage [3], and the expression of cell surface markers of T-cells and macrophages [4] and of degradative enzymes [5,6] have been described. When transplanted subcutaneously to normal syngeneic DBA/2 mice, less than ten cells of this highly agressive variant can grow, metastasize, and kill the host within a few weeks. Because of this agressiveness and the speed with which this tumor infiltrates liver, spleen, and lung, this tumor is very difficult to treat and represents a true challenge for the design of effective antimetastatic therapy strategies.

T-CELL-MEDIATED HOST IMMUNE RESPONSES TO ESb TUMOR CELLS

Tumor immunization/protection experiments revealed that the ESb line expresses a tumor-associated transplantation antigen (TATA), which can induce weak protective immunity [7] and which can activate specific cytotoxic T-lymphocytes (CTL) following in vivo sensitization and in vitro restimulation protocols [8]. Anti-ESb CTL had the same fine specificity as the protective immunity in vivo, and both were able to distinguish the metastatic variant from the parental tumor Eb [7]. The strength of the host antitumor response depended to a great extent on the site of tumor cell inoculation and thus on its microenvironment [2,9]. By far the strongest response was obtained in the pinna where as many as 5×10^4 life syngeneic ESb tumor cells could be regularly rejected. In virtually all other sites of the body progressive tumor growth rather than spontaneous rejections were observed. When we compared the immune status of tumor-specific T-cells in tumor-immune animals and tumor-bearing animals we found a difference: CTL precursor (CTLP) of tumor immune animals could be restimulated by the tumor antigen alone, whereas CTLP of tumor-bearing animals could not be activated by tumor cells alone.

TWO-SIGNAL ACTIVATION OF TUMOR-SPECIFIC CYTOLYTIC T-LYMPHOCYTES (CTL) FROM TUMOR-BEARING ANIMALS

When we tried to activate sensitized T-cells from tumor-bearing animals, we found that restimulation with ESb tumor cells together with additional lymphokines as cofactors allowed the activation of such T-lymphocytes. Neither the tumor antigen alone nor lymphokines alone were sufficient for CTL activation. We assume that a similar two-signal activation is achieved when the ESb tumor cells are coated with Newcastle disease virus (NDV) and as such are used for activation of tumor-specific CTLP.

In a further series of experiments we compared the tumor-specific T-cell response also at the clonal level when immunizing animals with virus-modified ESb cells or with nonmodified ESb cells. It could be shown that the modification with the virus resulted in a clonal amplification of tumor-specific CTLP. The virus modification thus led to both clonal amplification of tumor-specific T-cells and additional activation of CTLP to

CTL. Further studies in vivo revealed that NDV-modifed ESb cells had a greatly increased immunogenicity compared to ESb cells alone [10].

These in vitro findings provided a scientific basis for constructing a virus-modified tumor cell vaccine for postoperative immunotherapy experiments.

POSTOPERATIVE IMMUNOTHERAPY OF ESb MICROMETASTASES AFTER ACTIVE SPECIFIC IMMUNIZATION WITH NDV-MODIFIED ESb TUMOR CELLS

We have performed a large number of experiments using NDV-modified ESb tumor cells for postoperative immunotherapy in order to activate sensitized CTLP to CTL. The standard protocol was as follows: DBA/2 mice were inoculated with 5×10^4 ESb cells intradermally. When the tumor had reached a size of 5–7 mm diameter (usually 8–10 days after tumor transplantation), it was removed surgically. Surgery alone was found to be insufficient for therapy because the tumor had already spread to visceral organs (liver, spleen, lung). Adjuvant immunotherapy consisted of a single immunization after the operation with 2.5×10^7 10,000 R-irradiated ESb tumor cells either without modification or after modification with Newcastle disease virus. For virus modification we used 160 hemagglutinating units of the avirulent strain Ulster for 2.5×10^7 tumor cells. No therapeutic benefit was observed when animals were immunized after surgery with irradiated ESb tumor cells alone. Immunization with NDV virus alone had a minor effect in some animals. By far the best therapeutic results were obtained when we used NDV-modified ESb tumor cells for immunization where we observed on the average about 50% long-term survivors [11]. When the two components NDV and tumor cells were given seperately (subcutaneously and intramuscular) there was only 25% survival, thus indicating that the two components were optimal when being given together.

After having established the optimal conditions for the antimetastatic therapy effect we noticed the following therapeutic effects: 1) disappearance of micrometastases from visceral organs as ascertained by a sensitive bioassay in vivo, 2) life prolongation in virtually all animals when compared to controls (operated only), and 3) cures in about 50% of the treated animals. These animals were found to develop long-lasting systemic ESb specific immunity [12].

CONCLUSIONS

One of the important messages of this study is that active specific immunotherapy should be tried as an adjuvant therapy with modified tumor cells rather than with tumor cell preparations as such. Tumor cells can be modified in a variety of ways, for instance by certain chemical agents, by the use of viruses or bacterial products, or possibly by biological response modifiers as adjuvants. From our own experience with the described animal tumor system as well as from certain clinical trials using the ''ASI'' approach with colon cancer patients [13] or with melanoma patients [14], we conclude that it would be desirable to design a cancer treatment strategy that includes an adjuvant immunotherapy protocol. The aim would be to achieve immune control of minimal residual disease, a task for which the immune system should be ideally suited because of its specifity and location and because the immune system is capable of eliminating a small tumor burden.

In the study of Hoover et al. [15], it was shown that the majority of colon cancer patients after active specific immunization with autologous tumor cells and BCG responded to their own tumors by mounting a cell-mediated delayed hypersensitivity (DTH) skin reaction as well as a humoral immune response. It has recently been possible to immortalize activated B-cells from such patients and thereby isolate human monoclonal antibodies recognizing particular human tumor antigens on colon cancers [16]. This study has therefore shown that the immune system of cancer patients can be stimulated to react against their own cancers and that these express tumor-associated antigens recognizable in the autochthonous host. Because of this we think it is not too speculative to get such immune responses involved in an adjuvant immunotherapy protocol. To what extent such responses can be evoked generally in different types of human tumors remains to be seen when such a procedure may be extended to other cancer types.

From a theoretical point of view, we consider tumor-specific T-cells to be the best candidates to achieve long-lasting therapeutic effects because of their "memory" and their circulatory properties. The human body contains about 300×10^9 T-lymphocytes. Some of these have immune regulatory functions; others have immune surveillance effector functions. We think an optimal tumor vaccine would consist of autologous inactivated viable tumor cells to provide the correct tumor antigen against which T-cells of the cancer patient might have been sensitized. To achieve activation of these cells after recruitment to the site of the vaccine inoculation, unspecific immune activating agents such as bacteria, viruses, or others might be added. The correct dosage is an important factor since it was found in various experimental models [11,17,18] that such agents have a low dose optimum. An optimal vaccine furthermore should try to mimic as closely as possible a physiological situation such as a virus infection, so that the correct amounts of lymphokines are provided by the infiltrating host cells.

REFERENCES

1. Schirrmacher V, Shantz G, Clauer K, Komitowski D, Zimmermann H-P, Lohmann-Matthes ML: Int J Cancer 23:233–244, 1979.
2. Schirrmacher V, Fogel M., Russmann E, Bosslet K, Altevogt P, Beck L: Cancer Metastasis Rev 1:241–274, 1982.
3. Larizza L, Schirrmacher V, Pflüger E: In: J Exp Metastasis 160:1579–1584, 1984.
4. Larizza L, Schirrmacher V., Graf L, Pflüger E, Peres-Martinez M, Stöhr M: Int J Cancer 34:699–707, 1984.
5. Vlodavsky I, Fuks Z, Bar-Ner M, Ariav Y, Schirrmacher V: Cancer Res 43:2704–2711, 1983.
6. Kramer MD, Robinson P, Vlodavsky I, Barz D, Friberger P, Fuks Z, Schirrmacher V: Eur J Cancer Clin Oncol 21:307–316, 1985.
7. Bosslet K, Schirrmacher V, Shantz G: Int J Cancer 24:303–313, 1979.
8. Schirrmacher V, Bosslet K, Shantz G, Clauer K, Hübsch D: Int J Cancer 23:245–252, 1979.
9. Schirrmacher V, Bosslet K, Altevogt P, Rußmann E, Beck L, Fogel M: In Lapis K (ed): "Tumor Progression and Markers, Proc. IV. Meeting of EACR, Budapest 1981." Amsterdam: Kugler Publications, 1982, pp 155–164.
10. Schirrmacher V, Ahlert T, Heicapell R, Appelhans B, von Hoegen P: In Cancer Rev 5:19–49, 1986.
11. Heicappell R, Schirrmacher V, von Hoegen P, Ahlert T, Appelhans B: Int J Cancer 37:569–577, 1986.
12. Schirrmacher V, Heicappell R: Clin Exp Metastasis 5:147–156, 1987.
13. Hoover HC Jr, Surdyke MG, Dangel EB, Peters LC, Hanna MG: Cancer 55:1236–1243, 1985.
14. Cassel WA, Murray DR, Phillips HS: Cancer 52:856–860, 1983.
15. Hoover HC Jr, Surdyke M, Dangel R, Peters LC, Hanna MG Jr: Cancer Res 44:1671–1676, 1984.
16. Hanna MG, Hoover HC, Peters LC, Key KE, Haspel MV, McCabe RP, Potamo N: In Oldham R (ed): "Principles of Cancer Biotherapy." New York: Raven Press, 1988.
17. Hanna MG, Brandhorst JS, Peters LC: Cancer Immunol Immunother 7:165–173, 1979.
18. Yamaguchi H, Moriuchi T, Hosokawa M, Kobayashi H: Cancer Immunol Immunther 12:119, 1972.

Index

Abelson murine leukemia virus, 104; see also Leukemia viruses
Aberrant cytogenetic patterns, 43
Aberrant populations, 43
Adenocarcinoma. See specific types of carcinoma
Adhesion, of tumor cells, 161–166
Adhesion molecules, 275, 276, 278
Adult bovine aortic endothelial cells, 165
Agglutinins, 239
Allograft rejection, 88
alu sequences, 35
Alveolar macrophages, 89–90, 94
Ames assay, 151, 154
Aneuploid cells, 143–150
Aneuploidy, generation of, 21–28
Animal carcinomas. See specific types of carcinoma
Antibody production, 88
Antigamma interferon antibodies, 203
Antigenic heterogeneity, 147
Antigenicity, 143–150
Antimetastatic substances, 267–268
Antimyosin staining, 6
Antitumor activity, 87–102
Ascites, 202
Attachment assays, and human ovarian tumor cell, 257
Autoradiography, 129
Autosomal genes, 175
5-aza-CR, 176–177
Azacytidine, 159

*Bam*HI fragment, 34, 37
Basal cell carcinoma, 9
Basement membrane, 49, 84
  reconstituted, 261–269
Basement membrane collagenase, 137
Basement membrane matrix, 216, 219
  and human prostate, 219–227
Benign prostatic hyperplasia, 212
Benign tumors, 184–185
Biological response modifiers, 88, 91, 94, 99–100
  effect on CTL activity, 91–93, 99
  effect on macrophage-mediated cytotoxicity and cytostasis, 94
  effect on NK and LAK activities, 91
Bladder cancer cells, 176
B-N-Acetylglucosaminidase (B-NAG) assay, 254
Bovine aortic endothelial cells, 164
Bovine corneal endothelial cells, 252
Boyden chamber, 189, 224–226, 262, 263, 265
Brain-specific antigens, 161–166
Breast cancer, 40–41, 47, 139, 143–150, 263, 266
BRMs. See Biological response modifiers

B16 melanoma cells, 49, 51–52, 54, 75–86, 132, 238–239
  metastases, 140
  smear preparations of, 78

Cancer cells
  destruction of, 285–292
  human, 251–260
Carcinomas
  breast, 40–41
  central nervous system, 45–46
  colorectal, 115–126, 233, 235, 279–284
  liver, 105, 282
  lung, 127–133
  lymph nodes, 233–236
  mouse mammary, 22–28
  prostate, 189–231
  renal, 42–45
  see also Malignant tissues; Tumors, malignant
Cell adhesion molecules, 245–250
Cell-cell interaction, 1–12
Cell fusion. See Spontaneous fusion
Cell lines, 179–188
Cell motility, 245–250
Cells
  breast carcinoma, 143–150
  immune response of, 61–62
  incubation of B16 melanoma tumors, 78
  inflammatory, 151–155
Cell surface properties, 158–159
Cellular attachment, 251–260
Cellular genes, 19
Cellular morphology, 46
Cellular respiration, 104
Central nervous system tumors, 45–46
c-Ha-*ras* gene, 175–176
c-Ha-*ras* protein family, 187
Chemical carcinogens, 173–174
Chemotherapy, 55, 285
Chicken β-actin plasmid probe, 16, 17
Chick heart cultures, 179–180, 183
Chinese hamster cells, 174
Chloramphenicol acetyl transferase, 64–65, 71
Chondroitin sulfate proteoglycan, 115–126
Chondroitin sulfate-specific mouse monoclonal antibody (CS-56), 115–126
Chondroitinase ABC treatment, 119
  of tumor tissue, 118
Choriocarcinoma, 13–20
Chromosome, 7, 273–274
Chromosome aberrations, 39, 46, 47
CIRAS-1 cells, 128–133
Class II antigens, 168–169
Clonal heterogeneity, 75–76
Cloning, of ovarian cancer cells, 80–81

Clonogenicity, 158
CNS tumors. *See* Central nervous system tumors
Collagenase, 158, 261, 262, 264, 267
Collagenolysis, 50
Collagenolytic activity, 1–12, 116
Collagens, 175, 237–244
Colorectal cancer, 115–126, 233, 235, 279–284
Colorectal neoplasm, 280–281
    transplanted into nude mouse, 280–281
C1-LDT cells, 127–133
C127 cells, 182, 183, 187
Contact hypersensitivity, 169–170
Cranial-caudal growth gradient, 192, 193, 202
Cutaneous immune cells, 168–169
Cutaneous immunity, 167–171
Cytochalasin-induced heterokaryon formation, 147
Cytocidal action, 164
Cytogenetic heterogeneity, 39–48
Cytokeratins, 145
Cytolysis, 104
Cytometric analysis, 146–147
Cytosine, 173, 174
Cytospin, immunocytochemistry of, 78, 85
Cytostasis. *See* Macrophage cytostasis
Cytotoxic reactions, 163–164
Cytotoxicity, of mouse splenocytes, 165

Demethylation, 175, 176
Desmoplasia, 123
Desmosomes, 84
Diapedesis, 234
Diethylstilbestrol (DES), 189, 206–211
Dihydrotestosterone, 203
Diploid cells, 39
Diploid neoplastic cells, 145–147
DNA, 30
    in breast cancers, 146–147
    content in T-cell hybridomas, 273
    flow cytometry, 235
    foreign, 138–140
    methylation, 173–177
    ploidy, 235
    polymerase activity in prostate cancer, 206
    role in tumorigenic transformation, 30
    in study of tumor cell populations, 138–139
    transfection, 136–137, 180
        from squamous cell carcinoma, 31–37
DNA-mediated gene transfer, 64
Dot-blot analysis, 115–126
Double-stranded polyribonucleotides, 87–102
DU-145, 194, 195, 199, 201–203, 207, 210, 220, 222, 224, 225, 227
Duke's staging, 115–116, 121
Dynamic heterogeneity, 153

Effusion metastases, 144, 148
Ehrlich ascites tumor cells, 124
Elastinolysis, 50

Embryogenesis, 245–250
Embryonic diploid fibroblasts, 136
Endo-β-D-glucuronidase, 49–59
Endocytosis, 285
Endogenous lectins, 237–244
Endoglycosidase activity, 52–54
Endothelial cells
    differences among, 161–166
    sinusoidal, 271–272
Enografts, 191–192
Entactin, 261, 262
Env gene, 13
Enzyme activities, role in tumor metastasis, 49–59
Enzyme-generated oxygen metabolites, 154
Epithelial cell cultures, 212
    from human prostate, 212–216
Epithelial cells, 143–150
Epithelial/stromal cells
    in human prostates, 216–219
ERV3, 13–20
ESb micrometastases, 295
ESb tumor cells, 295
ESb tumor model system, 294
Ethyl methanesulfonate, 151–155
Extracellular matrix, 251–260
Extravasation process, 238

Fetuin, 239
Fibrinolysis, 50
Fibroblasts
    cultures, 2
    monolayers, 272
    response, heterogeneity of, 1–12
    subpopulations, 6
    10T1/2, 127–133
    tumor-associated, 5–6
Fibronectin, 145, 237–244
Fibronectinolysis, 50
Fibrotic tissues, of colorectal carcinoma, 122–123
Fischer rat fibroblastic cell lines, 179–187
Fischer rat FR3T3 cells, 181–182, 185
Fischer rat FR3T3C cells, 181
Flow cytometric analysis, 77
Flow cytometry, 39–48
Fucosylated glycoproteins, 116
Fusion. *See* Spontaneous fusion

Gamma-delta heterodimers, 169
Gel electrophoresis, two-dimensional, 219
Gene
    transfection, 128
    transfer, 29–38, 135
Genetic constitution, of tumor cells, 157–159
Genetic instability, 151–155
Genomic DNA, 159
Giemsa-banded karyotype, 200
Gingival fibroblast cell line, 7–8
Glial tumors, 46

Glioblastoma, 46
Glioma cells, 162–164
Glycoprotein, 239
    expression, 147
Glycosaminoglycans, 237–244
    chains, 116
Glycosidase activities, 256
Glycosyltransferases, 55
G^- phenotype, 180–181
G^+ phenotype, 180–181
G protein, 132
Granulocytes, 168
Guanidine-HCl, 124–125

Hapten, 169, 170
Ha-*ras* gene, 29–38, 37
HCC cells, 281
HeLa cells, 174
Heparan sulfate proteoglycans, 49–59, 261, 262
Heparin, 49–59
Heparinases, 267
Hepatic metastases, human colorectal carcinoma, 281–283
Hepatocytes, 272, 275
Hepatoma cells, 163
Heterogeneity, 21–28
    of endothelial cells, 161–166
Heterotransplantation, of human prostatic tumors, 190
Heterotypic aggregation, 238
Histocompatibility antigens, 168
Hodgkin's lymphoma, 40
Hoechst staining method, 22
Homotypic aggregation, 238
Host cell lysis, 50
H-*ras* oncogene, 136–137
    transcription, 127–133
Human breast cancer, 143–150
Human carcinomas. *See specific types of carcinoma*
Human endogenous provirus, 13–20
Human fibroblast cell lines, 7
Human fibrosarcoma cells, 264
Human gestational choriocarcinoma, 19
Hybrid cells, 21–28
Hybridoma cells, 193
Hydatidiform moles, 19
Hydrocarbon carcinogens, 174
Hydrolytic enzymes, 238, 259
Hyperplastic alveolar nodule (HAN) lines, 155
Hypomethylation, 174, 175

Immortalized cell lines, 136
Immune cells
    cutaneous, 168–169
    effector, 129
Immune surveillance, 61–73
Immunity, against tumors, 61–62

Immunoblotting, 248
Immunofluorescent labeling, 63, 248
Immunohistochemical localization, of CSPG, 119, 122
Immunohistochemistry, 75–86
Immunologic factors, influence on skin cancers, 167–171
Immunomodulators, 285
Immunomodulatory activities, 88, 90
Immunoprecipitation analyses, 248
Immunotherapy, 233
    postoperative, 293–296
Implantation, lung, 129–130, 132
Incubation, of B16 melanoma tumors, 78
Infiltration index, 275
Inflammatory cells, 151–155
Inoculation, of melanoma cells in mice survival data, 92
Interaction index, 275
Interferon-gamma, 87–102
Interferons, 71, 267–268
Intrasplenic injection, 189, 193, 194–203, 206, 279–284
Intratumoral heterogeneity, 44
Intravesical injection, of prostate cancer cells, 203
Invasive tumors. *See* Tumors, malignant, invasion into host tissues
I^- phenotype, 179–180
I^+ phenotype, 179–188
Irradiation therapy, 203
ISO-DALT system, 217–219

Kaplan-Meier survival curves, 90
Kaposi's sarcoma, 264
Keratinocytes, 167, 169, 170
KHT fibrosarcoma, 132

Laminin, 237–244, 261, 262, 267
Lamininolysis, 50
Langerhans' cells, 168–170
Lectin-binding sites, of endothelial cells, 161–166
Lectins, endogenous tumor cell, 237–244
Lesions, metastatic. *See* Tumors, malignant
Leukemia viruses, 61–73
Leukemias, 27, 39–40
Lewis lung carcinoma, 91–93
LFA-1, 271, 275–276, 278
L fibroblast cells, 27
Liposome-immunomodulator therapy, 288–289
Liposomes, 285
    containing immunomodulators, 287–288
    containing multiple immunomodulators, 289–290
    delivering signals to phagocytic cells, 286–287
Liver
    metastases, 103–113, 201, 271–284
    metastases of RAW117-H10 cells, 112
L929 fibroblasts, 163

Localization in situ, 75–86
LTRAT1 cells, 184
LTRs, 13–14
Lung
    carcinomas, 8, 10, 55, 89, 91–93
    colonization, 128
    DES and tumors, 211
    endothelial cells, 161
    fibroblasts, 161
    implantation, 129–130, 132
    metastases, 32–33, 81, 83, 85, 95
    tumors, 11, 157
Lung-derived tumor cells, 127–133
Lymphangiochemotherapy, 233
Lymphatic endothelium, 163
Lymphatic metastasis, 233–236
Lymph node cells, 169
Lymph node metastasis. See Tumors, malignant
Lymphocyte-mediated immune surveillance, 163–164
Lymphocytes, 168
Lymphoid cells, 168
Lymphoid tumor cells, 271
Lymphokine-activated killer, 87, 91, 93, 96–99
Lymphokines, 285
Lymphomas, 39–40
Lysis, 66–67
Lytic activity, 99

Macrophage, 104, 151, 168–169
    activation factors, 286
    cytolysis, 104
    tumoricidal activity, 87–90
    tumoristatic activity, 89–90, 97
Macrophage-conditioned media, 110
Macrophage cytostasis, 104–105
    in macrophage coculture, 105
    in macrophage-conditioned media, 105–106
Macrophage-released cytostatic factor, 103–113
Major histocompatibility complex antigens, 61–73
Malignancies. See Tumors, malignant
Malignant effusions, 148
Malignant tissues, 1–20
Mammary adenocarcinomas, 56, 136
Mammary carcinoma cells, 124
Mann-Whitney U-test, 90
Mast cells, 1–12, 168
MATRIGEL, 221–225, 263
    invasion, 266
MCDK cells, 184–185
Mechanical dispersion techniques, 147
Medulloblastoma, 46
Melanoma
    in vitro growth of B16 clones, 82
    in vivo metastatic potential, 82
    see also Tumors, malignant
Messenger RNA, 13–20
Metastasis, 237–244
    gene transfer in study of, 135–141
    selection model, 140
    treatment of, 87–102
    and tumor cell surface lectins, 237–244
Metastasis assays, 129
    experimental and spontaneous in prostate, 208
    in murine large cell lymphoma, 104
Metastatic cells, origin of, 127–128, 132
Metastatic efficiency, 127–133
Metastatic phenotypes, 29–38, 135–141
    and cellular interactions, 238–239
Metastatic potentials, 110, 124
    in colorectal carcinoma, 116
    of RAW117 cells, 110–112
Metastatic tumors. See Tumors, malignant
Metastatic variants, 75–86
Methylation patterns, 176–177
Methylpalmitate, 203
Methyltransferase, 173–177
Met-72, 75–76
Met 72/83 antigen, 75–86
MHC antigens. See Major histocompatibility complex antigens
Microenvironmental influences, on metastatic potential, 82–84
Microspectrophotometry, 146–147
Mitochondrial electron transport chain, 103–113
MLE cells, 181
Molecular genetics, 136–137
Moles, invasive, 18–19
Moloney leukemia virus, 110
    see also Leukemia viruses; Murine large cell lymphoma
Monoclonal antibodies, 62–63, 70
    in B16 melanoma tumors, 75
Mouse brain endothelial cells, 163
Mouse lymphatic endothelial cells, 165
Mouse mammary adenocarcinoma, 136
Mouse mammary tumor, 151–155
Mouse melanoma, 137
Mouse ovary endothelial cells, 163
Mouse pancreas, 181
mRNA expression, 13–20
Multilamellar vesicles, 287
Multinucleated cells, 145
Muramyl dipeptide, 286
Murine endothelial cell, 161–166
Murine large cell lymphoma, 103–113
Murine leukemia viruses. See Leukemia viruses
Murine mammary tumors, 157–159
Murine melanoma cells, 264
Murine melanomas, 79
Mutagenic macrophages, 151–155
    and mouse mammary tumors, 153
Mutations, and mammary tumors, 152–154

NADH dehydrogenase, 103–113
Natural killer activity, 87–91, 93, 95–99

Natural killer cells. *See* NK cells
N-CAM, 245-250
Neoplasia, 154
Neoplasm, 104
Neoplastic cells, 135-137, 173
    diploid, 143-150
Neoplastic populations, 151
Neural cell adhesion molecule, 245-250
Neuroepithelial cells, 245
Newcastle disease virus, 294-295
NIH 3T3 cells, 32
Nitrocellulose membrane, 118-120
NK-cell-mediated cytotoxicity
    inhibitory effect of DES on, 206-207
NK-cell-mediated lysis, 161-166
NK cells, 155, 161-166, 169
    inhibition, and prostate cancer, 209-210
    in lungs, 127-133
NMuMG cells, 185
Northern blot analysis, 128-129, 131
    of total cellular RNA, 63-64
Northern blot hybridization, 14, 15, 17
Nude mice, 173, 176-177, 185-187
    to investigate human colorectal cancer, 279-284
    to investigate human prostate cancer, 189-231

Oncogene, 29-38
    and invasive phenotypes, 179-188
    transfer of into nonmetastatic neoplastic cells, 136-137
    see also ras gene
OPAE antibody, 275
Orthotopic transplantation, 281
Ovarian metastases, 83, 85
Ovarian teratocarcinoma, 163
Ovarian tumors, 75, 79-81, 251-260

Paracrine growth factors, 112
Parental primary tumor, 127
PC-3, 194-203, 220, 224
Pearson's correlation coefficient, 90, 95
PEG-induced fusion, 27
Percoll gradient, 189, 212-216
Perilymphangitis, 235
Periprostatic injection, of prostate cancer cells, 203
Peritoneovenous shunting, 158
Pertussis toxin, 271
    effects, 277
    inhibition of invasion by, 274
Phagocytic cells, 285
Phosphatidylcholine, 287
Phospholipid vesicles, 285
Photoimmunology, 167-171
Plasmid DNA, 138
Plasmids, in transfection of cell lines, 180
Plasminogen activator, 267

Platelet activator, 267
Platelet aggregation, 50
Pleural effusion specimens, 148
Pol gene, 13
Poly (I,C)-LC, 87-102
Polysaccharides, 54
Portal venous injection, 202
Preclinical models, 87-102
Premature chromosome condensation, 40
Primary tumors, growth of, 135-141
Prostate cancer, 189-231
    DES and, 206-211
    DNA transfection and, 203-206
    epithelial cell cultures, 212-216
    epithelial/stromal cells, 216-219
    morphology of, 219-227
    nude mouse model in study of, 191-203
Protease output, 158
Protein phosphorylation, 132
Proteoglycanolysis, 50
Proteoglycans, 116
    dot-blot analysis of, 119, 123
Protooncogenes, 29-30
Proviral mRNA expression, 13-20
Pulmonary colonization, 157
Pulmonary macrophages, 94
Pulmonary metastases, 90
Pulmonary parenchymal mononuclear cells, 89

Radiation leukemia virus-induced tumors, 71
Radioactivity-labeled cells, 132
Radioimmunoassay, 77-78
Radiolabeled proteoglycans, 120
Radiotherapy, 55, 285
ras gene, 127-133, 137, 176, 187
    family, 30
ras transcription, 127-133
ras-transfected BW5147 cells, 273
Rat2 cells, 182, 184
RAW117-H10 cells, 103-113
    differentially expressed, 106-107, 108-110
    superinfection of, 104-105, 107-108, 109
Recurrence, of cancer. *See specific types of carcinoma*
Renal carcinoma, 42-45, 47, 282
Respiratory-inhibiting factors, 104, 112
    retinoblastoma tumors, 19
Retrovirus genomes, 13
Rhabdomyosarcoma, 19
RNA, 18
    in leukemia viruses, 63-64
    role in Northern blot analysis, 129-131
    tumor virus, 103-113
Rous sarcoma virus, 245, 247-249

Semliki Forest virus, 27
Sendai virus, 27
Serum enzyme, 49-59

Serum-free media, 189, 212, 215–216
Sex chromosome, 46
Sigmoid colon adenocarcinoma. *See* Colorectal cancer
Sinusoidal endothelial cells, 271–272
Skin cancers, 29–38, 167–171
^{35}S labeling, 116, 117–118, 120, 124
Southern blot analysis, 138
  of primary tumors and lung metastases, 139
Southern blot hybridization, 15, 29, 31
  with *ras* probes, 36
S phase, 146
SP1 clones, 137
SP1 tumor, 139
Splenocytes, 164
Spontaneous conversion, 179–188
Spontaneous fusion, 21–28
  in situ, 26
  in vitro, 23
  in vivo, 23
Squamous cell carcinoma, 29–38
^{38}S-sulfated proteoglycans, preparation of, 117–118
Staging, of colorectal carcinomas, 115–116, 121
Stromal-epithelial fractions, 212
Stromal fibroblasts, 8, 11
Stromal matrix, 144
Subcutaneous inoculations, 139
Subpopulations, 82
  androgen-dependent, 190
  androgen-resistant, 190
  diploid, 44
  metastatic, 21–28
  with metastatic potential, 82–85
  nonmetastatic, 21–28
  and primary tumor growth, 135–141
Suppressor cells, 168
Survival rates, from cancer. *See specific types of carcinoma*

T-cell, 93, 163, 294
  hybridoma, 271–272
  lymphoma, 136
  receptor genes, 168–169
T-cell-independent antigens, 191
  and prostate cancer, 191–192
Therapeutic activity, in tumor cells, 87–102
Thoracic X-irradiation macrophages, activation of, 290–291
Thy-1, 161
Tissue degradation, 1–2, 251–260
T lymphocytes, 168–170, 191
  cytolytic, 87–102
  cytolytic, from tumor-bearing animals, 294–295
  cytotoxic, 61–63, 293–296
  see also T-cell

trans activation, 61–73
Transfection
  experiments, 185
  of H-*ras* oncogene, 136–137
  of low- or noninvasive cells, 182
Translocation, 44
Tumor-associated fibroblasts, 7–8
Tumor-associated macrophages, in mouse mammary tumors, 153
Tumor-associated stromal fibroblasts, 9
Tumor cell, 4, 157, 271–278
  detachment, 245–250
  fibroblast interactions, 5–6
  genetic constitution of, 157–159
  host factors of, 157–159
  populations, growth analysis of, 138–139
Tumor-cell-conditioned media, 5
Tumor heterogeneity, 151–155, 173–177
Tumor necrosis factor, 145
Tumor vaccines, 293–296
Tumoricidal assays, 89
Tumoricidal macrophages, 285–292
Tumorigenic cells, 175
Tumorigenicity, 29–38, 123–124, 128, 180
Tumors, malignant, 21–28, 49–59
  breast, 40–44, 143–150
  central nervous system, 45–46
  colorectal, 279–284
  culturing of cells, 41
  heparanase inhibitors, 54–55
  immunohistochemistry of cryostat sections, 78–79
  invasion into host tissues, 1–12
  lung, 127–133
  lymph nodes, 233–236
  metastasis, 103–104
  prostate, 189–231
  renal, 42–45
  serum enzyme levels and, 55–57
  skin, 167–171
  see also specific carcinomas
Tunicamycin, 259–260
Tyrosine-isoleucine-glycine-serine-arginine, 267

Ultraviolet radiation, 30
Urological tumors, 251–260
UV radiation, 167–171

Vaccine, for postoperative immunotherapy, 293–296
Vascular endothelial cells, 161–166
Viral infection, 88
Virus-modified tumor cell vaccine, 293–296
Vitamin E, 155

Wilm's tumor, hepatoblastoma, 19

Xenografts, 191–192